Advances in Intelligent Systems and Computing

Volume 1312

AF862975

The series "Advances in Intelligent Systems and Computing" contains publications on theory, applications, and design methods of Intelligent Systems and Intelligent Computing. Virtually all disciplines such as engineering, natural sciences, computer and information science, ICT, economics, business, e-commerce, environment, healthcare, life science are covered. The list of topics spans all the areas of modern intelligent systems and computing such as: computational intelligence, soft computing including neural networks, fuzzy systems, evolutionary computing and the fusion of these paradigms, social intelligence, ambient intelligence, computational neuroscience, artificial life, virtual worlds and society, cognitive science and systems, Perception and Vision, DNA and immune based systems, self-organizing and adaptive systems, e-Learning and teaching, human-centered and human-centric computing, recommender systems, intelligent control, robotics and mechatronics including human-machine teaming, knowledge-based paradigms, learning paradigms, machine ethics, intelligent data analysis, knowledge management, intelligent agents, intelligent decision making and support, intelligent network security, trust management, interactive entertainment, Web intelligence and multimedia.

The publications within "Advances in Intelligent Systems and Computing" are primarily proceedings of important conferences, symposia and congresses. They cover significant recent developments in the field, both of a foundational and applicable character. An important characteristic feature of the series is the short publication time and world-wide distribution. This permits a rapid and broad dissemination of research results.

Indexed by DBLP, EI Compendex, INSPEC, WTI Frankfurt eG, zbMATH, Japanese Science and Technology Agency (JST), SCImago.

All books published in the series are submitted for consideration in Web of Science.

More information about this series at http://www.springer.com/series/11156

Siddhartha Bhattacharyya · Janmenjoy Nayak ·
Kolla Bhanu Prakash · Bighnaraj Naik ·
Ajith Abraham
Editors

International Conference on Intelligent and Smart Computing in Data Analytics

ISCDA 2020

Springer

Editors
Siddhartha Bhattacharyya
Rajnagar Mahavidyalaya
Rajnagar, Birbhum, India

Kolla Bhanu Prakash
Department of Computer Science
and Engineering
K. L. University
Vijayawada, India

Ajith Abraham
Machine Intelligence Research Labs
Auburn, AL, USA

Janmenjoy Nayak
Department of Computer Science
and Engineering
Aditya Institute of Technology
and Management (AITAM)
Srikakulam, India

Bighnaraj Naik
Department of Computer Applications
Veer Surendra Sai University of Technology
Sambalpur, India

ISSN 2194-5357 ISSN 2194-5365 (electronic)
Advances in Intelligent Systems and Computing
ISBN 978-981-33-6175-1 ISBN 978-981-33-6176-8 (eBook)
https://doi.org/10.1007/978-981-33-6176-8

This Springer imprint is published by the registered company Springer Nature Singapore Pte Ltd.
The registered company address is: 152 Beach Road, #21-01/04 Gateway East, Singapore 189721, Singapore

The editors would like to dedicate this book to those deceased and infected due to the ongoing COVID-19 pandemic.

Preface

The development of society and mankind through technological innovations and their sustainability is the ultimate aim of universities, industries and research institutes across the globe. The technological advances in the areas of artificial intelligence, data analytics, security and advanced computing will surely play a major role in building the knowledge society, focusing on socio-economic development of individuals.

The International Conference on Intelligent and Smart Computing in Data Analytics (ISCDA) organized by the Computer Science and Engineering Department of Koneru Lakshmaiah Education Foundation (KLEF) Deemed to be University, Vaddeswaram, Guntur, India, during 3–5 October 2020 is an international forum that has provided a platform for researchers, academicians as well as industrial professionals from all over the world to present their research results and development activities in the areas of smart computing, data analytics and data security. It has attracted **202** papers from various parts of the world. After a thorough double-blind peer review process, editors have selected **32** papers and were placed in the proceedings of ISCDA.

During the conference, **11** eminent academicians and researchers from different countries like the USA, Australia, Vietnam, Malaysia, the UK, Turkey and India have delivered keynote addresses to enlighten the participants.

The editors would like to acknowledge the support received from authors, reviewers, invited speakers, members of the advisory committee, members of the organizing committee and the members of programme committee, without whose support the quality and standards of the conference could not be maintained.

In addition to the above, we would like to express our sincere gratitude to '**Koneru Lakshmaiah Education Foundation (KLEF) Deemed to be University**,' for hosting this conference.

Birbhum, India — Siddhartha Bhattacharyya
Srikakulam, India — Janmenjoy Nayak
Vijayawada, India — Kolla Bhanu Prakash
Sambalpur, India — Bighnaraj Naik
Auburn, USA — Ajith Abraham

Acknowledgements

The theme and relevance of ISCDA2020 attracted more than 200 researchers/academicians around the globe which enabled us to select good quality papers and serve to demonstrate the popularity of the ISCDA2020 conference for sharing ideas and research findings with truly national and international communities. Thanks to all those who have contributed in producing such a comprehensive conference proceedings of ISCDA2020. The organizing committee believes and trusts that we have been true to the spirit of collegiality that members of ISCDA2020 value even as also maintaining an elevated standard as we have reviewed papers, provided feedback and presented a strong body of published work in this collection of proceedings. Thanks to all the members of the organizing committee for their heartfelt support and cooperation. We have been fortunate enough to work in cooperation with a brilliant international as well as national advisory board, reviewers and program and technical committee consisting of eminent academicians to call for papers, review papers and finalize papers to be included in the proceedings. We would like to express our heartfelt gratitude and obligations to the benign reviewers for sparing their valuable time, putting an effort to review the papers in a stipulated time and providing their valuable suggestions and appreciation in improvising the presentation, quality and content of this proceedings. The eminence of these papers is an accolade not only to the authors but also to the reviewers who have guided towards perfection. Last but not least, the editorial members of Springer Publishing deserve a special mention, and our sincere thanks to them not only for making our dream come true in the shape of this proceedings, but also for its hassle-free and in-time publication in the reputed Advances in Intelligent Systems and Computing, Springer. The ISCDA2020 conference and proceedings are a credit to a large group of people, and everyone should be proud of the outcome.

Contents

About the Editors

Siddhartha Bhattacharyya *FIET (UK)*, is currently Principal at Rajnagar Mahavidyalaya, Rajnagar, Birbhum, India. He was a Professor in CHRIST (Deemed to be University), Bangalore, India, from December 2019 to March, 2021. He served as a Senior Research Scientist at the Faculty of Electrical Engineering and Computer Science of VSB Technical University of Ostrava, Czech Republic, from October 2018 to April 2019. Prior to this, he was the Principal of RCC Institute of Information Technology, Kolkata, India. He is a co-author of 5 books and a co-editor of 75 books and has more than 300 research publications in international journals and conference proceedings to his credit. His research interests include soft computing, pattern recognition, multimedia data processing, hybrid intelligence and quantum computing.

Janmenjoy Nayak is working as Associate Professor, Aditya Institute of Technology and Management (AITAM), (An Autonomous Institution) Tekkali, K Kotturu, AP- 532201, India. He has published more than 100 research papers in various reputed peer-reviewed refereed journals, international conferences and book chapters. Being two times Gold Medallist in Computer Science in his career, he has been awarded with INSPIRE Research Fellowship from the Department of Science & Technology, Govt. of India (both as JRF and SRF level) and Best Researcher Award from Jawaharlal Nehru University of Technology, Kakinada, Andhra Pradesh, for the AY: 2018-19 and many more awards to his credit. He has edited 11 books and 8 special issues in various topics including data science, machine learning and soft computing with reputed International Publishers like Springer, Elsevier, Inderscience, etc. His area of interest includes data mining, nature-inspired algorithms and soft computing.

Dr. Kolla Bhanu Prakash is working as Professor and Research Group Head in CSE DEPARTMENT, K L University, VIJAYAWADA, Andhra Pradesh, India. He received his M.Sc. and M.Phil. in Physics from Acharya Nagarjuna University, Guntur, India, and M.E. and Ph.D. in Computer Science Engineering from Sathyabama University, Chennai, India. He has 15+ years of experience working in the academia, research, teaching and academic administration. His current research interests include deep learning, data science, smart grids, cyber-physical systems, cryptocurrency, blockchain technology and image processing. He is an IEEE senior member. He has reviewed more than 125 peer-reviewed journals which are indexed in Publons. He is Editor for 6 books in Elsevier, CRC Press, Springer, Wiley and De Gryuter publishers. He published 65 research papers, 6 patents, 8 books + 4 accepted. His Scopus h-index is 14. He is a frequent editorial board member and a TPC member in flagship conferences and refereed journals.

Dr. Bighnaraj Naik is Assistant Professor in the Department of Computer Application, Veer Surendra Sai University of Technology (Formerly UCE Burla), Odisha, India. He received his Ph.D. in Computer Science and Engineering, M.Tech. in Computer Science and Engineering and B.E. in Information Technology in 2016, 2009 and 2006, respectively. He has published more than 80 research papers in various reputed peer-reviewed journals, conferences and book chapters. He has edited more than 10 books from various publishers such as Elsevier, Springer and IGI Global. At present, he has more than ten years of teaching experience in the field of Computer Science and IT. He is a member of IEEE. His area of interest includes data mining, computational intelligence, and its applications. He has been serving as Guest Editor of various journal special issues from Elsevier, Springer and Inderscience.

Dr. Ajith Abraham is Director of Machine Intelligence Research Labs (MIR Labs), a Not-for-Profit Scientific Network for Innovation and Research Excellence connecting Industry and Academia. As Investigator/Co-Investigator, he has won research grants worth over 100+ Million US$ from Australia, USA, EU, Italy, Czech Republic, France, Malaysia and China. Dr. Abraham works in a multi-disciplinary environment involving machine intelligence, cyber-physical systems, Internet of things, network security, sensor networks, Web intelligence, Web services, data mining and applied to various real-world problems. In these areas, he has authored/co-authored more than 1400+ research publications out of which there are 100+ books covering various aspects of Computer Science. About 1100+ publications are indexed by Scopus and over 900+ are indexed by Thomson ISI Web of Science. He has 1100+ co-authors originating from 40+ countries. Dr. Abraham has more than 39,000+ academic citations (h-index of 95 as per google scholar).

Performance Analysis of Machine Learning Algorithms Over a Network Traffic

J. Varun, E. S. Vishnu Tejas, and T. G. Keerthan Kumar

Abstract The machine learning algorithms are becoming more potential in artificial intelligence. In order to evaluate network security and performance, the classification of network is very much essential. In recent decades, various software or products produce various network traffic with different parameter types and with different service as per necessity. Thereby, classification of the network traffic plays a major role to increase the performance of a network management. The traffic classification has become more vital study range especially with the evolution of machine learning techniques. Here, we considered few machine learning techniques like the support vector machine, random forest classifier, and multilayer perceptron which are used to classify the network traffic. We considered various parameters like Telnet, Ping, and Voice traffic flows simulated by distributed Internet traffic generator tool. Each host in the network was connected through an overlay network to an Open vSwitch (OVS). The OVS was connected to a Ryu controller which collected basic flow statistics between hosts. These statistics were then parsed by a Python traffic classification script which periodically output the learned traffic labels of each flow. After investigating different classification techniques, we found that multilayer perceptron was found to work much better than other classifiers techniques.

Keywords Machine learning · Network traffic · Performance · Supervised learning · Multilayer perception · Random forest classifier

J. Varun · E. S. Vishnu Tejas · T. G. Keerthan Kumar (✉)
Siddaganga Institute of Technology, Tumakuru, India
e-mail: keerthanswamy@gmail.com

J. Varun
e-mail: varu021999@gmail.com

E. S. Vishnu Tejas
e-mail: vishnutejas15@gmail.com

S. Bhattacharyya et al. (eds.), *International Conference on Intelligent and Smart Computing in Data Analytics*, Advances in Intelligent Systems and Computing 1312,
https://doi.org/10.1007/978-981-33-6176-8_1

1 Introduction

Classification of network traffic links in a network which is produced by various applications is a major step for the network analysis. The implementation of a very good application level project for classification of a network traffic over a few years is more challenging. More valuable data are collected from various network traffic analysis and particularly for security purposes like filtering traffic, identifying, and detecting malicious activities. Numerous network traffic classification methods have been established and applied over few areas to get solutions for various problems [1]. In recent years, there is a rapid development in intelligent devices over the networking area. The network traffic in the world is increasing day by day. Large datasets produce an enormous Internet traffic flows which are difficult to process and analyze. So, the concept of machine learning came into existence. Providing precise and appropriate Internet traffic-related data is more significant for numerous applications like admission control, anomaly detection, bandwidth allocation, and congestion control [2]. Machine learning helps to easily classify the datasets and helps to produce an accurate solution to the given problem. Classification and clustering of flows can help identify network hotspots and potential bottlenecks [3]. Software-defined networking (SDN) is an developing architecture; it will abstract normal functions of router and switches and which is manageable efficiently and more cost-effective than traditional network. Moreover, the SDN is adaptable, dynamic, making it idyllic for the high-bandwidth because of dynamic nature of recent applications. The SDN architecture separates the network into control functions and forwarding functions also called as control plane and data plane [4]. Although we are having many challenges in the current network for traffic classification, the machine learning helps to improve the network management to make the concept simple and easy to use for extracting the important statistical data of network traffic from switches or routers or systems. The reputation of network traffic classification is in resolving network problems like Denial of Service (DoS) attack and intrusion detection systems [5].

2 Literature Survey

In [6], the authors describe that the machine learning (ML) is used drastically in many applications that solve most of the difficult problems and enable the use of various automation technique in different areas. Basically, this is because of the availability of more and more data, the more improvements in machine learning techniques, and major evolution in computing proficiencies. Machine learning techniques are applied to many composite problems which arise while operating and managing a network. There are plenty of research works carried out in the network traffic classification by applying machine learning concepts. In this paper, author presents both the application of different machine learning algorithms in various key areas of networking across different network technologies. In [7], ML techniques are applied for different

Table 1 System requirements

1	Operating system	Ubuntu 18.04
2	RAM	4 GB
3	CPU	CORE i5
4	Programming language	PYTHON 3

vital problems in networking like the traffic prediction, the network intrusion, the congestion control, routing problems, resource and error management, Quality of service, and Quality of experience management and network security. In this survey paper, author describes the restrictions, disadvantages, challenges encountered, and future chances to advance machine learning in computer network area. It timely describes the influence of the design of machine learning for networking, that is assertive the limitations of network process, functioning, and management. In [8], the author describes network traffic classification using flow measurement which allows the workers to do more vital network administration. The stream accounting methods like NetFlow are considered as inadequate for classification needful additional packet-level information, host behavior examination, and focused computer hardware limiting their practical acceptance. In [9] in this paper for data classification, author proposes artificial neural regression for classification based on technical views and finally compares with various machine learning models. Table 1 gives font sizes of headings. Table captions should always be positioned above the tables.

3 Problem Specifications

The recent advances in networking area the usage of machine learning (ML) algorithms to solve problem like classification becomes more popular. The use of ML techniques in developing network traffic classification systems is not a new idea. The machine learning algorithms have more impact on network traffic classification [10], and in [11] we came to know that there are two machine learning methods that can be applied classify a network traffic. In [12], distributed Internet traffic generator manual helped us to create network traffic and also got the required dataset for our project. We came across by many papers and researches from which we came to know the working of machine learning algorithms and the use of each algorithm. Also, we came to know how a network transfers each data from source to destination, how a network traffic affects the flow of the data, how a noise or disturbance in the flow of network can create an issue. As the technology got upgraded, network and network-based technology also got upgraded. As there was a tremendous use of networks, there occurred many errors while flow of data. Network traffic is basically classified into three types. There was loss of data and the accuracy of data flow got decreased. So, we thought to use machine learning algorithms to study the network traffic and increase the accuracy of the data flow. Now, we can formally express the problem of traffic classification. The traffic classification includes each flow to an application, based on the features that have been mined from the given data. Let P is the n-dimensional random variable corresponding to the flow features. Let us consider a vector $P = (p_1, p_2, p_3, \ldots, p_{n-1}, p_n)$ comprising of the 'n' measured features which is associated to respective flow.

4 Implementation

Figure 1 shows the proposed model, and the network traffic collected from the real time environment acts as input data set that passed into the machine learning module. The proposed model uses different algorithms like support vector machine (SVM), random forest classifier, and multilayer perceptron. The network traffic is passed to the machine learning modules made up of three ML algorithms. The network is classified based on the parameters like Telnet, Ping, and voice traffic data and helps to classify the network based on the result. The result is based on the accuracy in which the data can be uploaded or downloaded form a protocol. The algorithm having the best accuracy will be having the best network traffic controller.

We used existing data set generated [14] using Tcpdump tool, and data set size is more than two million and stored in four CSV files. While choosing the appropriate datasets, we came across many parameters which were used to classify the network. So chose the dataset which were having more parameters and suitable for our model. The parameters are duration, protocol, service, state, upload of packets, download of packets, rate, s time to live protocol (sttl), d time to live (dttl), sload, dload, input packet (sinpkt), input packet (dinpkt), Jitter (sjit), Jitter (djit),

Fig. 1 Proposed model

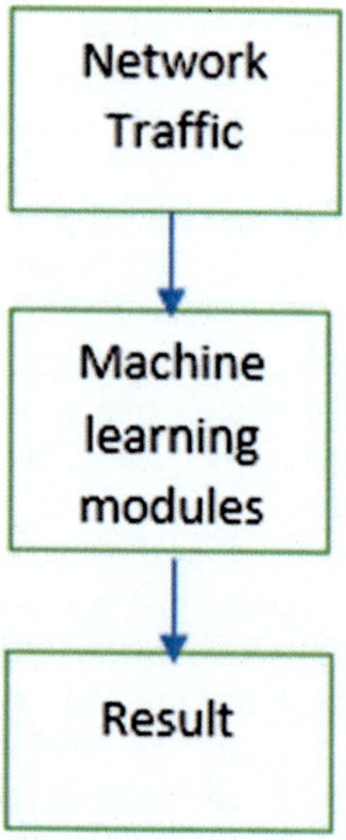

Windows Internet naming (swin), transfer control protocol (stcpb, dtcpb), tcprtt, mean square error (smeansz, dmeansz), transition depth (trans_depth), ct_srv_src, ct_state_ttl, ct_dst_ltm, file transfer protocol (is_ftp_login), the hypertext transfer protocol (ct_flw_http_mthd). The Feature selection method used to reduce the quantity of attributes uses the automatic choice of attributes in the given data, by inclusion or by exclusion of data without modifying the data, so we can select minimum subset. Here, we used hybrid future selection methods for the existing data set [14], it uses two phases. In the initial phase, we do the analyses of sample domain and in next phase improve the samples to take the finest outcome.

Response of the source (response_body_len), each and every parameter have their own criteria of distinguishing the network such as the size of the data packet, which protocol it uses, time taken or duration of the data packet took to reach its destination. These parameters helped to classify the network based on accuracy.

4.1 The Dataset

The dataset we used to train our machine learning models are taken by the Cyber Range Lab of the Australian Center for Cyber Security (ACCS). The people who made the data set used the recent developed tool called the IXIA Perfect Storm tool which is used to generate a hybrid real modern normal activities and synthetic contemporary network traffic behaviors. The main reason that we chose the dataset was because it uses as features the fields contained in PCAP files. PCAP files are derived from the Wireshark software. Wireshark software helps in analyzing the networks based on their behavior. This means that the system can be applied in real situations, using as input packets captured in the network with Tcpdump.

4.2 The Supervised Learning

The supervised learning is also known as labeling learning technique. These are the algorithms consisting of a well set of trained datasets which are known as inputs and outputs used to build the required system model which learns relationship between the input and output. After training the system, when a new input is given to the system, the trained model helps to get a related or accurate required output. In this techniques, cluster of decision rules can be used find the outcome.

4.3 The Multilayer Perceptron (MLP)

The MLP is a form of feed-forward neural network. It helps to generate a set of outputs from a set of inputs. It has been characterized into different layers of input nodes which are connected as directed graph between the inputs and outputs layer. Multilayer perceptron also uses back propagation for training a well-defined networking system. MLP is also known as deep learning method. MLP is mostly used in solving complicated problems which require supervised learning to get accurate solution to the problem. It is also used in speech recognition, image recognition, and machine translation, where w tells about the vector of weights, x tells about the vector of inputs, b tells about the bias, and Phi tells about the non-linear activation function. The model was compiled with an optimizer and a categorical cross-entropy loss function and trained in batches of 150 instances for 150 iterations. So, the datasets were iterated for 150 times. After each iteration, we came to know that the accuracy was gradually increasing and the mean square was gradually decreasing.

4.4 The Random Forest Classifier

The random forest classifier is a type of supervised learning algorithms. It is used to distinguish both classification and regression. A forest consists of trees. It is said that if the trees in the forest are more, then more robust is the forest [13]. The random forest is used widely in the networking field. It is useful in many of application like image processing, engine recommendations, and to predict medical diseases. It uses the base of Boruta algorithm equation, which helps to select important features in dataset.

Mathematically,

$$\mathrm{RFfi}_i = (\Sigma_{j \in \text{all trees}} \mathrm{normfi}_{ij})/T \tag{1}$$

where RFfi(i) tells about the significance of the feature represented as 'i', which is calculated from all the trees in the random forest algorithm. normfi(ij) tells about the normalized feature importance for 'i' in the tree 'j' of the random forest, and T denotes the total number of trees in the random forest.

- fi denotes the frequency of the label i at the node.
- normfi is used to find the importance feature of i in the given node j and also characterizes the similar data in the given dataset.

The framework that we used after trying several variants which like thousand estimators and five is the depth of a tree. The random forest classifier algorithm gives us with better accuracy results of 81.336% accuracy. Generally, our opinion was to use the algorithm to its extinct to get accurate results, and it was easy to apply and execute faster than other algorithms.

4.5 The Support Vector Machine (SVM)

In machine learning algorithms, the support vector machine is more popular, which is useful to analyze the data for both classification and regression. SVM is also a supervised learning which accepts the data and sorts it into different categories. The support vector network (SVN) is also referred as support vector machine, it plays a major role in the fields of networking. It is used to classify networks based on the protocols and port number. Equation (3) is used to represent hypothesis function 'h' as all the point above or on the hyperplane that will be classified as class +1, and the class −1 is classified for all the point below the hyperplane.

$$h(x_i) = \begin{cases} +1 \text{ if} w \cdot x + b \geq 0 \\ -1 \text{ if} w \cdot x + b < 0 \end{cases} \tag{2}$$

The support vector machine models used calculate decision boundaries between the labeled data, and same is called as the hyperplane. The points or arguments near to these hyperplanes are known as the extreme points, and the algorithm is going to choose these decision boundaries by setting up many margins which helps to differentiate the hyperplanes. The real-world data can be classified as one-dimensional data and multi-dimensional data, and all one-dimensional or multi-dimensional data sets are need not always linear separable. Data set is present in multi-dimensional datasets. While executing the datasets eventually, the SVM took more time to execute, but gradually the time would increase exponentially with more data as SVM tends to cross-calculate each point with the rest of the data. Comparing to the other two algorithms, the time was in a much higher scale.

5 The Performance Evaluation and Results

Table 1 shows the system requirements considered for performance evaluation. We used a well-configured system consisting of 4 GB RAM, Ubuntu 18.04 operating system. We used Python as our primary programming language which also helped machine learning algorithms to give appropriate results. In Ubuntu, we installed SciKit, Tensor flow Backend, Panda, and Matplotlib functions to implement our project.

5.1 The Accuracy

Accuracy is the method for evaluating classification models. It is the fraction of prediction in which the models have got right solutions. It can be defined as number of exact predictions versus total number of predictions. For binary classifications,

Table 2 Accuracy table for various algorithms

Algorithms	Accuracy (%)
Support vector machine	76.101
Multilayer perceptron	83.96
Random forest classifier	81.336

accuracy can also be calculated as follows: The accurateness can be represented by the mathematical formal (TP + TN) / (TP + TN + FP + FN). In which, FN represents false negatives. TP is true positives; FP is false positives, and TN is true negatives. For respectable classifiers, The TPR and TNR both would be closer to 100%. So, the accuracy changes for different algorithms as given in Table 2.

As we can see from Table 2 and the accuracy graph in Fig. 2, the multi-layer perceptron feed-forward algorithm gives the best performance among other algorithms.

Figure 3 shows the confusion matrix: As we can see the matrix provided as with only about 1.4% false positive classifications and above matrix, it is differentiated as true positive classification and false positive classification. We have used best-effort traffic which consists of both normal data packets and less errored data packets. So it represents that the most of the data packets are normal which true positive classification is and only some data packets are errored data packet which are false positive classification.

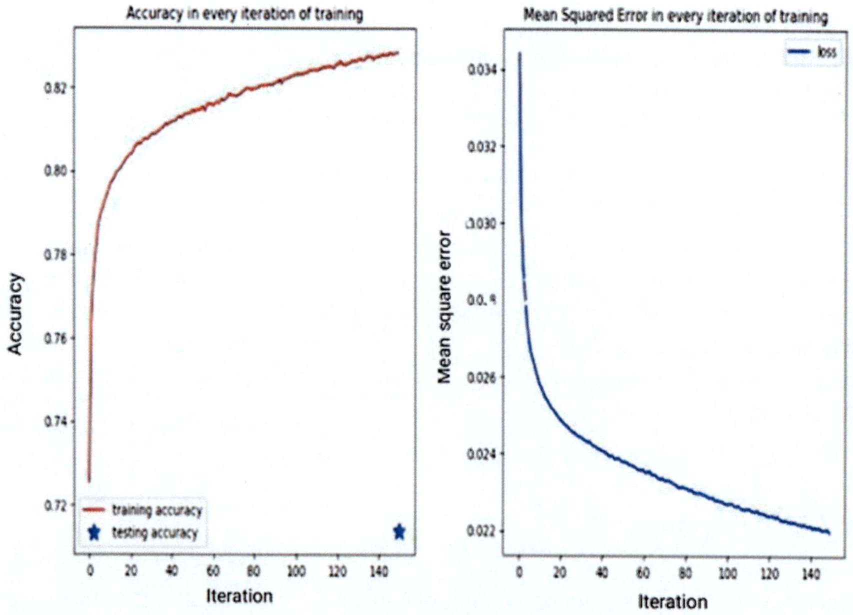

Fig. 2 Accuracy graph

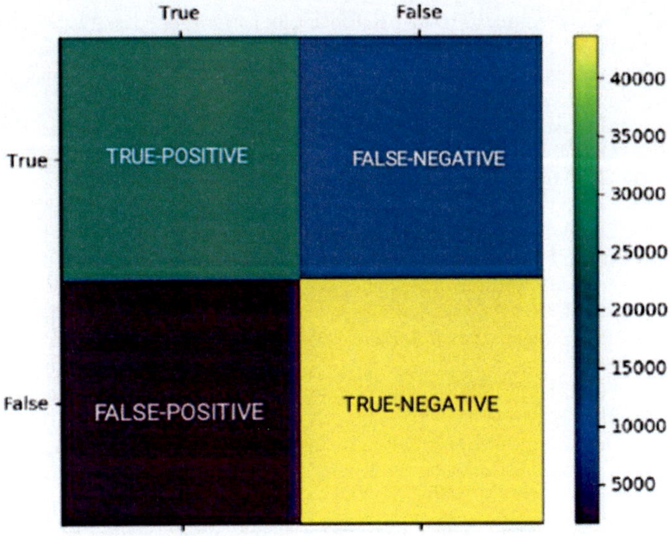

Fig. 3 Confusion matrix

6 Conclusion and Future Work

In this paper, we have used the existing data set and selected a few ML algorithms like the support vector machine (SVM), the random forest classifier, and a multilayer perceptron for network traffic classification. The final result analysis shows the accuracy of various ML algorithms against the unique data set. The support vector machine algorithm gave an accuracy of 76.101%, the random forest classifier gives an accuracy of 81.336%, and the multilayer perceptron gives an accuracy of 83.96%. It is used to minimize the use of external controllers to classify the network traffic. In future, we are planning to apply this model for real-time data, and we compare the cross-validation method with other techniques.

References

1. Goss RG, Nitschke GS (2013) Automated network application classification: a competitive learning approach. In: 2013 IEEE symposium on computational intelligence for communication systems and networks (CIComms), Singapore, 2013, pp 45–52. https://doi.org/10.1109/CICommS.2013.6582853
2. Wang W et al (2018)A network traffic flow prediction with deep learning approach for large-scale metropolitan area network. In: NOMS 2018—2018 IEEE/ifip network operations and management symposium, Taipei, 2018, pp 1–9. https://doi.org/10.1109/NOMS.2018.8406252.
3. Angra S, Ahuja S (2017)Machine learning and its applications: a review. In: 2017 international conference on big data analytics and computational intelligence (ICBDAC), Chirala, 2017, pp 57–60. https://doi.org/10.1109/ICBDACI.2017.8070809

4. Shastry N, Keerthan Kumar TG (2020) Enhancing the performance of software-defined wireless mesh network. In: Bindhu V, Chen J, Tavares J (eds) International conference on communication, computing and electronics systems. Lecture notes in electrical engineering, vol 637. Springer, Singapore
5. Anagha MJ, Lepakshi R, Goutham V, Thavish V, Keerthan Kumar TG (2020) Packet injection and Dos attack controller software(PDACS) module to handle attacks in software defined network. In: 2020 fourth international conference on computing methodologies and communication (ICCMC), Erode, India, 2020, pp 966–970. https://doi.org/10.1109/ICCMC48092.2020.ICCMC-000179
6. Lavrač N, Škrlj B, Robnik-Šikonja M (2020) Propositionalization and embeddings: two sides of the same coin. Mach Learn. https://doi.org/10.1007/s10994-020-05890-8
7. Musumeci F et al (2019) An overview on application of machine learning techniques in optical networks. IEEE Commun. Surv. Tutorials 21(2): 1383–1408. https://doi.org/10.1109/COMST.2018.2880039
8. Dainotti A, Pescapè A, Claffy KC (2012) Issues and future directions in traffic classification. IEEE Network 26(1):35–40
9. Dreiseit S, Ohno-Machado L (2002) Logistic regression and artificial neural network classification models: a methodology review. J Biomed Inform 35(5–6):352–359. ISSN: 1532-0464. https://doi.org/10.1016/S1532-0464(03)00034-0
10. Jun L, Shunyi Z, Yanqing L, Zailong Z (2007) Internet traffic classification using machine learning. In: 2007 second international conference on communications and networking in China, Shanghai, 2007, pp 239–243. https://doi.org/10.1109/CHINACOM.2007.4469372
11. Dashevskiy M, Luo Z (2012) Two methods for reliable classification of network traffic. Prog Artif Intell 1:223–234. https://doi.org/10.1007/s13748-012-0019-5. https://www.unsw.adfa.edu.au/unsw-canberra-cyber/cybersecurity/ADFA-NB15-Datasets/
12. Avallone S, Guadagno S, Emma D, Pescape A,. Ventre G (2004) D-ITG distributed Internet traffic generator. In: First international conference on the quantitative evaluation of systems, 2004. QEST 2004. Proceedings, Enschede, The Netherlands, 2004, pp 316–317. https://doi.org/10.1109/QEST.2004.1348045
13. Keerthan Kumar TG, Shubha C, Sushma SA (2019) Random forest algorithm for soil fertility prediction and grading using machine learning. Int J Innov Technol Explor Eng (IJITEE) 9(1). ISSN: 2278-3075. https://doi.org/10.35940/ijitee.L3609.119119
14. Kärkkäinen T (2014) On cross-validation for MLP model evaluation. In: Fränti P, Brown G, Loog M, Escolano F, Pelillo M (eds) Structural, syntactic, and statistical pattern recognition. S+SSPR 2014. Lecture Notes in Computer Science, vol 8621. Springer, Berlin, Heidelberg. https://doi.org/10.1007/978-3-662-44415-3_30

Binary PSO-Based Feature Selection and Neural Network for Parkinson's Disease Prediction

K. Naga Sireesha, Babitha Donepudi, and Vamsidhar Enireddy

Abstract The Parkinson's disease which affects the nervous condition influences the life of the patients and their family members. The study has shown that the prevalence is more in developed countries, as more elderly people are found in their population. It has been also found out that the men are affected more than the women. In this paper, binary particle swarm optimization which is a swarm-based algorithm is used for selecting the best feature subset. Support vector machine, logistic regression, support vector machine using stochastic gradient descent, and neural networks are used for classification. A classification accuracy of 89.74% is achieved using PSO-NN, while this rate is 87.69% in PSO-SGD, 86.67% in PSO-LR, and 81.54% in PSO-SVM. Thus, application of neural networks gave the best accurate prediction of disease.

Keywords Feature selection · Logistic regression · Parkinson's disease · Particle swarm optimization · Support vector machine

1 Introduction

The neurological disorder, Parkinson's Disease (PD) influences the standard life of the patients and their family members. It has become more prevalent in the developed countries and in the countries where there are more elderly people in their population. In a study done in the US, they have found that by there will be one million cases alone in the country, and it will be around ten million worldwide. The

K. Naga Sireesha
Department of Computer Science, St. Joseph's College for Women (A), Visakhapatnam, India
e-mail: vnsiri@gmail.com

B. Donepudi · V. Enireddy (✉)
Department of Computer Science and Engineering, Koneru Lakshmaiah Education Foundation, Vaddeswaram, India
e-mail: enireddy.vamsidhar@gmail.com

B. Donepudi
e-mail: donepudi.babitha@gmail.com

S. Bhattacharyya et al. (eds.), *International Conference on Intelligent and Smart Computing in Data Analytics*, Advances in Intelligent Systems and Computing 1312,
https://doi.org/10.1007/978-981-33-6176-8_2

women are less affected than the men, and the possibility is around 1.5 times higher in men [1]. The disorder symptoms include slow movement, shivering, body stiffness, impaired balance and unable to hold things. As the sickness advances, patients may encounter trouble in imperative assignments, for example, strolling, discourse, gulping, and biting, passionate changes, and sleep disorder. PD side effects happen gradually, and in certain individuals, the illness advances quicker than others. It has also been observed that the intensity of the symptom's changes from individual to individual and does not make a similar impact [2]. Although there is no treatment strategy to dispense with this illness totally, sedate medication is employed to lessen the signs found in the initial stages. To identify this disorder, the methods such as vocal analysis and walking are widely used [3]. Non-linear problems are solved using Support Vector Machine (SVM), which uses supervised algorithm for learning and gives an effective results for prediction. Another machine learning algorithm we used is Logistic Regression (LR) and is the better algorithm which can be applied for binary classification. Neural networks were also applied in our study to predict the PD disease. The dataset utilized in the investigation is acquired from 31 individuals having 195 instances with 22 attributes [4]. Inspired by the natural behavior of animals, Swarm Intelligence (SI) has become a popular study to solve the complex problems. This type of systems comprises commonly of a population of generally straightforward specialists associating just locally with themselves and with their condition, without having global information in relation to their personal state and their condition of the surroundings. It has wide applications in clustering and classification which are mostly used in the data mining techniques. Ant Colony Optimization (ACO) and Particle Swarm Optimization (PSO) are the two principle swarm intelligence algorithms mostly used for optimization. Ant colony optimization mostly used for discrete functions and particle swarm optimization for continuous functions. PSO is a population-based search algorithm and is initialized with a population of random solutions, called particles [5]. PSO uses particles to represent the population for finding a solution as it is a population-based search algorithm. Not at all like in the other developmental calculation procedures, every particle in PSO is additionally connected with a velocity. Particles fly through the pursuit space with velocities which are powerfully balanced by their authentic practices. Along these lines, the particles tend to fly toward the better inquiry territory through the span of search process. PSO has demonstrated better performance in unsupervised learning algorithms like clustering techniques.

The favorable circumstances of PSO over different metaheuristics are that they can be easily implemented, less parameters to tune, high-efficient memory abilities due to previous best value and global best value, and each particle updates itself using the information gathered from the best particle.

In this paper, binary PSO is used along with the mutual information in finding the best feature subset.

2 Methodology

The Parkinson's dataset is prepared by gathering the data from 188 patients with Parkinson's disease in which 107 are men and 81 are women, the ages ranging from 33 to 87 years, and this data is available in the UCI website [6]. This data is downloaded, and then, it is imported into our working directory. The entire research is performed in the Jupyter notebook and Python environment. The data is already class labeled with the target feature named as "target," which predicts whether a person has Parkinson's or not. The data then pre-processed, and data normalization is applied so that all the attribute values fall within the same range. Normalization is obtained by transforming the data and scaling the data to have values between 0 and 1. If the data is not normalized, then it results in biased results. Then, we apply different classification algorithms on this data by computing the optimal values for our own custom objective function. All the classifiers will then be evaluated based on model evaluation metrics. The metrics include classification accuracy, recall, precision, and $F1$-Score. Particle swarm optimization is applied on all the algorithms we perform in this study. We used the optimizer Binary Particle Swarm Optimization (Binary PSO) to perform feature subset selection to improve classifier performance. The definition of the collection of feature subsets is to be able to find the best features that are appropriate for the task of classification. The location of the particles is represented in two terms for a Binary PSO: 1 or 0 (on or off). If we have an n-dimensional particle, then its position can be defined at that time as: $P = [p_1, p_2, p_3, \ldots, p_n]$, where p_i belongs to 0, 1

The objective function is:

$$f(X) = \alpha(1 - P) + (1 - \alpha)\left(1 - \frac{N_f}{N_t}\right) \quad (1)$$

where α, hyper parameter with the intent of deciding on the trade-off between the output of the classifier and the dimension of the subset of features with respect to the total number of features. We would then prepare a classifier utilizing positions obtained by running different cases of the calculations which we need to apply. We can think about the presentation when we're utilizing all the features. Another significance is the ability to select the best features or dimensionality reduction on our information. This improves the classification accuracy and accelerates the model. In this study, several machine learning algorithms like PSO-SVM, PSO-LR, PSO-SGD, and PSO-NN models are compared with each other to find the best model which could accurately predict the PD disease. The hyper parameters are set arbitrarily. The performance of the model is calculated using the parameters like the accuracy, precision, recall, $F1$ score parameters (Fig. 1).

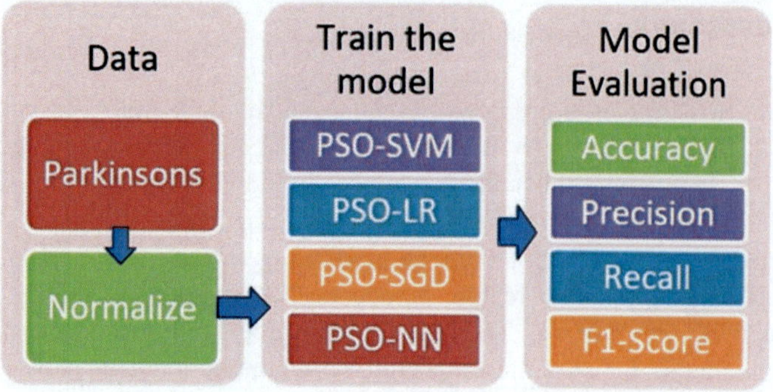

Fig. 1 Process flow of the methodology implemented

2.1 Neural Networks

These networks are developed such that they impersonate the activities of a human cerebrum to perceive connections between huge measures of data. They have interconnections between the nodes. A perceptron is nothing but a node in the neural network which is like multiple linear regression. The multi-layer perceptron consists of a input layer, hidden layer, and a output layer. The network can have more than one hidden layer [7]. The number of input neurons indicates the number of input features, and number of output layer neurons represents the number of output features. An activation function is used, and a network can have more than one activation function: one at hidden layer and other at output layer. The input weights can be tuned using different methods to reduce the errors. There are other parameters based on the model of the neural network which can tuned to obtain better results. The neural networks are very popular and used in many applications. In this network, the weights are updated using the formula. W represents the weight; i represents the input layer; j to represent the hidden layer and k the output layer. Activation function employed is the Sigmoid function and

$$\omega_{jk}(t+1) = \omega_{jk}(t) + \underbrace{\alpha\delta_k z_j + \eta\left[\omega_{jk}(t) - \omega_{jk}(t-1)\right]}_{\Delta\omega_{jk}(t+1)} \tag{2}$$

$$w_{ij}(t+1) = w_{ij}(t) + \underbrace{\alpha\delta_j x_i + \eta\left[w_{ij}(t) - w_{ij}(t-1)\right]}_{\Delta w_{ij}(t+1)} \tag{3}$$

The learning rate α to be chosen between 0.001 and 0.1. Momentum factor helps in achieving a quicker convergence.

3 Results and Discussions

We created an instance of binary PSO optimizer to mask all the variables in the Parkinson's dataset. Then, for each particle, the objective function is computed, and the classifier is trained by k-fold cross-validation, and the cross-validation score is assessed as the performance measure. The same procedure is repeated for the whole swarm and for the number of iterations arbitrarily chosen. Once the classifier is optimized, it returns the best cost and position of the particle selected.

The classification accuracy of the logistic regression when all the features in the dataset are used is 83.95%, whereas when the best subset features selected by the particle swarm optimizer are used, then the classification accuracy increased to 86.67%. Thus, there is an increase of approximately 3% improvement in the classification accuracy.

The classification accuracy of the SVM using SGD when all the features in the dataset are used is 54%, whereas when the best subset features selected by the particle swarm optimizer are used, then the classification accuracy increased to 87.69%. Thus, there is an increase of approximately 33% improvement in the classification accuracy.

The classification accuracy of the SVM when all the features in the dataset are used is 75.4%, whereas when the best subset features selected by the particle swarm optimizer are used, then the classification accuracy increased to 81.54%. Thus, there is an increase of approximately 6% improvement in the classification accuracy.

The neural network model is performed for 100 iterations, and all the costs are computed. The iterations are plotted on the X-axis, and the costs are plotted on the Y-axis. The best cost obtained is 0.25. After 50 iterations, the classifier already has reached the convergence point (Fig. 2).

The above bar chart shows the comparison between the models developed in this study based on the performance accuracy. The algorithms are plotted on the X-axis, whereas the percentage of accuracy is plotted on the Y-axis. The value of the accuracy is labeled above the bar of the respective algorithm. Of all the models developed, PS0-NN has the highest predictive performance with accuracy of 89.74%, whereas the least accurate model is PSO-SVM with 81.54% when compared with other models.

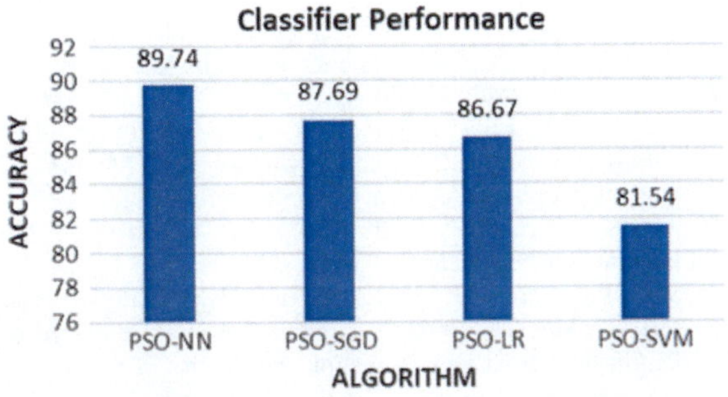

Fig. 2 Classification accuracy obtained for different classifiers

Table 1 Accuracy, precision, recall and F-1 score values obtained for different classifiers

Algorithm	Accuracy	Precision	Recall	$F1$-Score
PSO-NN	89.74	92	85	87
PSO-SGD	87.69	93	73	74
PSO-LR	86.67	86	79	84
PSO-SVM	81.54	89	75	87

Table 1 shows the comparison among the classifier models. These models are compared using the performance metrics like accuracy, recall, precision, and $F1$-Score. It shows that PSO-NN model has highest accuracy and also the precision, recall, and $F1$-Score. Some models with low accuracy may sometimes have good precision or recall. Thus, in disease prediction, it is mandatory to have an accurate prediction of the disease.

4 Conclusion

An accurate diagnosis is very useful for the doctors to treat the patients and not only that the early diagnosis helps to save the life of a human being. Many optimization algorithms are developed in the literature. These algorithms can help to find the optimal features so that the redundancy and the complexity of the classification algorithm can be reduced. In this paper, particle swarm optimization which is swarm optimization is used to predict the Parkinson's disease. Binary swarm optimization is used for finding the classification accuracy, and this has provided a satisfactory result. The best model PSO-NN achieved a classification accuracy of 89.74%, while this rate is 87.69% in PSO-SGD, 86.67% in PSO-LR, and 81.54% in PSO-SVM. Thus, application of neural networks gave the best accurate prediction of disease.

References

1. https://parkinson.org/Understanding-Parkinsons/Causes-andStatistics/Statistics
2. https://www.worldpdcoalition.org/page/AboutParkinson
3. Liu X, Fu H, PSO-based support vector machine with cuckoo search technique for clinical disease diagnoses. Sci World J 2014, Article ID 548483
4. https://ftp.ics.uci.edu/pub/machine-learning-databases/
5. Kennedy J, Eberhart R (1995) Particle swarm optimization. In: Proceedings of the IEEE international conference on neural networks, vol 4, pp 1942–1948
6. Sakar CO, Serbes G, Gunduz A, Tunc HC, Nizam H, Sakar BE, Tutuncu M, Aydin T, Isenkul ME, Apaydin H (2008) A comparative analysis of speech signal processing algorithms for Parkinson's disease classification and the use of the tunable Q-factor wavelet transform. Appl Soft Comput
7. Pal SK, Mitra S (1992) Multilayer perceptron, fuzzy sets, and classification. IEEE Trans Neural Networks 3(5):683–697

An Evolutionary-Based Additive Tree for Enhanced Disease Prediction

Babitha Donepudi, M. R. Narasingarao, and Vamsidhar Enireddy

Abstract The increased usage of machine learning in healthcare applications requires the highly accurate decision support models which are good in predictive performance and intuitive explanation. Although the models like additive tree could balance both the factors, it can be further enhanced by applying the evolutionary methods. This paper thus provides a decision support system by introducing an enhanced additive tree which could provide an accurate disease prediction in the medical domain. Along with good increase in accuracy, it also scales down the nodes in the tree by performing dimensionality reduction. The proposed model is also as accurate as the linear classifier algorithms and ensemble models.

Keywords Additive tree (ADT) · Extremely randomized trees (EXT) · Machine learning · Multi-layer perceptron (MLP) · Support vector machine (SVM) · Particle swarm optimization (PSO)

1 Introduction

Disease prediction in medical domain is a crucial machine learning application for almost a decade. Any misprediction or false outcome generated by the classifier models could result in huge loss which is linked to the patient's health or life. Thus, the model developed must be highly accurate and easily understandable by the medical practitioners and users. This paper builds a simple model which can be applied to any healthcare application to provide most accurate predictions.

Additive tree is a type of ensemble model which bridges the classification and regression tree (CART) [1] and gradient boosting [2]. It can be inferred as a highly interpretable decision tree which is as accurate as the gradient boosting models. In this work, we propose a hybrid methodology that combines the self-exploratory learning functionality of the PSO [3] with the ADT classifier. Feature space performs a vital

B. Donepudi (✉) · M. R. Narasingarao · V. Enireddy
Department of Computer Science and Engineering, Koneru Lakshmaiah Education Foundation, Guntur 522502, India
e-mail: donepudi.babitha@gmail.com

S. Bhattacharyya et al. (eds.), *International Conference on Intelligent and Smart Computing in Data Analytics*, Advances in Intelligent Systems and Computing 1312,
https://doi.org/10.1007/978-981-33-6176-8_3

role in the classifier's predictive efficiency. Therefore, we develop a multi-objective optimization to achieve the best accuracy with minimum quantity of significant features.

2 Related Work

Luna et al. [4] developed an additive tree model which is as interpretable as decision tree and as accurate as gradient boosting methods. However, the ensemble methods outperformed the additive tree at the cost of interpretability. Research done by Cervante et al. [5] shows that binary PSO can be employed for feature selection on decision tree and can be evaluated the selected feature subsets based on predictive accuracy. Kaucha et al. [6] applied several image processing techniques on CT scan images to detect lung cancer at an early stage. The collected outcomes are categorized utilizing the SVM.

Research performed by Valupadasu and Chunduri [7] developed a multi-layer perceptron model which aids the doctors in early detection of cardiovascular disease. Wavelet transformation is applied for feature extraction, and the ECG features extracted are used by MLP classification. The extra trees were applied by Zafari et al. [8] to construct a kernel which is then used for classification using SVM. They analyzed that SVM with extra trees as kernel outperforms the general SVM Kernels.

Sweety and Jiji [9] proposed a hybrid algorithm to detect Alzheimer disease by applying PSO for feature extraction. The MRI images of brain are used, and then, decision tree classifier is used to detect the disease. Dogo et al. [10] performed a comparative analysis on several stochastic gradient algorithms by applying convolution neural networks on several image datasets and evaluated them on metrics like loss and accuracy.

3 Methodology

Three benchmark datasets from UCI and PMLB are used in our experiments. The UCI-Parkinson's dataset, DS1, has 195 instances of 24 variables. The main goal is to discriminate the healthy people from those suffering from Parkinson's. The target feature is "status," i.e., to classify whether a person has Parkinson's disease or not. DS1 contains the biomedical voice profile of the people. Like DS1, the dataset DS2, which is collected from PMLB-Hepatitis dataset, is also medium sized with 155 observations of 20 features. It is binary classed, and the motive is to detect if a person has Hepatitis or not. DS3 is fetched from UCI-Heart disease dataset. It contains 303 instances of 14 variables. The classification task is to find whether a person has heart disease or not. The class labels are binary and featured under the name "target." Thus, all the classification tasks are binary class classification and related to disease prediction in medical domain. Our aim is to find a generalized classifier which can

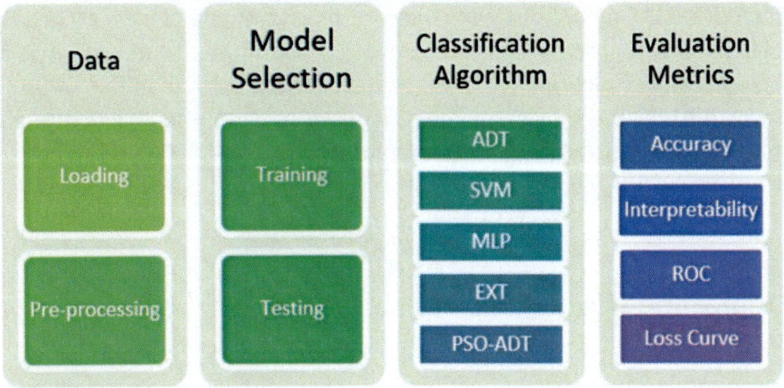

Fig. 1 Phases of classification task

handle all datasets of healthcare satisfying the evaluation criteria as mentioned in Fig. 1.

The data is pre-processed by performing dimensionality reduction. In the model selection phase, the available data is divided into train and test sets using the K-fold cross-validation. Now, each algorithm in the next phase is trained using every training set of the datasets and validated with the test set. In this paper, PSO is applied for feature selection in building the classifier model PSO-ADT. The multi-objective fitness function we applied is:

$$f(D) = \beta(1 - A) + (1 - \beta)(1 - Nf/N_t) \tag{1}$$

where D is the set of attributes in dataset, and β is a hyperparameter which determines the fine balance between classification accuracy (A) and the size of the subset of features (N_f) over the whole range of features (N_t).

Algorithm: Proposed method PSO-ADT

Input: Swarm size, data, dimensions, arbitrary parameters, maximum iterations, Fitness function.
Output: Final subset, Accuracy, Additive Tree.

1. Creating Initial Population.
2. Train Additive Tree and evaluate the Objective function in Eq. (1).
3. Find personal and global best values of all the particles in the swarm.
4. Update all the particles location and velocity.
5. Stop in case of observing termination criteria.
6. Generate next generation and Go to Step 2.

In the PSO-ADT model, the parameters of the swarm are chosen arbitrarily. The number of particles chosen is 30 and the stopping condition as the maximum iterations as 5. The objective function is then evaluated for each particle in the swarm, and it is performed to the whole swarm. The proposed model is first trained to gain the optimum subset of attributes. The test tuples are then validated on the classifier to get the testing accuracy.

4 Results and Discussions

Classification algorithms are trained on the selected datasets, and their respective models were developed as shown in Fig. 2. It can be stated that ADT gives a satisfactory result which balances both the accuracy and interpretability. But it can be further improved by applying swarm intelligence to obtain the best possible features which boosts up the accuracy.

The mean values of personal best cost and the neighborhood cost of the optimizer are plotted in Fig. 3. Binary PSO is applied on DS1 to select the relevant features which can enhance the accuracy of the classifier. The objective function is computed for each particle, and it is applied to the whole swarm. The loss values are found for each iteration. The best position and cost of the particle itself and its neighbors are also considered while optimizing the fitness function. Thus, out of the 24 features of DS1, PSO selected the 16 features, thus hiking the accuracy from 87.18% (on full set) to 92.31% (on best subset). The best cost thus obtained is 0.142. The same procedure is used for the other two datasets, and the proposed algorithm is implemented on the features selected. Once the hybrid models are developed, they can be compared with the simple ADT model with respect to both the evaluation metrics we consider.

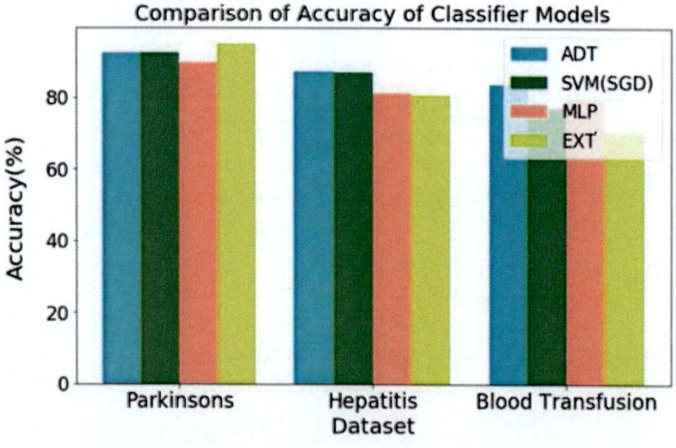

Fig. 2 Bar chart comparing several classifier models developed on three datasets

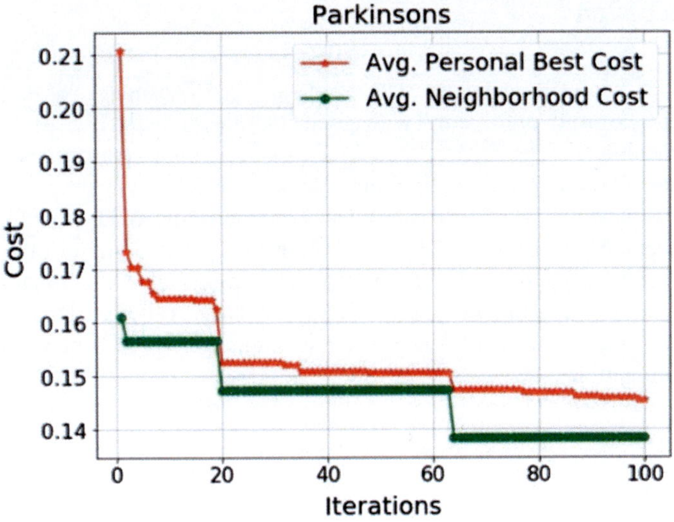

Fig. 3 Cost history of PSO applied on DS1

Table 1 displays the comparison between ADT and PSO-ADT evaluated on different measures. It can be depicted that there is an increase in accuracy in PSO-ADT on all the datasets. However, sensitivity has fluctuated slightly, whereas the $F1$-score has increased. On average, there is an increase of 2% of $F1$-score in all the three cases. The features have almost decreased to its half size in the latter model in all the scenarios. Thus, the length of the feature set and the range of decision nodes has decreased when applying PSO-ADT.

Table 1 Model evaluation of ADT versus PSO-ADT

Dataset	Model	Sensitivity (%)	Accuracy (%)	$F1$-score (%)	Features selected	Decision nodes
DS1	ADT	91	87	93	24	13
	PSO-ADT	93	92	95	16	9
DS2	ADT	99	84	90	20	17
	PSO-ADT	93	87	93	13	13
DS3	ADT	91	82	85	14	29
	PSO-ADT	91	84	86	8	19

5 Conclusion

In this paper, we recommended a state-of-the-art classifier model PSO-ADT which can provide accurate predictions with good interpretation for high-stake applications like healthcare. The model is evaluated by comparing its performance accuracy against other classifiers trained. In terms of interpretability, comparison is done with ADT based on split nodes created and variety of features used. Thus, PSO-ADT can be implemented as a generalized classification model for any kind of application in healthcare to provide reliable predictions. However, this research can be further improved by applying this model on multi-class datasets. It can also be improved by applying the advanced swarm intelligence algorithms which may give further accurate predictions.

References

1. Xie T, Li R, Zhang X, Zhou B, Wang Z (2019) Research on heartbeat classification algorithm based on CART decision tree. In: 8th international symposium on next generation electronics (ISNE), Zhengzhou, China, pp 1–3
2. Wen Z, He B, Kotagiri R, Lu S, Shi J (2018) Efficient gradient boosted decision tree training on GPUs. In: 2018 IEEE international parallel and distributed processing symposium (IPDPS), Vancouver, BC, pp 234–243
3. Hamed E, Anushya A, Alzoubi R, Vincy BSA, Balawneh DA (2017) An analysis of particle swarm optimization for feature selection on medical data. In: 2017 international conference on energy, communication, data analytics and soft computing (ICECDS), Chennai, pp 227–231
4. Luna J, Gennatas, Efstathios et al (2019) Building more accurate decision trees with the additive tree. In: Proceedings of the national academy of sciences
5. Cervante L, Xue B, Zhang M, Shang L (2012) Binary particle swarm optimisation for feature selection: a Filter based approach. In: IEEE Congress on evolutionary computation, Brisbane, QLD, pp 1-8
6. Kaucha DP, Prasad PWC, Alsadoon A, Elchouemi A, Sreedharan S (2017) Early detection of lung cancer using SVM classifier in biomedical image processing. In: 2017 IEEE international conference on power, control, signals and instrumentation engineering (ICPCSI), Chennai, pp 3143–3148
7. Valupadasu R, Chunduri BRR (2019) Automatic classification of cardiac disorders using MLP algorithm. In: 2019 prognostics and system health management conference, Paris, pp 253–257
8. Zafari A, Zurita-Milla R, Izquierdo-Verdiguier E (2019) Land cover classification using extremely randomized trees: a kernel perspective. In: IEEE geoscience and remote sensing letters, pp 1–5
9. Sweety ME, Jiji GW (2014) Detection of Alzheimer disease in brain images using PSO and decision tree approach. In: 2014 IEEE international conference on advanced communications, control and computing technologies, Ramanathapuram, pp 1305–1309
10. Dogo EM, Afolabi OJ, Nwulu NI, Twala B, Aigbavboa CO (2018) A comparative analysis of gradient descent-based optimization algorithms on convolutional neural networks. In: 2018 international conference on computational techniques, electronics and mechanical systems (CTEMS), Belgaum, India, pp 92–99

Novel Defense Framework for Cross-layer Attacks in Cognitive Radio Networks

Ganesh Davanam, T. Pavan Kumar, and M. Sunil Kumar

Abstract Cognitive radio networks are the self-configuring and mainly solve the problem of spectrum utilization. Cognitive radio networks always try to identify Occupied or un-occupied channels for transmission. Cognitive radio networks (CRN's) are an enabling technology for multiple features like dynamic spectrum access, spectrum sharing, and dynamic allocation. The existing research of security issues in CRN's mainly considers attacks in individual layers and provides significant solutions but attacker cannot propagates his attacks in single layer. In this work, we designed a cross-layer attack solution, where attackers attack two different layers at a time. The attacks we considered are report false sensing data (RFSD) attack in physical layer and small backoff window (SBW) attack in MAC layer. Simulation results shows that our proposed solutions perform in reducing these two attacks and significantly reduce the attack probability and increase channel utilization by primary users.

Keywords Cross-layer attacks · Framework · Security · Cognitive radios · Trust fusion

1 Introduction

Today, wireless communication systems are very important in human life. Wide range of applications and services of wireless communications are going to change the world more in future. The growth and usage of wireless communication systems increased rapidly across the world which led to the main problems of wireless communications, which are the scarcity of radio resources like power, frequency, and time. At present, the frequency spectrum's less availability, the need of reuse

G. Davanam (✉) · T. Pavan Kumar
Department of Computer Science and Engineering, Koneru Lakshmaiah Educational Foundation, Vaddeswaram, AP, India
e-mail: dgani05@gmail.com

G. Davanam · M. Sunil Kumar
Department of Computer Science and Engineering, Sree Vidyanikethan Engineering College (Autonomous), Tirupati, AP, India

S. Bhattacharyya et al. (eds.), *International Conference on Intelligent and Smart Computing in Data Analytics*, Advances in Intelligent Systems and Computing 1312,
https://doi.org/10.1007/978-981-33-6176-8_4

of the frequency have also gained great importance. There is a necessity to design, improve, and upgrade the wireless communication systems if we need to attain the improvement of communications.

In wireless communications, the resources must be utilized properly or else it may cause a issue scarcity of resources, which need to be solved. The spectrum is a major resource, and it should be allocated such that it is not going to be wasted. Static spectrum allocation and dynamic spectrum allocation can be said as the types of the allocation methods. The static spectrum allocation has given many successful applications the required spectrum they needed, but a situation was faced, where the spectrum [1] which was available has became insufficient for the emerging technologies, as the available applications left no space for them. We can also say that the spectrum is left unutilized. The main concept behind the working of a cognitive radio is the reuse or using this unutilized spectrum in an optimal way. We can solve these issues by using CRN's. Cognitive radio's have capability that to be aware of its environment. Mitola was the first person to introduce cognitive radio. The CR should need adaptability, sensing, flexibility, agility. Cognitive radio networks are formed by connecting all the cognitive radios. These cognitive radios try to sense the spectrum and try to figure out the white spaces in it.

Cognition, awareness, adaptability are the basic features of CRN's. The performance of a system can be made as optimal only by processing the information that we obtain from the environment, and this process is known as cognition. The process of finding whether a spectrum is available for communication or not that is sensing the environment which is known as awareness. A dynamic system which can reconfigure its parameters [2] is a cognitive radio system. The issues like utilization of unused spectrum and the less availability of the spectrum can be solved by using the dynamic accessing property of the spectrum of a cognitive radio [3]. As these networks are dynamic, open, flexible, there are chances that they can be exploited. These networks are vulnerable to attacks. Hence providing them with security is of a big and a complicated task. The cognitive cycle can be represented as shown in Fig. 1.

1.1 AI for Cognitive Radio Networks

Cognitive radio (CR) is the emerging technology for providing many applications [4] like self-organizing networks, spectrum markets, dynamic spectrum access, and so on. The cognitive radio designs can be implemented by using AI techniques [5] which help in improving the factors such as security, robustness, stability, responsiveness of a cognitive radio [6]. The three main things that should be in cognitive radio are: observation, reconfiguration, and cognition.

- Observation: It is the process of collecting the characteristics of the radio and information about the environment.
- Reconfiguration: The process of changing a radio's operating parameters.

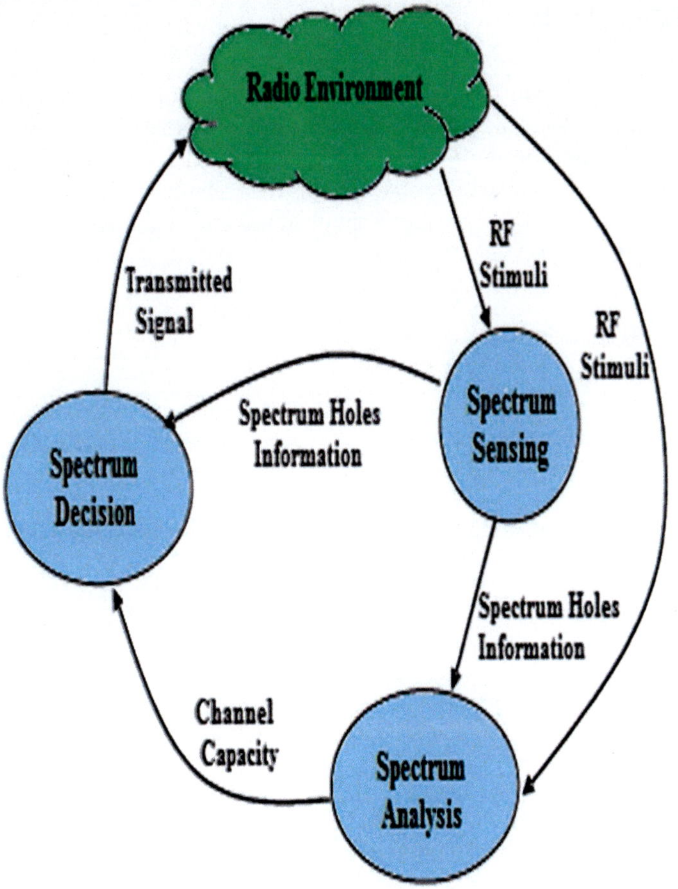

Fig. 1 Cognitive cycle

- Cognition: The process of analyzing the radio characteristics and environment, making decisions of actions, noting the impact of these actions on radio is done here.

These three can be combined to form an element called cognitive engine (CE). In a CR, the tasks of cognition are taken care by this engine [7]. The process starts by taking the input from environment; now, the analysis and classification of the situation are done by CE [8].

2 Related Works

The cognition in a radio can be viewed in application of artificial intelligence to the radio domain [8]. This paper presents a view on different types of techniques [9] used for implementing the design of a cognitive radio and providing security against attacks on cognitive radios like sensing data falsification attack, primary user emulation attack, etc. The table representing attacks and their existing solutions are given in Table 1.

Table 1 Traditional attacks and their existing solutions

Attack	Solution	Contributions
Primary user Emulation attack	Yardstick-based Threshold Allocation	N. Sureka, K. Gunaseelan, "Detection, Defense against Primary User Emulation Attack in Dynamic Cognitive Radio Networks", 2019
Objective function attack	Differential game-based approach	Guangsheng Feng, Junyu Lin, Qian Zhao, Huiqiang Wang, Hongwu Lyu "A Differential Game Based Approach Against Objective Function Attack in Cognitive Networks" 2018
Jamming attack	Boundary node detection	Saurabh, S., & Rustogi, R., "Tracing Jammed Area in Wireless Ad-hoc Network using Boundary Node Detection", 2018
Spectrum sensing falsification data attack	q-out-of-m rule scheme	Ngomane, I., Velempini, M., and Dlamini, S. V.," The detection of the spectrum sensing data falsification attack in cognitive radio ad hoc networks", (2018)
Hello attack	Symmetric key algorithms	Shekhar raj., Dr. O.P. Sahu., "Counter measures to security threats/Attacks on different protocol layers in cognitive radio networks", 2017
Sinkhole attack	Hop count-based sinkhole attack detection algorithm	Sejaphala, L., Velempini, M., and Dlamini, S. V. HCOBASAA: "Countermeasure Against Sinkhole Attacks in Software-Defined Wireless Sensor Cognitive Radio Networks". 2018
Sybil attack	Session key certificate	D. Srinivas Reddy, Dr. V. Bapuji, Dr. A. Govardhan and Prof. SSVN Sarma" Sybil Attack Detection Technique Using Session Key Certificate in Vehicular Ad Hoc Networks", 2017
Lion attack	Particle swarm optimization (PSO)	Shekhar raj., Dr. O. P. Sahu., "Counter measures to security threats/Attacks on different protocol layers in cognitive radio networks", 2017

3 Attack Models

3.1 PHY Layer Attack Model

The report false sensing attack (RFSD) that occurs in PHY layer mainly uses the collaborative spectrum sensing reports to mislead the resultant users. In collaborative spectrum sensing, the sensing reports from the several secondary users are considered to make a final decision of a primary user presence in the spectrum. Now, if "on" is the result of the fusion center that gives a clarity that attack is accomplished. The honest secondary users sensing reports characteristics can be seen now. In every stage of sensing, the sensing energy of a ith client can be denoted as E_i and it's distribution is

$$E_i \sim \begin{cases} \chi^2_{2m}, H_0 \\ \chi^2_{2m}(2\gamma_i),\ H_1 \end{cases} \tag{1}$$

where χ specifies chi-square allocation, $m =$ time band width, $\gamma_i =$ signal to noise ratio, H_0 represents primary user is absent, and H_1 represents main user which is available. Let G_0 represents sincere coverage, and G_1 represents untruthful coverage. An attacker reports correct Em value if it is above the threshold, i.e., Em $\geq \xi$ and dishonestly report if and if it is below threshold, i.e., Em $< \xi$ he reports wrong value Em + Δ (because primary user is not present), where $\xi =$ threshold and $\Delta =$ bias which attacker adds.

3.2 Defense Scheme

There is a three step procedure. In this scheme, at primary step, the presence of primary user is find out by using the sensing reports given by each node by the fusion center. Which is done by using a hypothesis test 1 for each node? The Neyman Pearson lemma is of the form:

$$\prod_{i=1, i\neq j}^{N} \frac{P(E_i = e_i | H_1)}{P(E_i = e_i | H_0)} \tag{2}$$

where η is the threshold value for examination 1. In second step, if the result of test 1 is H_0, then only we perform test 2 to find out if the node (j) is lying.

$$\frac{P\left(E_j = e_j | G_1, H_0\right)}{P\left(E_j = e_j | G_0, H_0\right)} \tag{3}$$

3.3 MAC Layer Attack Model

In order to start the transmission of the data packets by a inferior user, it need to stay for some length of time known as distributed inter frame space (DIFS). DIFS means the length of the time upto which a channel must remain idle after that time completes a secondary user can use that channel to transmit the data. A interval [0, CW] is used to distribute uniformly this backoff time. Contention window is the representation of CW. If the transmission becomes successful, then the CW will be again set to minimum value.

3.4 Defense Scheme

The cramer-von Mises (C-M) test is used as defense scheme. The difference between distributive functions is used here to find the malicious users, where a window size is observed, and it is examined whether it follows the distribution of the original window size or not. In the first step, for each and every node, the observed window size is calculated

$$x_i = \frac{t_i - t_{i-1} - T_{\text{DIFS}} - T_o}{\delta} \tag{4}$$

where t_{i-1} = last transmission end time, T_o = time taken between last transmission end time and current time of packet, and t_i = current time of packet. A cumulative distribution can be made, and it is denoted by F_1. Now, the difference can be evaluated between cumulative functions is calculated as θ. Let $\times 1, \ldots, xK$ be the K observations, and $y_1, \ldots, y_L$ be the L sample data of real distribution. Then, the θ can be calculated as:

$$\theta = \frac{KL}{(K+L)^2}\left(\sum_{i=1}^{K} \text{sgn}(F_0(x_i) - F_1(x_i))[F_0(x_i) - F_1(x_i)]^2 \right. \\ \left. + \sum_{j=1}^{L} \text{sgn}(F_0(y_j) - F_1(y_j))[F_0(y_j)\ (6) - F_1(y_j)]^2 \right) \tag{5}$$

A value "D" defined as max $\{\theta, 0\}$ is used to find the trust value. The trust value π_2 is calculated by

$$\pi_2 = e^{-D^2} \tag{6}$$

If the value of θ becomes negative, then we can say that original window size is less than the backoff window size. D takes the value of zero, and the trust value becomes 1.

3.5 Cross-Layer Attack

The utilization of the channel can be reduced easily by using a cross layer attack. The attack which is considered here is: Firstly, the RFSD assault occurs in physical layer, and secondly, the small backoff window (SBW) assault occurs in medium access control layer [15]. These both attacks take a relationship of "OR." The attack probability P_1 is used by attackers to perform RFSD attack and P_2 to perform SBW attack on their corresponding layers. These attack probabilities are the values which are optimal and chosen by the attackers carefully.

3.6 Cross-Layer Defense

The section shows a cross-layer defense framework, and it is represented as (Fig. 2).

The parts of the above represented framework are:

- SLMTC: Single-layer monitoring and trust calculation: The part of the framework where the trust values of nodes in individual layers are calculated.
- Trust fusion: The trust values from individual layers are considered, and a final trust value T is calculated from all the available nodes in the network.
- Anomalous recognition: After calculating the final test value for a node, it is considered, and the node is classified whether it is malicious or not is done here.

The CTM—cross-layer trust manager is obtained by combining trust fusion and abnormal detection parts of the defense framework. The goal of the trust fusion is to determine how much a node I can be trusted by the CTM. The final trust value can be calculated as:

$$T = w_1\pi_1 + w_2\pi_2 \tag{7}$$

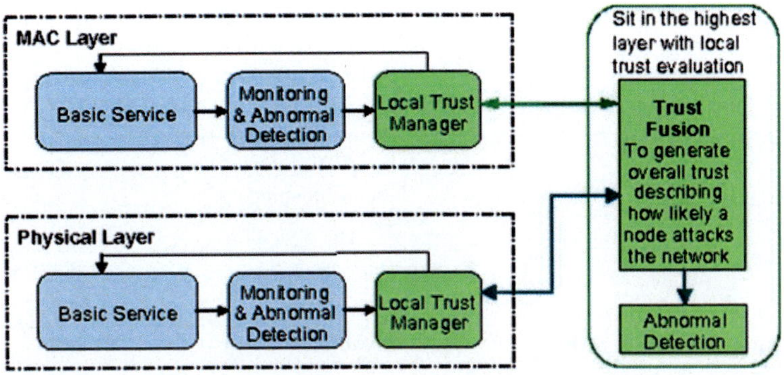

Fig. 2 Cross-layer defense framework for CRN's

where w_1 is the level with which the CTM trusts the PHY layer results, and w_2 is the level with which the CTM trusts the MAC layer results. π_1 and π_2 are the individual layer trust values. The weights are derived by using variance values. The weights are calculated as:

$$w_1 = \frac{v_2}{v_1 + v_2}, \; w_2 = \frac{v_1}{v_1 + v_2}. \tag{8}$$

A heuristic method is used here to find the values of variances. Let v_j represents the variances with $j = 1, 2$, and v_j^i denotes the sequence of variances $\left\{\pi_j^i(1) \ldots \pi_j^i(M)\right\}$, where M is current detection round; I is node number; j is layer number. The variance is calculated as:

$$v_j = \frac{1}{c_j} \sum_{i, 1 \leq i \leq N \& \frac{v_j^i}{v_j^m} \leq \rho} v_j^i \tag{9}$$

where c_j is the count of nodes who satisfy the condition $\frac{v_j^i}{v_j^m} \leq \rho$, and ρ is the threshold value for finding which variances doesn't satisfy normal nodes variances. After the calculation of the final trust value for a node if it is less than the threshold value λ_3, it is considered as malicious.

4 Results

4.1 Simulation Setup

For the simulation initially, we consider a wireless CRN with 10 nodes, Let $N = 10$ out of which two secondary users are not trusted, and they do not collude. The main important parameters we have considered are listed in Table 2.

Table 2 Simulation parameters

S. No.	Parameter	Description
1	Cognitive radio nodes	10
2	Bandwidth product	6
3	Transmission power	300 MW
4	Noise level	−125 bBm
5	Loss factor	4
6	Backoff window size	64–512
7	Threshold value	1.25

4.2 Results

Figure 3 illustrates the defense mechanism we are following in the physical layer, and the considered parameters are attack probability in X-axis and channel availability in Y-axis. When there is no attacker the performance in the physical layer is considerably good but when two attackers are there, then the performance automatically degrades. When the attackers are there and the defense mechanism defined in our work is used, then performance is automatically good. The above graph shows an evident result about the physical layer defense mechanism in our work is considerably very good. When assault chance is 0, and control accessibility will be 1.

Figure 4 illustrates the defense mechanism we are following in the MAC layer, and the considered parameters are attack probability in X-axis and transmission probability in Y-axis. When there is no attacker, then the performance in the MAC layer is excellent but when two attackers are there, then the performance automatically degrades, and it reaches to the attack probability of 1(all nodes are not useful and attacked). The above graph shows an evident result about the MAC layer defense mechanism in our work which is considerably very good. When assault chance is 0 and control accessibility will be 1.

From these two simulations, the following observations are noted in physical and MAC layers.

- When there is no security, the channel accessibility in attack probability increases and physical layer decreases significantly.
- Physical layer performance is good, and there is a more chance of attacks in this layer than in MAC layer.

Fig. 3 Physical layer attack and defense scheme

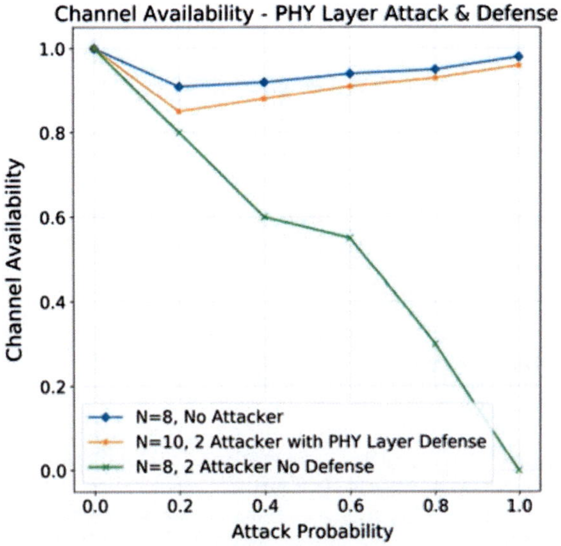

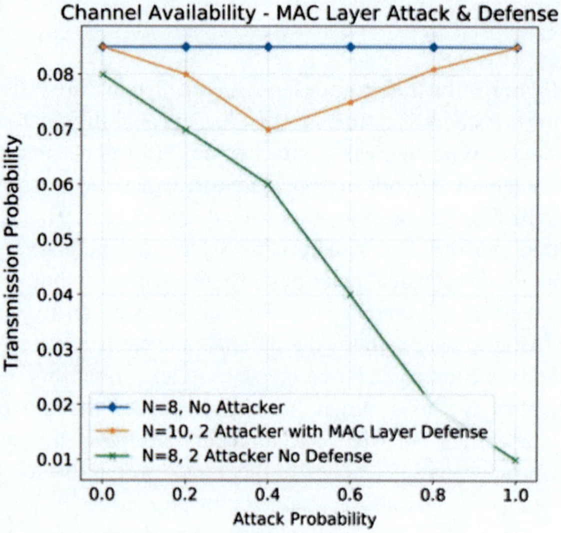

Fig. 4 MAC layer attack and defense scheme

- From the simulation, it is observed that the optimal assault chance is 0.5, and the utmost performance deprivation is 16.42%.
- In MAC layer, defense attack chance is 0.8, and the maximum performance decrease is 8.72%.

5 Conclusion

This work gives a significant solution to cross-layer attacks in cognitive radio networks. When secondary user attacks in one layer, his attack strength is very less compared to coordination in multiple layers. The layers we have considered are physical, MAC, and the attacks are RFSD (Physical) and SBW (MAC) layers. The Trust fusion mechanism demonstrated in this work works provides solution for abnormal users detection in physical and MAC layers and cross- layer trust management schemes. Finally, this concept of cross-layer trust management schemes can also be useful to remaining attacks in other layers of CRN's.

References

1. Ganesh D, Pavan Kumar T (2018) A survey on advances in security threats and its counter measures in cognitive radio networks. Int J Eng Technol 7(2.8):372–378
2. . Sureka N, Gunaseelan K (2019) Detection& defense against primary user emulation attack in dynamic cognitive radio networks. In: Fifth international conference on science technology engineering and mathematics (ICONSTEM), 2019, pp 505–510

3. Feng G et al (2018) A differential game based approach against objective function attack in cognitive networks. Chin J Electron 27(4):879–888
4. Saurabh S, Rustogi R (2018) Tracing Jammed area in wireless ad-hoc network using boundary node detection. In: IEEE international conference on advanced networks and telecommunications systems (ANTS), 2018, pp 1–4
5. Velempini NM, Dlamini SV (2018) The detection of the spectrum sensing data falsification attack in cognitive radio Ad Hoc networks. In: Conference on information communications technology and society (ICTAS)
6. Raj S, Sahu OP (2017) Counter measures to security threats/Attacks on different protocol layers in cognitive radio networks. In: International conference on smart technology for smart nation, 2017, pp 1076–1082
7. Sejaphala L, Velempini M, Dlamini SV (2018):HCOBASAA: countermeasure against sinkhole attacks in software-defined wireless sensor cognitive radio networks. In: International conference on advances in big data, computing and data communication systems (icABCD), 2018
8. Srinivas Reddy D, Bapuji V, Govardhan A, Sarma SSVN (2017) Sybil attack detection technique using session key certificate in vehicular Ad Hoc networks. In: International conference on algorithms, methodology, models and applications in emerging technologies (ICAMMAET), 2017
9. Wang W, (Lindsay) Sun Y, Li H, Han Z (2010) Cross layer attack and defense in cognitive radio networks. In: IEEE Globecom 2010 proceedings

Texture Based Image Retrieval Using GLCM and LBP

Bably Dolly and Deepa Raj

Abstract In the technical period, things will enrich it every day, one of which is content-based image retrieval. The comparative study of texture-dependent algorithms based on a spatial domain with feature extraction and distance metrics was explored in this paper. Texture attribute extraction uses the gray level co-occurrence matrix and local binary pattern for statistical analysis. The correlation test shows that contrast, correlation, energy, entropy, and homogeneity feature of gray level co-occurrence matrix and local binary pattern features taken from the LBP histogram have a significant correlation. For the study of the gray level co-occurrence vector and local binary pattern on content-based image retrieval system, the precision, accuracy, and recall as well as F-score are measured.

Keywords CBIR · Feature extraction · GLCM · LBP

1 Introduction

The texture function is one of the essential aspects of extracting related images from a dataset in the content base image recovery framework. Therefore, one of the major research fields of computer vision is to locate the resemblance of images. In this paper, texture-based feature extraction techniques used in CBIR are discussed. According to authors [1], their research paper focuses on increasing accuracy of identifying texture by the rotational invariant feature of the texture of the liver image dataset by utilizing the Gabor filter technique with multi-scale Gabor rotation-invariant local binary method. As per authors [2], to extract the texture-based features, Local Binary Pattern (LBP) is an efficient technique and focuses on modeling a median sampling regulation with the description of the group of gradient LBP descriptors. It attempted to provide a feature prototype mapping system based on training and to create a frame based on texture differentiation using the multi-resolution hybrid algorithm of four gradient LBP identifiers in the next stage. According to this, LBP is efficient to use to the

B. Dolly (✉) · D. Raj
Department of Computer Science, Babasaheb Bhimrao Ambedkar University, Lucknow, Uttar Pradesh, India
e-mail: dolly0105@gmail.com

S. Bhattacharyya et al. (eds.), *International Conference on Intelligent and Smart Computing in Data Analytics*, Advances in Intelligent Systems and Computing 1312,
https://doi.org/10.1007/978-981-33-6176-8_5

extraction of features based on the statistical approach. The authors [3] in their research paper proposed the method of automated cervical cancer detection system by utilizing the multiple texture-based feature methods which are used to extraction of relevant information from a single cell of image. The author uses GLCM, LBP, DWT, Laws (laws texture energy measures), and first-order histogram. Authors [4] proposed an optical solution based on the aging of the permeable paper for feature extraction. The author used the Co-occurrence Matrix of Gray Level (GLCM) and collected the amount of features of the texture. For going through each aspect of the texture-based feature extraction techniques, this paper relies on the analysis of the GLCM, LBP techniques to check the effectiveness of each method for similar image retrieval.

2 Theoretical Background

Texture has been one of the most significant attributes which have been utilized to order. It tends to be described by textural primitives as unit components and neighborhoods in which the association and connections between the properties of these natives are defined. Various techniques that were intended for a specific application have been proposed in the previous papers. In any case, there is by all accounts no broad technique or a conventional methodology that is valuable in a large set of images.

2.1 Gray Level Co-occurrence Matrixes (GLCM)

The Co-occurrence Matrix of the Gray Level (GLCM)) is one of the measurable strategies to remove highlights dependent on the analysing texture. GLCM is a grid characterizing two measurements between sets of pixels for joint probabilities with a separation in a provided guidance. Various examinations have been done by scientist in contrast ways by using this technique in an alternate territory of uses like the clinical picture, satellite picture, etc. GLCM used to calculate special dependency of gray level in an image. The matrix size is $M \times M$, where the image uses m as the number of gray levels. Co-occurrence matrix is constituted in four special orientations (0°, 45°, 90°, and 135°). Resultant GLCM matrix is average of all the orientation. This gives various properties like perfection, normality, coarseness, and invariant. GLCM matrix can be generated by using this mechanism depicted in Fig. 1 in 0°. Same method is applied for each orientation. By considering the second-order statistic approach, it is likewise tended to as Special Gray Dependence Matrix (SGLDM), where the investigation is accomplished for certain extraordinary relations for sets of pixels.

There are 14 highlights to be characterized by the Haralick in GLCM for the arrangement dependent on texture features. As these highlights are amazingly

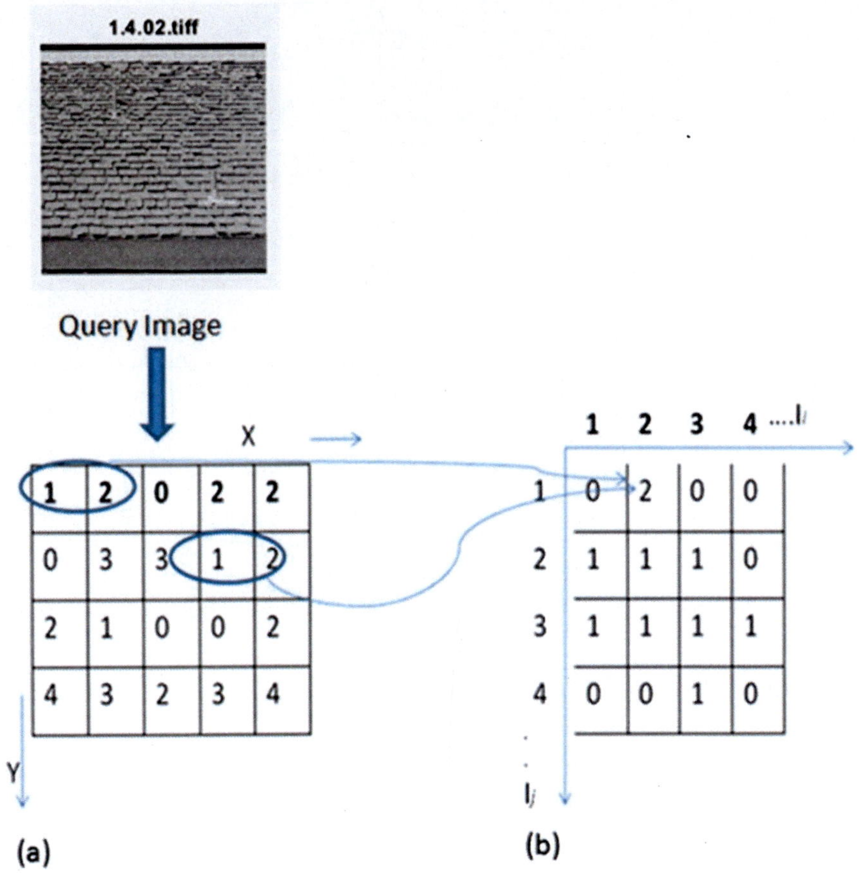

Fig. 1 GLCM matrix of an image

connected, such a large number of researchers utilized the four to five highlights in their exploration work [5]. It is better than the LBP concerning that it has great execution as for preparing time and multifaceted nature. However, for a lot of dataset GLCM is not vastly improved. The second-order statistic, GLCM, gives the relationship in between a reference pixel $P(i, j)$ and its neighborhood pixel at different angles and distances

$$\text{Contrast}(F1) = \sum_{i=0}^{n-1}\sum_{j=0}^{n-1}(i - j)^2$$

$$\text{Entropy}(F5) = \sum_{i=0}^{n-1}\sum_{j=0}^{n-1} m(i, j)(-\ln(m(i, j)))$$

$$\text{Energy}(F3) = \sqrt{\sum_{i=0}^{n-1}\sum_{j=0}^{n-1} m^2(i, j)}$$

$$\text{Homogeneity}(F4) = \sum_{i=0}^{n-1}\sum_{j=0}^{n-1} m(i, j)/1 + (i - j)^2$$

$$\text{Correlation}(F2) = \sum_{i=0}^{n-1}\sum_{j=0}^{n-1} [(ij)m(i, j) - \mu_x\mu_y]/\sigma_x\sigma_y$$

These are five features from GLCM matrix. In the above formula, the range of gray levels in the input image, denoted by n. Euclidean distance is calculated for GLCM as per the following formula:

$$\text{Euclidean Distance} = \sqrt{(F_{q1} - F_1)^2 + (F_{q2} - F_2)^2 + (F_{q3} - F_3)^2 + (F_{q4} - F_4)^2 + (F_{q5} - F_5)^2}$$

2.2 *Local Binary Patterns (LBP)*

LBP the most useful texture analyses offered by Ojala et al. [6] in 1966, which is a gGray scale-invariant surface estimated by the computations from the investigation of a 3 × 3 neighborhood district over a deepest (focal) pixel? LBP is identified with auxiliary strategies and factual techniques. The benefit of local binary patterns is that they are utilized to join both the basic and factual strategies to develop the exhibition regarding the surface investigation. It is anything but difficult to execute, and its expense of calculation is low, and it is likewise invariant as for changes in monotonic enlightenment. With these advantages, it additionally has a few disadvantages as it is touchy as for the turn gives long histograms of the picture and which bring about decline peculiarity and furthermore requires heaps of room. The data-dependent on the extracted texture is being restricted if there is a modest quantity of unique help and furthermore loses data identified with the nearby surface in view of by thinking about the indication of constraints of the neighborhood's pixel. It is very touchy regarding blurring and noise [7]. The result of LBP can be expressed as mentioned below:

$$\text{LBP}_{\text{p,r}}(x_c, y_c) = \sum_{n=0}^{7} \partial(g_n - g_c)2^n$$

where g_c is located at (x_c, y_c) and the values of eight adjacent pixels with the radius "*r*," and the number of the entire neighborhood is the size of the central pixel which

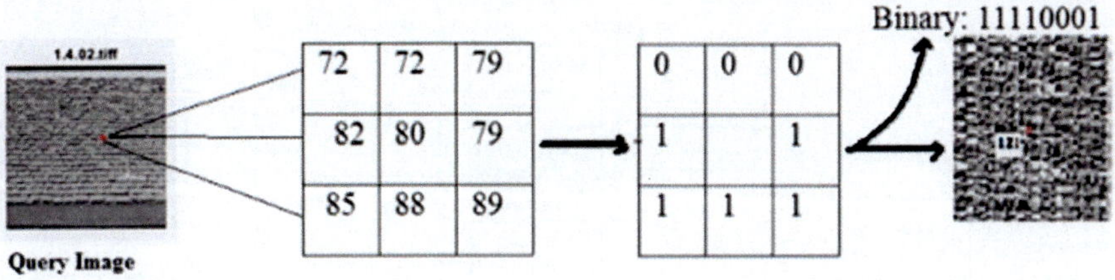

Fig. 2 Representation of LBP operator algorithm

is "*p*," and the ∂() function is represented as:

$$\partial(x) = \begin{cases} 1 & \text{if } x > 0, \\ 0 & \text{otherwise} \end{cases}$$

LBP matrix calculation method [8] is shown in Fig. 2. The histogram of the LBP followed as texture descriptor.

3 Experimental Results

For comparative analysis, sets of images are taken from the Internet. The database [9] consists of 18 gray images having the same category with different textures of wall tiles. They are in the TIFF format with a size of 256 pixels. There are mainly two steps followed for the retrieval of alike images and the comparative study. In the first step, scan all the images from the original dataset placed in Fig. 4 for feature ex-traction vectors and applied reprocessing methods as a 2D median filter is used to reduce the noises. In a software archive, the derived features are stored. The second step is to take the query image and collect the features using the above methods. The final steps are to retrieve related and most alike images from the dataset of features by using the GLCM and LBP as per requirement for analyzing the effectiveness of different methods. The block diagram of comparison of GLCM and LBP-based image retrieval (shown in Fig. 3), to start with MATLAB has been taken to extract feature vectors of input image as well as dataset image through GLCM and LBP separately, then evaluate the score based on Euclidean distance and mapped the input image to dataset images with respect to generated score and shows the top N-similar images. This process was done for both GLCM and LBP. On the basis of top N images retrieved through GLCM and LBP separately, there has been done the comparison of GLCM and LBP via statistical parameters—precision, recall, and F-score.

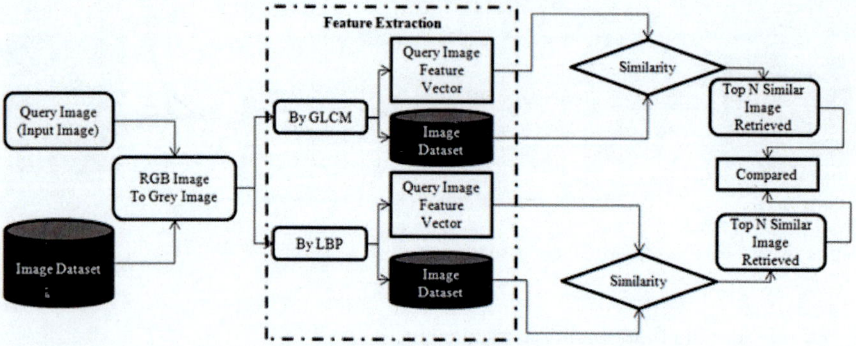

Fig. 3 Block diagram of comparison of GLCM and LBP-based image retrieval

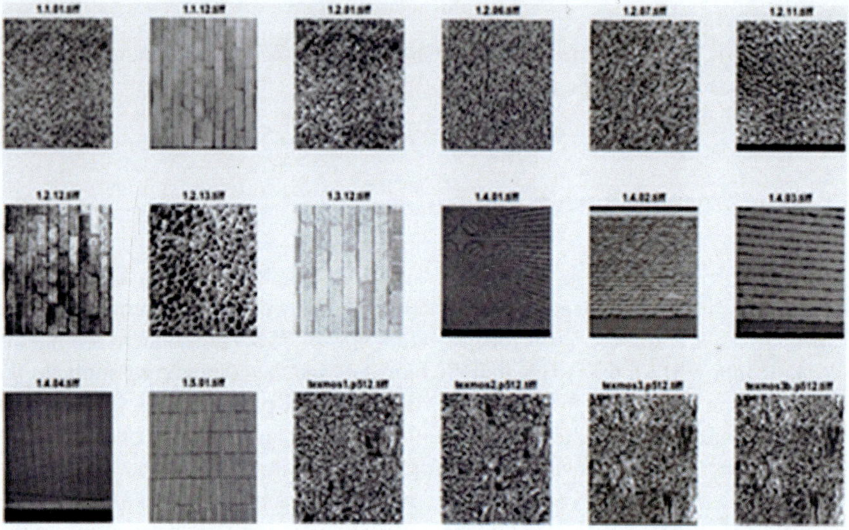

Fig. 4 Original dataset of images

3.1 Statistical Analysis

Three statistical parameters P as precision, R as recall, and Fs as F-score measure are used to check the efficiency of the GLCM and LBP algorithm. The F-score rating, which is a single value, offers the total effectiveness of image retrieval. For checking efficiency texture algorithm, five features F_1, F_2, F_3, F_4, and F_5 for images of the dataset are extracted using the GLCM approach. These are contrast, correlation, energy, homogeneity, and entropy as per the given formula as above mentioned. It is displayed in Table 1, and in the same way extracting the features of LBP, $F_n = [F_1, F_2, F_3, F_4, \ldots, F_n]$, five feature has been taken and depicted in Table 2.

Score is estimated by the Euclidian distance formula:

Table 1 Features using GLCM

S. No.	Dataset image	F_1	F_2	F_3	F_4	F_5
1	1.1.01	3.68	0.34	0.03	0.53	0.09
2	1.1.12	1.08	0.49	0.16	0.75	0.64
3	1.2.01	7.00	0.33	0.02	0.47	0.00
4	1.2.06	7.77	0.26	0.02	0.45	0.00
5	1.2.07	7.31	0.31	0.02	0.47	0.00
6	1.2.11	6.12	0.45	0.02	0.51	0.00
7	1.2.12	4.94	0.53	0.03	0.56	0.00
8	1.2.13	4.27	0.59	0.03	0.57	0.00
9	1.3.12	0.61	0.66	0.19	0.79	0.88
10	1.4.01	0.70	0.67	0.14	0.77	0.96
11	1.4.02	1.17	0.76	0.11	0.78	0.68
12	1.4.03	0.59	0.82	0.26	0.85	0.79
13	1.4.04	0.25	0.86	0.24	0.88	0.99
14	1.5.01	0.27	0.45	0.53	0.90	0.96
15	te1	7.16	0.32	0.02	0.48	0.00
16	te2	7.22	0.31	0.02	0.47	0.00
17	te3	6.88	0.35	0.02	0.48	0.00
18	te3b	6.85	0.35	0.02	0.48	0.00

$$\text{Euclidian Distance} = \sqrt{\sum_{1}^{n}(F_q - F_n)^2}$$

where n denotes the number of extracted feature, from each image dataset for every feature extraction. F_q and F_n denote the feature of Query image [10] (Qimage) and feature of every selected image in the dataset, respectively. The Euclidian distance is considered as a scorecard for each image as per the query image. The score of LBP and score of GLCM are depicted in Table 3. By seeing Table 3, the score of each image in the dataset has been generated. The efficacy of image recovery is focused mostly on scorecard generated for the set of images. The retrieval of a similar image from the dataset is based on scorecard produce for every image in the dataset through GLCM and LBP, respectively. On the basis of the scorecard of images in the dataset based on the query images for GLCM, the similar retrieved image can be seen in Fig. 5; in the same way, the similar images from the dataset can be for LBP are displayed in Fig. 6. On the basis of scorecard of GLCM and LBP, precision, recall, and F-score are calculated and shown in Table 4. The line graph of GLCM and LBP (shown in Fig. 7), with blue and brown lines having the nodes for precision, recall, and F-score.

Table 2 Features using LBP

S. No.	Images	F_1	F_2	F_3	F_4	F_5
	QImage	0.29	0.25	0.14	0.29	0.41
1	1.1.01	0.17	0.26	0.24	0.39	0.52
2	1.1.12	0.28	0.30	0.20	0.29	0.33
3	1.2.01	0.17	0.27	0.23	0.39	0.50
4	1.2.06	0.23	0.29	0.20	0.33	0.45
5	1.2.07	0.19	0.25	0.24	0.42	0.41
6	1.2.11	0.20	0.26	0.24	0.37	0.39
7	1.2.12	0.27	0.30	0.19	0.28	0.32
8	1.2.13	0.18	0.24	0.17	0.30	0.57
9	1.3.12	0.28	0.27	0.22	0.28	0.34
10	1.4.01	0.28	0.26	0.16	0.25	0.39
11	1.4.02	0.29	0.25	0.14	0.29	0.41
12	1.4.03	0.33	0.28	0.14	0.18	0.25
13	1.4.04	0.33	0.27	0.15	0.17	0.19
14	1.5.01	0.30	0.26	0.15	0.26	0.32
15	te1	0.19	0.27	0.20	0.35	0.49
16	te2	0.19	0.28	0.19	0.34	0.48
17	te3	0.19	0.27	0.20	0.36	0.49
18	te3b	0.19	0.27	0.20	0.36	0.49

for both GLCM and LBP. By going through the graph, it is depicted that GLCM has the higher value as per statistical parameter than the LBP. This shows the betterment result of image retrieval approach regarding GLCM and LBP.

4 Conclusion

An overview of extraction of its function using GLCM and LBP is provided in this article. The assessment measure for a content-based image retrieval process is being used to determine how many obtained images fulfilled the purpose of the user query. The experimental result confirms that the GLCM method achieves Precision, recall, and F-score are higher compared to LBP, and it is more successful than LBP. Retrieving rate for GLCM is better as per comparison to LBP for similar images according to the query image. This comparative analysis will be beneficial for the researcher to select the better approach for evaluated basic feature vectors based on the LBP and GLCM.

Table 3 Euclidian distance (Score) for GLCM and LBP

S. No.	Image of dataset	Score	
		GLCM	LBP
1	1.1.01.tiff'	2.63	0.34
2	1.1.12.tiff'	0.30	0.13
3	1.2.01.tiff'	5.90	0.33
4	1.2.06.tiff'	6.67	0.20
5	1.2.07.tiff'	6.21	0.27
6	1.2.11.tiff'	5.02	0.22
7	1.2.12.tiff'	3.85	0.14
8	1.2.13.tiff'	3.19	0.34
9	1.3.12.tiff'	0.61	0.17
10	1.4.01.tiff'	0.56	0.07
11	1.4.02.tiff'	0.00	0.00
12	1.4.03.tiff'	0.61	0.27
13	1.4.04.tiff'	0.99	0.33
14	1.5.01.tiff'	1.08	0.11
15	te1.tiff	6.05	0.25
16	te2.tiff	6.12	0.23
17	te3.tiff	5.77	0.25
18	te3b.tiff	5.75	0.25

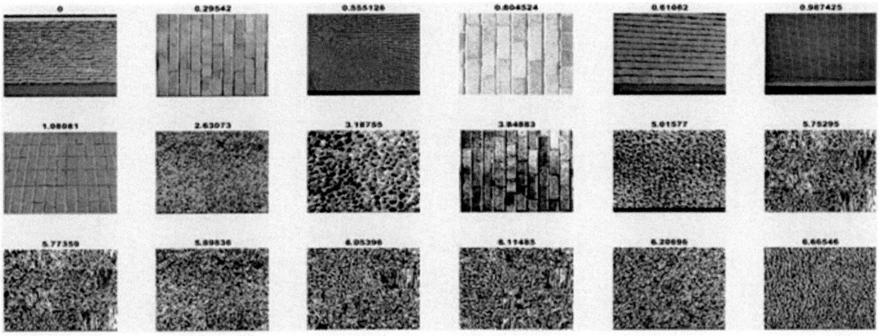

Fig. 5 Retrieved images using GLCM

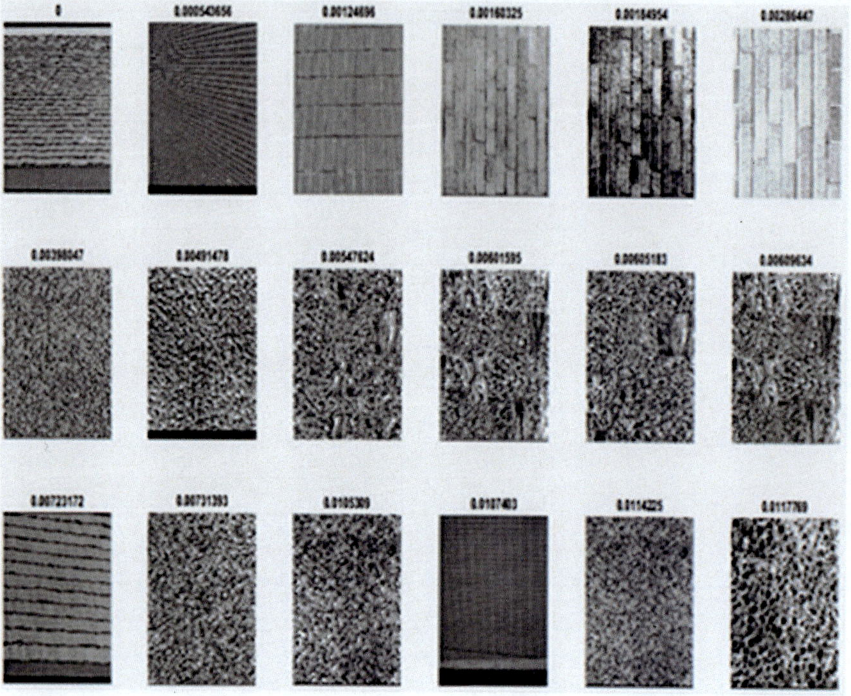

Fig. 6 Retrieved images using LBP

Table 4 Precision, recall, and F-score for GLCM and LBP

Feature extraction technique	GLCM	LBP
Precision	0.8	0.6
Recall	0.875	0.75
F-score	0.831	0.72

Fig. 7 Graphical representation of precision, recall, and F-score for GLCM and LBP

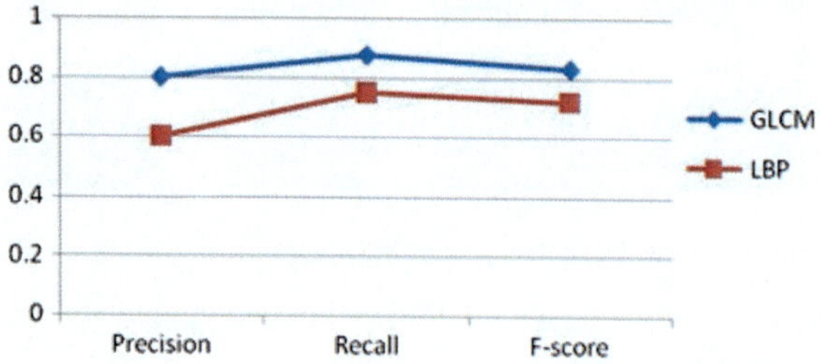

Reference

1. Ramamoorthy S et al (2015) Texture feature extraction using MGRLBP method for medical image classification. Article in Advances in Intelligent Systems and Computing
2. Ji L, Ren Y, Liu G et al (2017) Training-based gradient LBP feature models for multiresolution texture classification. IEEE Trans Cybernet 1:2168–2267
3. Arya M et al (2015) Texture-based feature extraction of smear images for the detection of cervical cancer. IET Res J ISSN 1751-8644, pp 1–11
4. Li S et al (June 2017) Aging feature extraction of oil-impregnated insulating paper using image texture analysis. IEEE Trans Dielectr Electr Insulat 24(3):1636–1645
5. Alsmadi MK (2017) An efficient similarity measure for content based image retrieval using Memetic algorithm. Egypt J Basic Appl Sci 4:112–122
6. Ojala T et al (1996) A comparative study of textures measures with classification based on featured distributions. Pattern Recogn 29(1):51–57
7. Humeau-Heurtier A (2019) Texture feature extraction methods: a survey. IEEE Access 7
8. Zhou S-R et al (2012) LPQ and LBP based Gabor filter for face representation. Neurocomputing, pp 1–5
9. Image Dataset used for texture analysis: Brodetz database
10. Bably Dolly DR (December 2019) Color based image retrieval by combining various features. Int J Eng Adv Technol 9(2): 454–460 ISSN: 2249-8958 (Online)

Design and Development of Bayesian Optimization Algorithms for Big Data Classification Based on MapReduce Framework

Chitrakant Banchhor and N. Srinivasu

Abstract The handling of big data refers efficient management of processing and storage requirements of very large volume of structured and an unstructured data of association. The basic approach for big data classification using naïve Bayes classifier is extended with correlation among the attributes so that it becomes a dependent hypothesis, and it is named as correlative naïve Bayes classifier (CNB). The optimization algorithms such as cuckoo search and grey wolf optimization are integrated with the correlative naïve Bayes classifier, and significant performance improvement is achieved. This model is called as cuckoo grey wolf correlative naïve Bayes classifier (CGCNB). The further performance improvements are achieved by incorporating fuzzy theory termed as fuzzy correlative naïve Bayes classifier (FCNB) and holoentropy theory termed as Holoentropy correlative naïve Bayes classifier (HCNB), respectively. FCNB and HCNB classifiers are comparatively analyzed with CNB and CGCNB and achieved noticeable performance by analyzing with accuracy, sensitivity and specificity analysis.

Keywords MapReduce · Correlative naive Bayes classifier · Classification · Big data · Holoentropy

1 Introduction

There are quintillions bytes of data created and generated every day and certainly require the big data classification [1]. The word big data is more appropriate nowadays because of frequent occurrences of the vast amount of data collection and processing activities [2, 3]. The information from the available large datasets can be extracted with more precisely although the analysis and knowledge extraction

C. Banchhor (✉)
School of Computer Engineering and Technology, Dr. VishwanathKarad MIT World Peace University, Pune, Maharashtra, India
e-mail: cobanchhor@gmail.com

N. Srinivasu
Department of Computer Science and Engineering, KoneruLakshmaiah Education Foundation, Vaddeswaram, AP, India

S. Bhattacharyya et al. (eds.), *International Conference on Intelligent and Smart Computing in Data Analytics*, Advances in Intelligent Systems and Computing 1312,
https://doi.org/10.1007/978-981-33-6176-8_6

from large databases are enhanced [4, 5]. There are two major categories of the data mining schemes: clustering and classification. The big data classification process is achieved by various classifiers like naïve Bayes classifiers, support vector machine and extreme learning machines [6, 7].

The main contribution of this research is improvement of enhanced classification strategies using fuzzy, Holoentropy, cuckoo search and grey wolf optimization integrated with correlative NB classifier for the big data classification.

2 Correlative Naive Bayes Classifier (CNB)

One of the highly utilized classifier is naïve Bayes classifier; the typical classifier is adopted with MapReduce framework and used for big data classification [8]. At the initial phase of the training process, the input data are arranged in different groups on the basis of number of classes.

$$\text{CNB}_{Q\times m} = \left\{\mu_{Q\times m}, \sigma_{Q\times m}, R_{Q\times 1}\right\} \tag{1}$$

where $\mu_{Q\times m}$ is the mean to be calculated, $\sigma_{Q\times m}$ is specified as variance, $R_{Q\times 1}$ denotes correlation function, and it is illustrated in vector form. Testing data result is represented using the following equation:

$$C = \arg_{q=i,\ldots,Q}^{\text{Max}}\left[P\left(C_q\right) \times P(X|C_q)\right] \times R^q \tag{2}$$

The equation shown in (2) is used to indicate that the highest posterior value is only selected as consequential class.

3 Cuckoo Grey Wolf Optimization with Correlative Naïve Bayes Classifier (CGCNB)

The integrated CGWO and CNB classifier with MapReduce framework are named as Cuckoo Grey wolf correlative naïve bayes classifier along with MapReduce structure method (CGCNB-MRP). CGWO is the integration of cuckoo search algorithm and grey wolf Optimization (GWO) [9, 10]. The block diagram of developed model for big data classification is depicted in Fig. 1.

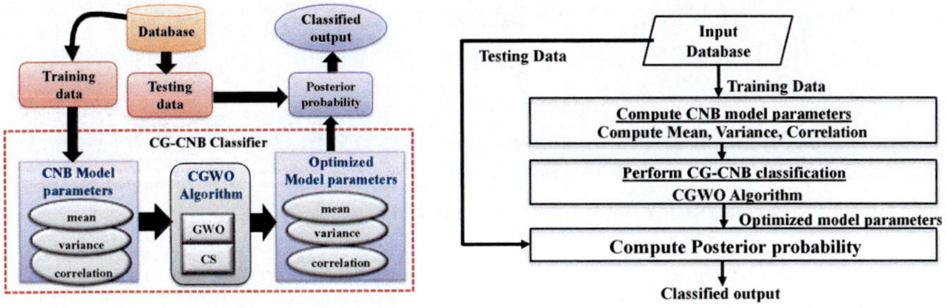

(a) Block diagram (b) Flow chart

Fig. 1 Control and data flow of CGCNB-MRP classifier

4 Fuzzy Correlative Naive Bayes Classifier (FCNB)

One more extension of CNB classifier is inclusion of fuzzy theory, and it is named as FCNB [11]. FCNB classifier is shown in the following equation:,

$$\mu_q^s = \frac{\left|m_q^s\right|}{d}. \tag{3}$$

The term μ_q^s represents membership degree of symbol sth in the qth element of training model. The whole incidence of sth symbol in qth element is represented by the term $\left|m_q^s\right|$, and d is utilized for representing data sample in attribute.

Each data sample is classified into number of classes let it be called as K. It is represented as follows:

$$\mu_c^k = \frac{\left|m^k\right|}{d} \tag{4}$$

Here, whole incidence of Kth class in ground truth information is represented by $\left|m^k\right|$. The outcome of FCNB classifier is represented as below:

$$\text{FCNB} = \{\mu_q^k, \mu_c^k, C\} \tag{5}$$

In the testing stage of developed FCNB classifier, testing sample is classified into the appropriate classes by the use of posterior probability of naïve Bayes, fuzzy membership degree and a correlation factor among attributes. The output of FCNB is expressed as below equation:

$$G = \arg_{k=1 \text{ to } K}^{\text{Max}} P(g_k|X) * C^k \tag{6}$$

The term here represented as $P(g_k \mid X)$ denoted as posterior probability by using test data **X** for given class $\mathbf{g_k}$. The expression $\mathbf{C^k}$ signifies correlation for class **K**.

5 Holoentropy Using Correlative Naïve Bayes Classifier for a Big Data Classification (HCNB)

The new classification technique called as HCNB is introduced through combining existing CNB classifier with holoentropy function [12]. The handling is based on the holoentropy estimation for each attribute using the following formula:

$$H_v^b = F \times T(ib) \tag{7}$$

Here, F represents the weight function, and $T(i_b)$ is the entropy. The formulae for the weight function and entropy are described in the following equations.

$$F = 2\left[1 - \frac{1}{1 + \exp(-T(i_b))}\right] \tag{8}$$

$$T(i_b) = -\sum_{b=1}^{M(i_b)} P_b \times \log P_b \tag{9}$$

Here, $M(i_b)$ is the unique value of the attribute vector i_b. The training phase of the HCNB based on the training data samples produces the result in the following vector form:

$$\text{HCNB}_{a\times s} = \left\{\mu_{a\times s}, \sigma^2_{a\times s}, C_{a\times 1}, H_{a\times s}\right\} \tag{10}$$

Here, $\mu_{a\times s}$ and $\sigma^2_{a\times s}$ represent the computed mean value and computed variance value between the attributes ***a*** and ***s***, respectively. Also, the correlation is represented by C_{ax1}, and holoentropy function is represented using $H_{a\times s}$. The individual class is selected by estimating posterior probability independently during a testing phase, which can be represented by below expression:

$$P(Y|k_v) = \prod_{b=1}^{s} P(Y = y_b|k_v) \tag{11}$$

where y_b illustrates yth data of bth element, and k_v indicates vth class number. The block diagram of the HCNB classifier is depicted in Fig. 2.

6 Results and Discussion

The implementation is done using JAVA, and the performance of the proposed classifiers is evaluated using two datasets, namely localization dataset [13] and skin dataset [14].

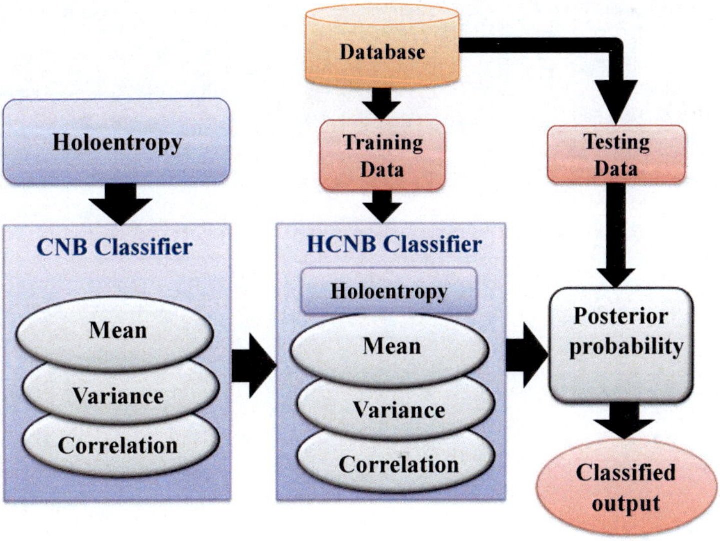

Fig. 2 Block diagram of HCNB classifier

6.1 Performance Evaluation

In this section, performances of developed methods are evaluated. The results of performance analysis based on sensitivity, specificity and accuracy with number of mappers 2, 3, 4 and 5 for skin dataset and localization data are shown in Figs. 3 and 4, respectively, for CNB classifier. In the similar ways, Figs. 5 and 6 show the

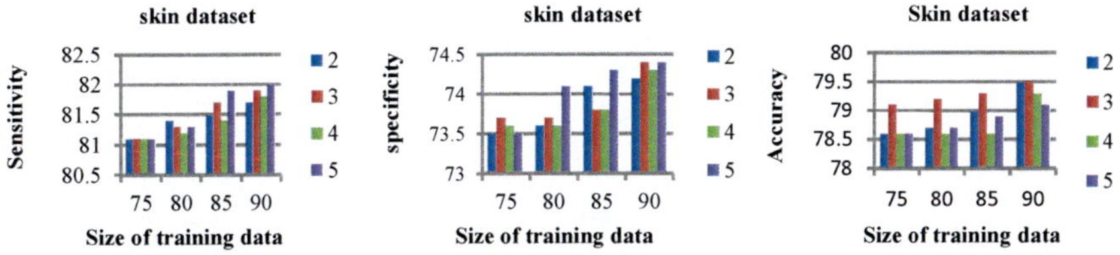

Fig. 3 Sensitivity, specificity and accuracy analysis of CNB classifier on skin dataset

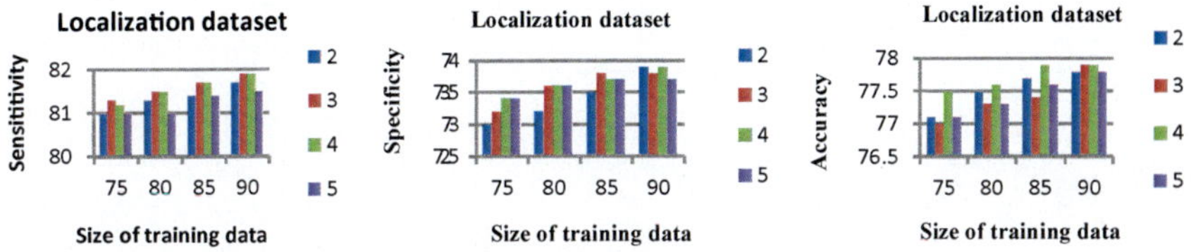

Fig. 4 Sensitivity, specificity and accuracy analysis CNB classifier on localization dataset

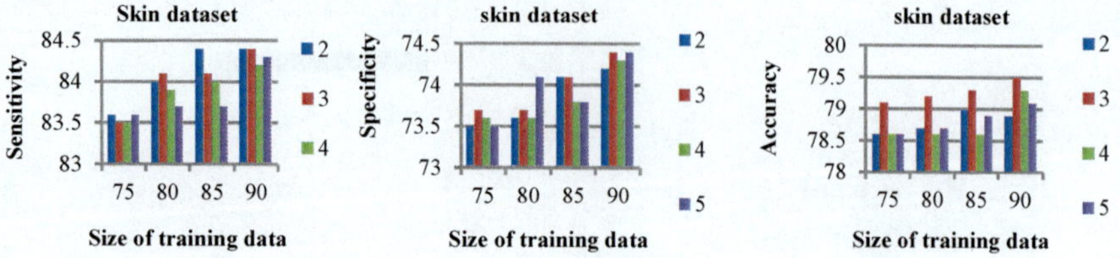

Fig. 5 Sensitivity, specificity and accuracy analysis CGCNB classifier on skin dataset

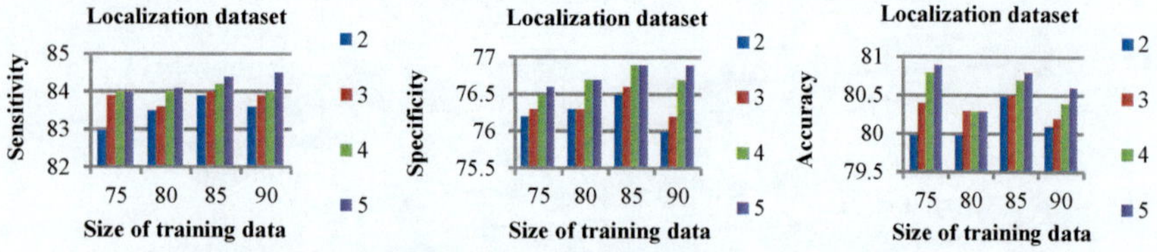

Fig. 6 Sensitivity, specificity and accuracy analysis CGCNB classifier on localization dataset

performance analysis of CGCNB classifier on skin data and localization data, respectively. In comparison with CNB, the CGCNB classifier has significant improvement in performance using sensitivity, accuracy and specificity analysis. Table 1 shows the comparative analysis of HCNB, CGCNB and CNB classifiers.

The holoentropy based proposed method for big data classification with MapReduce framework also shows comparatively performance improvements as compare to CNB and CGCNB classifiers based on the accuracy, sensitivity and specificity analysis on skin data and localization datasets with varying number of mappers and percentages of training data.

Table 1 Comparative analysis of HCNB with CNB and CGCNB

Datasets	Metrics (%)	Training = 75%		
		CNB	CGCNB	HCNB
Skin dataset	Accuracy	77.4994	80.5052	93.5965
	Sensitivity	81.1845	83.9789	94.3369
	Specificity	73.4195	76.5403	84
Localization dataset	Accuracy	76.0377	78.5795	80.5779
	Sensitivity	81.1186	83.5103	81.2108
	Specificity	71.2844	73.6079	84

7 Conclusion

This paper focused on big data classification based on different functions incorporated with mapreduce framework. The basic model is correlative naïve Bayes classifier, and later, it is integrated with optimization algorithms like cuckoo search and grey wolf optimization. The adoption of fuzzy theory with correlative naïve Bayes classifier with membership degree of attributes included in the dataset provides performance achievements comparatively with CNB and CGCNB classifiers. From simulation outcomes, developed models, such as FCNB, HCNB and CGCNB classifier demonstrates enhanced performance in localization and a skin segmentation databases. The future work includes the development of the model with incorporation of the deep learning method for further performance enhancement.

References

1. Wu X et al (2014) Data mining with big data. IEEE Trans Knowl Data Eng. https://doi.org/10.1109/TKDE.2013.109
2. Minelli M, Chambers M, Dhiraj A (2013) Big data, big analytics: emerging business intelligence and analytic trends for today's businesses, 1st ed. Wiley Publishing
3. Marx V (2013) The big challenges of big data. Nature. https://doi.org/10.1038/498255a
4. He H, Garcia EA (2009) Learning from imbalanced data. IEEE Trans Knowl Data Eng. https://doi.org/10.1109/TKDE.2008.239
5. López V et al (2015) Cost-sensitive linguistic fuzzy rule based classification systems under the MapReduce framework for imbalanced big data. Fuzzy Sets Syst. https://doi.org/10.1016/j.fss.2014.01.015
6. Huang GB, Zhu QY, Siew CK (2006). Extreme Learning Machine: Theory and Applications. https://doi.org/10.1016/j.neucom.2005.12.126
7. Santafe G, Lozano JA, Larranaga P (2006) Bayesian model averaging of naive Bayes for clustering. IEEE Trans Syst Man Cybernet Pt B (Cybernetics)https://doi.org/10.1109/TSMCB.2006.874132
8. C. Banchhor, N. Srinivasu (2016) CNB-MRF: adapting correlative Naive Bayes classifier and MapReduce framework for big data classification. In: International review on computers and software (IRECOS). https://doi.org/10.15866/irecos.v11i11.10116
9. ChitrakantBanchhor NS (2020) Integrating Cuckoo search-Grey wolf optimization and Correlative Naive Bayes classifier with Map Reduce model for big data classification. Data Knowl Eng. https://doi.org/10.1016/j.datak.2019.101788
10. Sampathkumar A et al (2020) An efficient hybrid methodology for detection of cancer-causing gene using CSC for micro array data. J Ambient Intell Human Comput. https://doi.org/10.1007/s12652-020-01731-7
11. ChitrakantBanchhor NS (2018) FCNB: fuzzy correlative Naive Bayes classifier with MapReduce framework for big data classification. J Intell Syst. https://doi.org/10.1515/jisys-2018-0020
12. ChitrakantBanchhor NS (2019) Holoentropy based Correlative Naive Bayes classifier and MapReduce model for classifying the big data. Evol Intel. https://doi.org/10.1007/s12065-019-00276-9
13. UCI Machine Learning Repository for Localization dataset https://archive.ics.uci.edu/ml/datasets/Localization+Data+for+Person+Activity. Accessed Oct 2017
14. UCI Machine Learning Repository for Skin segmentation dataset https://archive.ics.uci.edu/ml/datasets/skin+segmentation. Accessed Oct 2017

An IoT-Based BLYNK Server Application for Infant Monitoring Alert System to Detect Crying and Wetness of a Baby

P. Bhasha, T. Pavan Kumar, K. Khaja Baseer, and V. Jyothsna

Abstract The amount of employability among men and women had raised a lot in comparison with olden days. With this increase in employability, the amount of care taken by the parents toward their infants had also decreased. But, in childhood stage, children need proper rest and sleep for proper health and body growth. Thus, most of parents send their infants to their grandparent's house, and some may taught of living their babies at baby care houses. But all the people cannot keep nanny, and also, it is always difficult for the parents to keep trust on some strangers to look after their baby. But, in any of the cases, parents may not continuously monitor the situations and conditions of their babies. Therefore, an IoT-based baby monitoring system has been introduced which can be made available at affordable cost and works efficient in real time. The system is developed using Node MCU microcontroller, a speaker and a sound sensor module. The sound sensor module detects the babies cry and executed according to the action provided. The BLYNK application server is used to send the notifications to the registered parent's mobile number as alert message regarding their kids status.

Keywords Node MCU microcontroller · BLYNK android application · Wetness and sound detection · Alert message notification

1 Introduction

In India, percentage of working men and women had raised drastically when compared to olden days [1]. The percent of employability has increased among men and women. Due to this work burden, parents are not getting sufficient time to look after their infants in their early and later stages. Once the children grow up,

P. Bhasha (✉) · T. Pavan Kumar
Department of CSE, Koneru Lakshmaiah Education Foundation, Vaddeswaram, Guntur, AP, India
e-mail: basha.chanti@gmail.com

K. K. Baseer · V. Jyothsna
Department of Information Technology, Sree Vidyanikethan Engineering College (Autonomous), Tirupati, AP, India

S. Bhattacharyya et al. (eds.), *International Conference on Intelligent and Smart Computing in Data Analytics*, Advances in Intelligent Systems and Computing 1312,
https://doi.org/10.1007/978-981-33-6176-8_7

it is not a big problem to look after them, because they can do their own work and will not depend on their parents for all the works. Due to this situation, most of the parents wish to propel their babies to their grandparent's home. This will reduce the burden to the parents, but there is a risk in doing that because grandparents are aged people. But all the families are not affordable to keep a caretaker. Considering these issues facing by the parents, a baby monitoring system has been developed through which parents can feel comfortable even by leaving their infants in their home and involve in their work at home. Comparable to Arduino, Node MCU is more useful microcontroller because Node MCU is inbuilt Wi-Fi-enabled microcontroller [2]. For detecting the baby cry, a sound sensor is used. Baby cry is compared with a preloaded cry. If it matches, then microcontroller plays the songs using speaker to stop the cry of the baby and to fall asleep again. And an alert message will be sent to the parents or caretaker registered email ID or to the registered mobile number. By seeing this alert, parent can know the present situation of the baby [3]. Thus, the proposed baby monitoring system will help the parent to stay comfort wherever they are and helps to do their work without any issues. Alert messages will notify the parents or caretakers at each and every point of time so that they can look after their baby. The cost of this model is around 950 rupees and makes it more usable by most of the parents.

2 Related Work

The system consists of an Arduino UNO microcontroller that is inbuilt with a Wi-Fi module. When the baby is awake from the sleep then the MCU generates the notification, and DC motor will swing the cradle [4]. It will make the baby to fall asleep again. And the mic present in the system will detect the babies' cry, the input received through the microphone module is amplified, and to stop the cry of the baby, the system will play the preloaded songs, and cradle is swinging already with help of DC motor. The DHT11 sensor measures the temperature, and if temperature rises more than 39° with respect to room temperature, it sends the message to the node MCU which notifies the Blynk which in turn notifies the parent [5]. And wetness is measured basing on two electrodes moisture holding substrate. In this way, wetness will be detected and sends the message to node MCU, and it notifies the Blynk server for alerting the parents. And also, this system can turn on or turn off the fan present in the room if the parents are allowed to do so. So that baby will feel comfort. Thus, this system helps the parents to take care the baby remotely [6]. These authors mainly focused on developing the smart baby monitoring system based on IoT technology and radar technology [7]. Also, obstacle detection in the path of the baby is also provided using the ultrasonic sensors. The main view of this system is to solve the problems faced by the caretakers and also to secure the baby from entering into danger zone [8]. Here, danger zone refers to the zone where there are obstacles in the path of the baby. This alert generation is done based upon ultrasonic sensors. Here, the ultrasonic sensors used are the waterproof sensors. And this sensor is placed on the baby as a simple locket. As soon as the baby enters the danger zone, alert messages will be sent to the caretaker or the parents through mobile number or using different buzzers [9]. The authors proposed a system that processed using image processing techniques which use the different Python libraries for proper working of the system. This system is mainly developed for detecting three types of things. The activities which are performed on Raspberry Pi B+ microcontroller can perform many operations as its connectivity is much better than Arduino or other microcontroller. For sending the pictures of the baby, a pi camera is used in the system. This camera captures the pictures of the baby when baby starts crying and sends the snaps to the parents through email. If the baby's position is abnormal, the system will send an alert to the parent about the abnormality [10]. The authors proposed the real-time and low-cost efficient system. They proposed a new algorithm for taking care of the babies. The NodeMCU is used to connect and read data from the sensors and uploading into the AdaFruit MQTT server through Wi-Fi [11]. This system is mainly having cradle-like architecture. It will swing accordingly whenever the baby starts crying. A mini fan is provided at the top of the cradle to give exposure to air for the baby. The fan and cradle swings can be altered either remotely or manually through MQTT mobile application server. The user can get notifications through the IFTTT server once the baby cry is detected [12]. If the room temperature changes, the notification will be raised. If the room temperature exceeds 28 °C, the fan will be turned on automatically. The data which is captured by the sensors is stored in MQTT server through the Internet [13].

3 The Proposed Architecture of Baby Monitoring System

The basic idea of the proposed baby monitoring system using IoT technology is to provide the main functionalities like detect the baby cry and play songs, detection of wetness, send alert messages to the parent, turning on or turning off the fans. Figure 1 shows the architecture of baby monitoring system and how the components are connected to each other into a device. The sensors are used for detection. These are connected to the microcontroller as inputs. The sensor data is taken as input by the microcontroller. It processes the data according to the code uploaded and then gives output in the form of voice and alert messages to the parents.

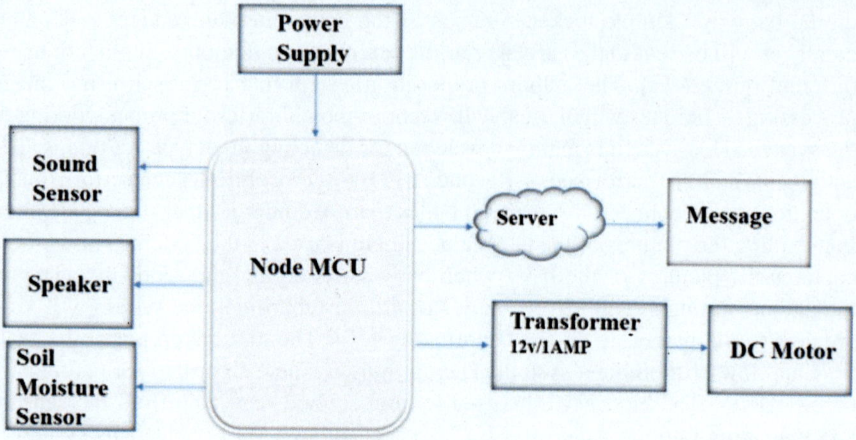

Fig. 1 Architecture of baby monitoring system

3.1 Baby Cry Detection Algorithm

1. Start
2. Initialize pin numbers.
3. Set the pin modes (input/output)
4. Read sound sensor value
5. If value>100
   5.1 Play songs using speaker
   5.2 Send alert notification to parent
6. Else
   6.1 Do Nothing
7. End.

3.2 Wetness Detection Algorithm

Wetness near the baby is detected by using the soil moisture sensor. If wetness value is 1, then it means that diaper needs to be changed. This alert will be sent to the registered users using Blynk application.

Algorithm

1. Start
2. If sensor value equals to 1
   2.1 Wetness detected and sends the notification to the Blynk
3. Else
   3.1 Do nothing
4. End

4 Experimental Results

The baby monitoring system has a sound sensor, which is used for detecting the baby cry. The data generated through sensors is sent to the microcontroller for further processing of information. This sound sensor works based on the sound absorbed [5]. If the sound absorbed is greater than 100 decibels, then it is noticed as the baby cry. As the baby is cried, the speaker present in the system plays the songs which are preloaded into the microcontroller. And an alert message will be sent by the microcontroller to the registered users for their registered mail or to the registered mobile number. By using the soil moisture, sensor wetness near the baby is detected, and an alert for the parent is sent. These alerts and monitoring of baby are done using Blynk android application. Figure 2 shows the developed baby monitoring with all the sensors and hardware connected.

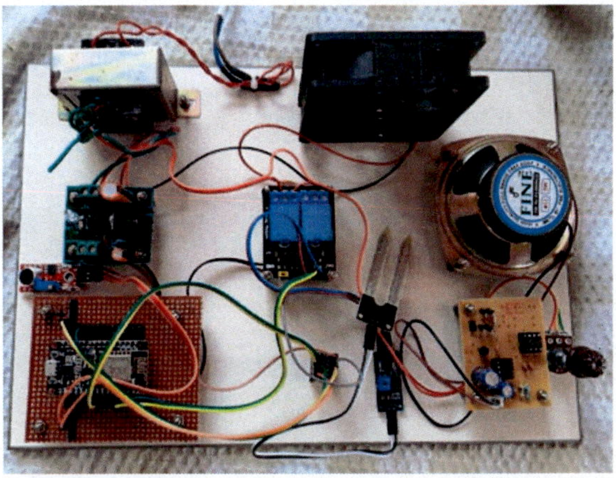

Fig. 2 Baby supervising system

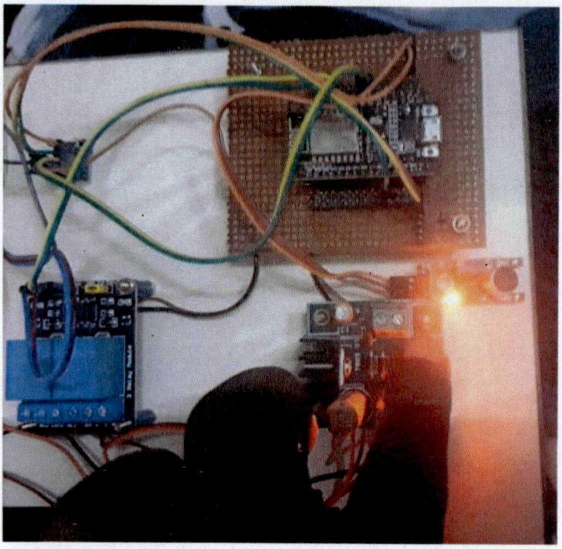

Fig. 3 When baby crying sound detect

4.1 Noise Detection by the System

As shown in Fig. 3 when the sound sensor absorbs the sound, i.e., greater than the threshold value, an LED will be blinked in the system.

Figure 4 shows the user interface of the Blynk application when an alert is sent to the registered users, about the generated noise.

4.2 Playing Songs

As shown in Fig. 5, when baby is crying, songs can be played in the system by controlling the system using Blynk app.

4.3 Wetness Detection

As shown in Fig. 6, when wetness is detected near the baby by soil moisture sensor, an LED will be blinked. Figure 7 shows the user interface of Blynk app when wetness is detected.

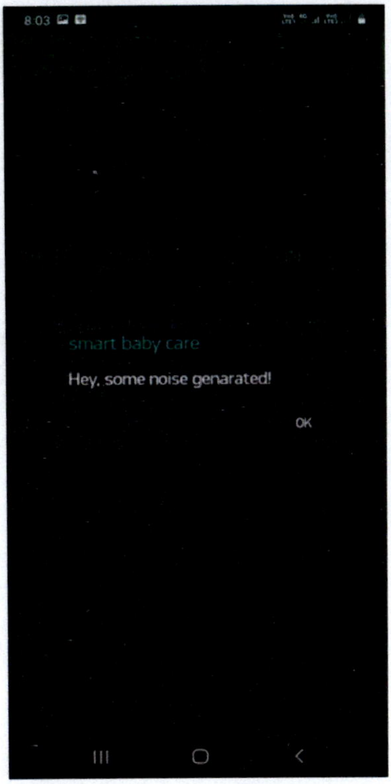

Fig. 4 Alert notification of noise in Blynk app

4.4 Turning on the Fan

As shown in Fig. 8, through Blynk app, user can turn on the fan. Figure 9 shows the user interface of Blynk app when fan button is turned on.

5 Conclusions and Future Work

Earlier, there are baby monitoring systems available but without the parents or care-taker's involvement. This makes the risk factor at baby's end. To overcome this, with the help of technology, a parent interactive baby monitoring system has been developed with which parent can track the baby from any place. This system sends the alert notifications to the parent whenever baby cries. And the speaker present in the system will play the songs to stop the baby's cry. And whenever there is wetness detected, then an alert notification will be sent to the parents. And all these alert notifications are sent using Blynk Android application. The main objective of this system is to provide the baby monitoring with reasonable price so that it will be affordable by all the people. This project is very useful for parents who are employed. This

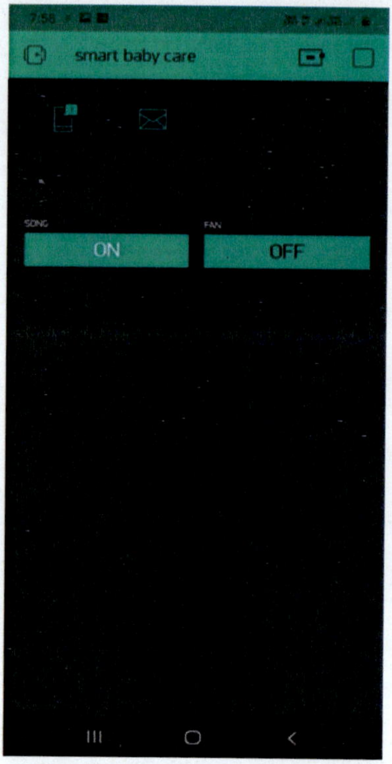

Fig. 5 Playing Song through Blynk App

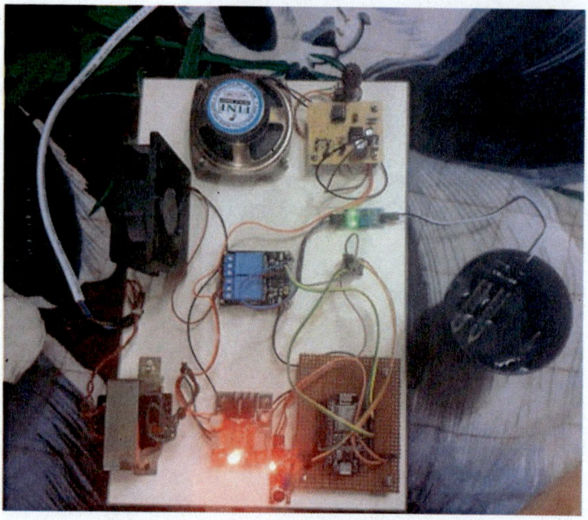

Fig. 6 When wetness is detected

Fig. 7 Alert notification for wetness

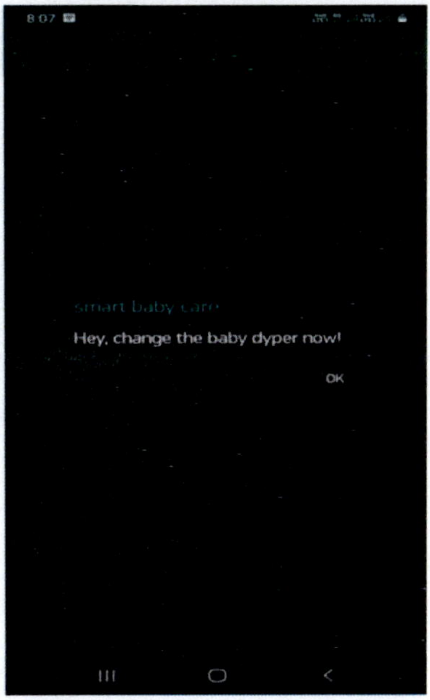

Fig. 8 When fan is in on state

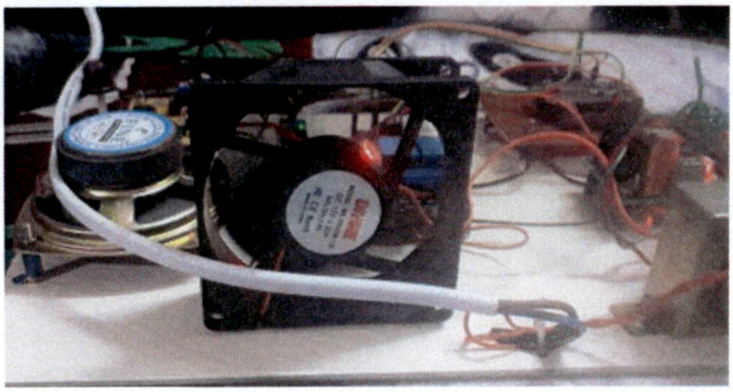

baby monitoring system reduces the burden to the parent, and they can perform their tasks properly. Due to the affordable cost of this system, it is more usable by most of the families. With this system, parents can take care of their baby remotely as this system can detect the baby cry and play songs to calm the baby and sleep again. This system sends the alert notification to the parent's mobile. Parents can turn on or turn off the fan or AC in the baby's room. All these futures of this baby monitoring system make it more usable. The system developed is of moderate budget. It can be reduced in future with much more enhanced functionalities and technologies in spite of assumption that reduction in cost makes compromise of performance. The enhancement of this system may by adding features like equipping a camera into the system, detecting the temperature of the baby, detecting the pulse rate of the baby and monitoring the baby's weight for medical analysis.

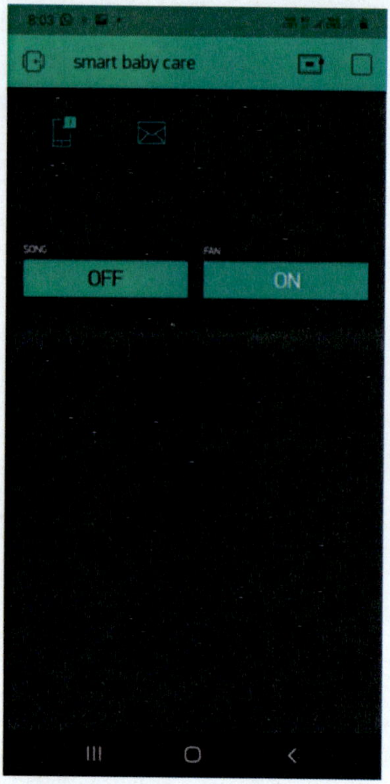

Fig. 9 Blynk app when fan is turned on

References

1. https://en.wikipedia.org/wiki/NodeMCU
2. Ishak DNFM, Mahadi M, Jamil A, Ambar R, Arduino based infant monitoring system. In: International research and innovation summit (IRIS2017)
3. Borkar M, Kenkre N, Patke H (2017) An innovative approach for infant monitoring system using pulse rate and oxygen level. Int J Comput Appl (0975–8887) 160(5)
4. Jabbar WA, Hamid SNIS, Almohammedi AA, Ramli RM, Ali MAH (2019) IoT-BBMS: Internet of Things-based Baby Monitoring System for Smart Cradle. IEEE vol. 7
5. https://www.elprocus.com/sound-sensor-working-and-its-applications/
6. Nazar NN, Kabeer MM, Shasna MA, Navami Krishna UA, Ashok N (2019) Infant cradle monitoring system using IoT. Int J Adv Res Comput Commun Eng 8(4)
7. Symon AF, Hassan N, Rashid H, Ahmed IU, Taslim Reza SM (2017) Design and development of a smart baby monitoring system based on Raspberry Pi and Pi Camera. In: Proceedings of the 2017 4th international conference on advances in electrical engineering 28–30 September, 2017
8. Horne RSC (2019) Sudden infant death syndrome: current perspectives. Int Med J 49(4):433–438
9. Badgujar D, Sawant N, Kundande D (2019) Smart and secure IoT based child monitoring system. Int Res J Eng Technol (IRJET) 6(11)
10. Dubey YK, Damke S (2019) Baby monitoring system using image processing and IoT. Int J Eng Adv Technol (IJEAT) 8(6)

11. Firmansyah R, Widodo A, Romadhon AD, Hudha MS, Saputra PPS, Lestari NA (2019) The prototype of infant incubator monitoring system based on the internet of things using NodeMCU ESP8266. Seminar Nasional Fisika (SNF) 2018, IOP Conf Ser: J Phys: Conf Ser 1171: 012015
12. Patil SP, Mhetre MR (2014) Intelligent baby monitoring system. ITSI Trans Electr Electron Eng 2(1)
13. Rajesh G, ArunLakshman R, Hari Prasad L, Chandira Mouli R (2014) Baby monitoring system using wireless sensor networks. ICTACT J Commun Technol 5(3):963–969

Analysis of DEAP Dataset for Emotion Recognition

Sujata Kulkarni and Prakashgoud R. Patil

Abstract In affective computing, emotion classification has a significant role and renders many applications in the areas like neuroscience, entertainment, neuromarketing, and education. These applications comprise classification of neurological disorder, false detection, recognition of stress and pain level, and finding level of attention. The traditional methods used for emotion recognition are facial expressions or voice tone. However, the outcomes of facial signs and verbal language can indicate the unfair and unclear results. Hence, investigators have started the usage of EEG (Encephalogram) method for analyzing the brain signals to recognize the various emotions. EEG-based emotion recognition has an ability to modify the way that we detect some health disorders. Brain signals reveal variations in electrical potential as a result of communication among thousands of neurons. This research article includes analysis of human affective state using DEAP- "Dataset for Emotion Analysis using Physiological Signals". It is a multimodal dataset, where 40 channels are used, 32 subjects participated, and 40 one-minute video pieces of music was shown to them. The participants evaluated each music video with respect to Valence, Arousal, Dominance, and Likings.

Keywords EEG · Emotions · Physiological signals · Valence · Arousal · Dominance · Liking · Classification

1 Introduction

Electroencephalography (EEG) is a popular method in neuro-imaging to capture the brain signals. It has the capability to measure the variations in voltages produced by the communication between neurons. These brain signals are classified into five frequency bands, and they are: delta (0.5–3 Hz), theta (4–7 Hz), alpha (8–13 Hz)

S. Kulkarni (✉) · P. R. Patil
KLE Technological University, Hubli, Karnataka, India
e-mail: sujatakulkarni@kletech.ac.in

P. R. Patil
e-mail: prpatilji@gmail.com

S. Bhattacharyya et al. (eds.), *International Conference on Intelligent and Smart Computing in Data Analytics*, Advances in Intelligent Systems and Computing 1312,
https://doi.org/10.1007/978-981-33-6176-8_8

beta (14–30 Hz), and gamma >30 Hz. Each of these brainwaves related some activity similar to thinking, meditation, learning, alertness, moving parts of body, or sleeping. Electroencephalography-based brain–computer interface is attaining attraction in the application areas of affective computing for the interpretation of human state of mind. [1]. But machine have significant role in human–computer interaction to recognize the emotions. It is really tough to look EEG signal and find state of human.

We commonly look at facial expressions, voice tone, and body language to understand the emotions. Higher than this, sometimes the facial expressions may lead to inconsistency. For instance in [2], the author noticed that persons smile in the course of negative emotional involvements. In view of this, physiological signals are central to recognize these emotions correctly. Less attention is given to physiological signals, due to comparative difficulty in classifying the data with particular emotion, and it needs heavy machines to record the data. But, one cannot overlook the significance of emotion detection using physiological signals, as the author assess the discomfort based on the variations in the heart rate[3]. Emotions are ever-present, and they are vital part of human being. They have a good role in daily activities and communications. Recognizing moods by computers has experienced a good development in the area of brain–computer interface.

This paper discusses an experiment conducted on the DEAP dataset comprises of physiological data for emotions. Aim is to apply two of classification machine learning algorithm and compare the results. Only in specific applications, machine learning algorithms perform better than Artificial Neural Networks and Deep Neural Networks.

Figure 1 shows the two-dimensional valence and arousal mode. Any emotion can be abstracted from the degree of valence and arousal from this circumplex model of emotion [4].

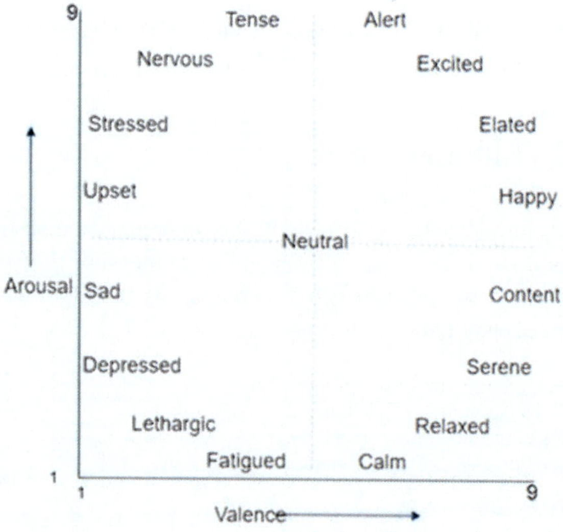

Fig. 1 Circumplex model with valence dimension on the *x*-axis and arousal dimension on the y-axis

Table 1 Contents of each participant file

Name	Size	Description
Data	40 × 80 × 8064	Video/trial × Channel × Data
Label	40 × 4	Video/trial × Label (Valence, Arousal, Dominance, Liking)

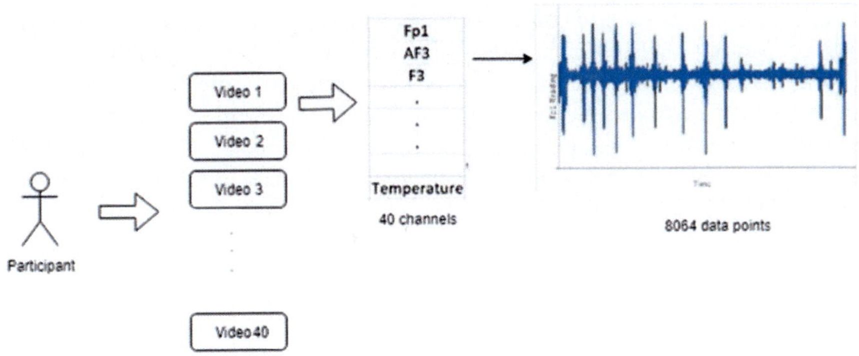

Fig. 2 Structure of feature vector used for training

DEAP [2] comprises data, created on Valence–Arousal emotion model represented in Fig. 1. It also includes series of peripheral data such as eye ocular movements (EOG), muscle-movement, GSR, breathing, blood pressure, and temperature. The data is collected from 32 EEG channels based on the international standard placement of electrodes 10–20 system [5], and eight channels for peripheral physiological data were used. For our analysis, peripheral data is not used. The sampling rate used to record the signals is 512 Hz, then after preprocessing down-sampled to 128 Hz. Table 1 shows the two arrays present in all participant file.

Figure 2 shows the structure of DEAP dataset used in the work to conduct training of data.

The result of this analysis has resulted in the following methodological contributions:

- All 32 files of DEAP dataset are united into a new large dataset.
- Visualization of DEAP dataset.
- To find the good classification technique for identification of emotion.
- Accuracy of KNN and SVM classification algorithms for EEG data.

Section 2 focuses on the work carried out in the area. Section 3 explains how the exploratory analysis of the data is done. Section 4 explains the results followed by conclusion and results in Sect. 5.

2 Related Work

The EEG signal-based research has many applications in its domain. These signals are usually used for recognizing stress as discussed in [6, 7], and they advise a strong connection between stress and EEG signals. The author in [8] applied Hilbert–Huang transform (HHT) to eliminate artifacts and accomplish cleaning. Hilbert–Huang transform is used for time–frequency analysis, and it abstracts the intrinsic mode functions (IMFs) which yields good Hilbert transforms. Using the Hilbert transformation, the IMF provides speedy frequencies as a function of time. The authors in [9] explained the usage of fast Fourier transform to identify the best means to sooth stress, and got a 76% precision. The author [10] shows that EEG signals can be used to function the robotic arms in the field of motor imagery. The author in [11] elucidated the means to recognize and differentiate the various brain waves of subject while performing task. In the article [12], the author discusses how to identify the early processing of dynamic region of the brain. The author in [13] explains the intrinsic noise present in the EEG data and proposed a method for strong representations of EEG data. The article [14, 15] describes EEG-based sleep pattern analysis, which has resulted in the development of sleep enhancement mobile applications. Fascinating point here is that CNN were used to extract time-invariant structures and bidirectional LSTM to routinely predict the different stages of sleep change from EEG epoch data.

The article [16] explains the classifier IClabel, and it runs on MATLAB, which has improved the existing classifiers. EEG signals are used for the detection of neurological disorder. The paper [17] discusses how these signals play a vital role to prevent the seizure and its type prediction. Different machine learning techniques were applied to detect the epileptic seizure. Many more articles describe the success in the range of 50–85% by different classification algorithms. The result of the model is extremely dependent on the feature extraction phase not on classification technique complexity [18].

2.1 Foundations

Principle Component Analysis: It is a well-known dimensional reduction method to lessen the number of training features. In the process of reducing the dimension, it tries to keep the original information and hence maintains the patterns. This technique is an experimental tool for data analysis. By summarizing the features, it reduces the training time and improves the performance. PCA steps are: Divide the dataset into two portions: class labels and the features. There are four labels and 8064 features. These features have to be minimized. Mean and covariance matrix are calculated. The formula for calculating the required number of different covariance is: $(n!/2*(n - 2))!$. The covariance matrix for 'n' features is calculate which is an $n \times n$ matrix.

The second step of PCA is to find eigenvectors and eigenvalues. It needs to find the determinant of n x n matrix to zero. Resolving this equation one can obtain the eigenvalues and the eigenvector. The third step is to keep the eigenvectors in the decreasing order of eigenvalues. The vector with smallest eigenvalue gives the least information. The top 20 vectors form our feature space.

KNN Classifier: KNN finds the distance between new data point and all the data points, chooses the K number of nearest points to the new data, and elects the most common label in case of classification. Euclidean distance is used for any dimensional space. The performance of this algorithm depends on the value of K. The performance of KNN decreases as the size of date increases. The model is created to check the different values of k ranging from 2 to 50 with a tenfold cross-validation from.

Support Vector Machines: This classification model works based on the use of hyperplanes. With the help of kernels, the algorithm is capable to transform the data, and uses these transformations to find best boundary among the outputs. In this algorithm, the EEG data points are plotted in the space. SVM belongs to p-complete problem, because it can be executed in a polynomial time. The vector w and the bias b are estimated during the training of a model.

3 Procedure

The foremost step to understand the data is to carry out an exploratory data analysis, where the data analysis is useful for establishing a base on which prediction models are built. The main goal to carry out an analysis is to find what methods have to be applied to standardize and extract the facts and figures from the data. In turn, this helps in determining improved methodologies while realizing predictive models. It is possible to execute different classifications for the four different classes of valence, arousal, dominance, and liking. The participants evaluated each of these video pieces and rated in the gauge of 1–9. Hence, one-hot encoding is helpful, by categorizing these values above 5 and below 5.

The pre-processed dataset is given in the system of pickle file. When these files are loaded, they give two separate arrays termed as labels and data. The labels were encoded to four separate files, individually demonstrating an emotion. The actual data and labels are separated in different files. All separation of data and labels are done prior to the cross-validation. Algorithms applied and resulted in the range of 53 to 70%.

In the "DEAP data" set, the video trials are one-minute duration, and it has not mentioned properly where exactly the emotion occurs within the one minute. Beside this, PCA is used to reduce the features, but the performance is not effective due to the variation of signals. Hence to improve the performance, segmentation of the signal and adaptation of change in calculating feature is required.

4 Results

The normal distribution (Gaussian distribution) of all 32 participant's score of four different emotions are shown in Figs. 3, 4, 5, and 6. From the histogram, it is noticed that the distribution is symmetric around 5, which signifies that, about the videos, maximum of the participants have mixed emotional state. The data in Fig. 6 is skewed toward 9; hence the dual classification model might produce improved results. One more key observation noticed is that most of participants have given integer ratings, and therefore, the spikes are present at integer values. The normal ratings for our different class of 32 participants are considered. The reduced with succeeding video trials and kept on decreasing (Table 2).

The results shown in the above table tells us that considering only EEG data does not perform well. The author [19] says that it should be combined with peripheral data also to get higher results. Even after features are reduces, there is no significant improvement in all our emotion results. With this, a question arises in the mind "Only

Fig. 3 Normal distributions of valence frequency ratings

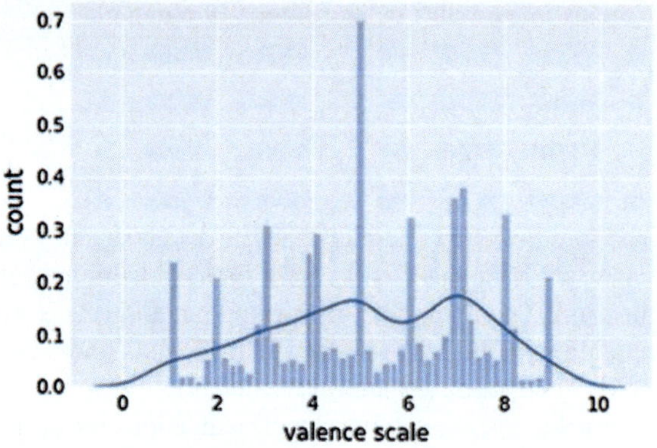

Fig. 4 Normal distributions of arousal frequency ratings

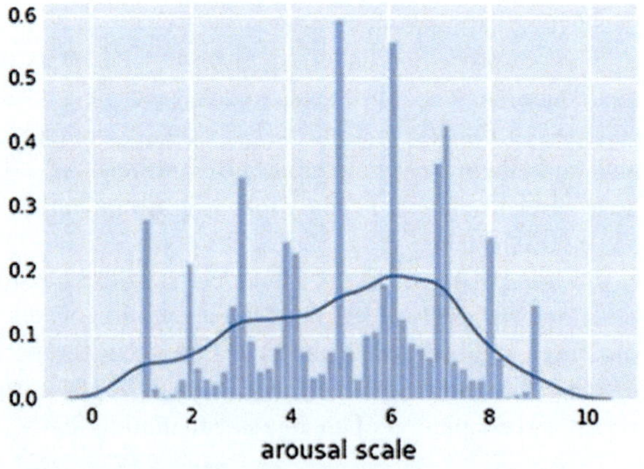

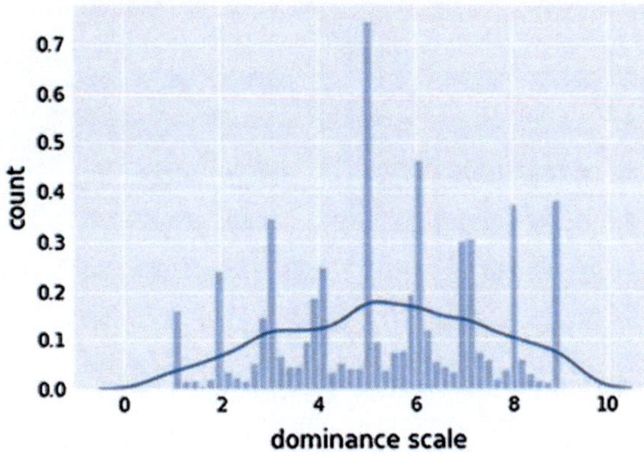

Fig. 5 Normal distributions of dominance frequency ratings

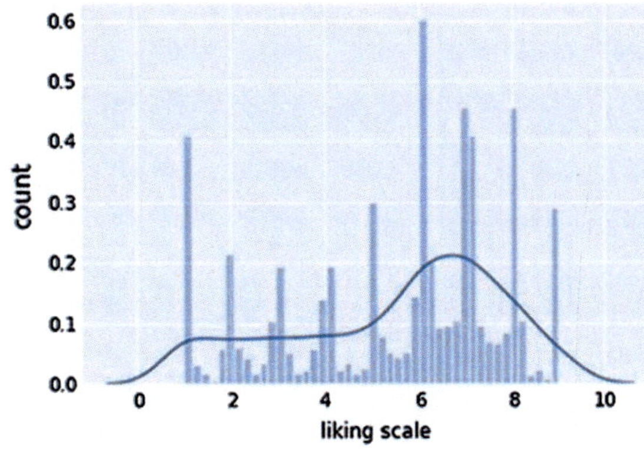

Fig. 6 Normal distributions of liking frequency ratings

Table 2 Results

Classification	Dimension	Accuracy	Precision	Recall	$F1$-score
KNN	Valence	64	65	83	73
	Arousal	56	66	69	67
	Dominance	68	72	88	79
	Liking	65	68	94	79
SVM	Valence	66	65	100	79
	Arousal	65	65	99	79
	Dominance	70	70	99	82
	Liking	70	70	100	82

using EEG data is it not possible to deduce good results for emotions?" It is an initial point to perform further experiments.

Figures 7, 8, 9, and 10 show the accuracy.

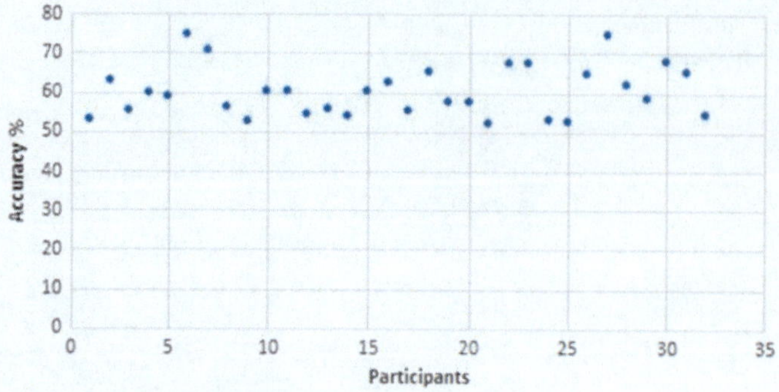

Fig. 7 Individual accuracy for Valence

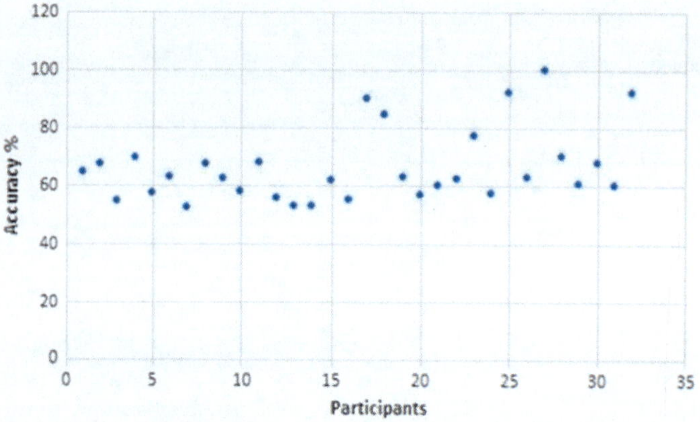

Fig. 8 Individual accuracy for Arousal

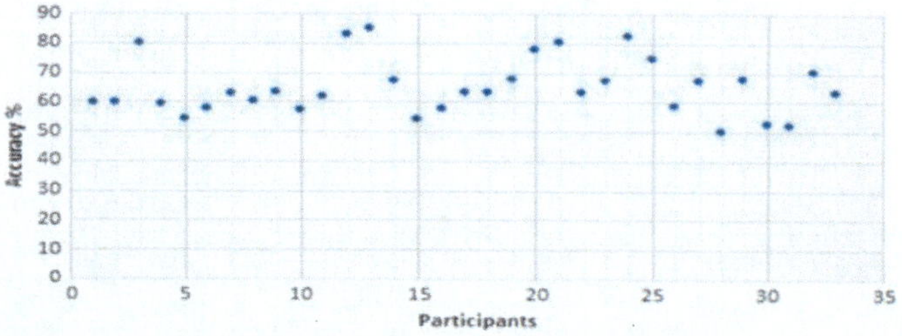

Fig. 9 Individual accuracy for Dominance

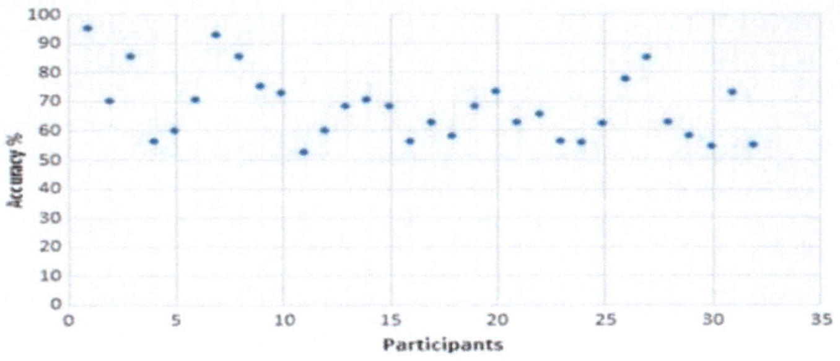

Fig. 10 Individual accuracy for Liking

5 Conclusions and Discussions

The main aim of the study was to learn how neurophysiological tools help an individual to feel emotions. Explored DEAP EEG dataset. The following are the observations made from the study: The signals are in the time domain; for better accuracy, the features have to be extracted in the frequency domain; beside this, PCA is used to reduce the features, but the performance is not effective due to the variation of signals. Hence to improve the performance, segmentation of the signal and adaptation of change in calculating feature is required. With this, a question arises in the mind "Only using EEG data, is it not possible to deduce good results for emotions?" It is an initial point to perform further experiments.

References

1. Koelstra S, Muhl C, Soleymani M, Lee J-S, Yazdani A, Ebrahimi T, Pun T, Nijholt A, Patras I (2012) Deap: a database for emotion analysis; using physiological signals. IEEE Trans Affect Comput 3(1):18–31
2. Ekman P (1989) The argument and evidence about universals in facial expressions. Hand-book of social psychophysiology, pp 143–164
3. Lindh V, Wiklund U, Hakansson S (1999) Heel lancing in term new-born infants: an evaluation of pain by frequency domain analysis of heart rate variability. Pain 80(1–2):143–148
4. Posner J, Russell JA, Peterson BS (2005) The circumplex model of affect: an integrative approach to affective neuroscience, cognitive development, and psychopathology. DevPsychopathol 17(3)
5. Klem GH, Lu¨ders HO, Jasper H, Elger C et al (1999) The ten-twenty electrode system of the international federation. Electroencephalogr Clin Neurophysiol 52(3): 3–6
6. Vanitha V, Krishnan P (2016) Real time stress detection system based on EEG signals
7. Liao C-Y, Chen R-C, Tai S-K (2018) Emotion stress detection using eeg signal and deep learning technologies. In: 2018 IEEE international conference on applied system invention (ICASI). IEEE, New York, pp 90–93
8. Koelstra S et al (2011) Deep: a database for emotion analysis; using physiological signals. IEEE Trans Affect Comput 3:18–31
9. Bazgir O, Mohammadi Z, Habib SAH, Emotion recognition with machine learning using eeg signals. IEEE

10. Jia W et al (2012) Electroencephalography (eeg)-based instinctive brain-control of a quadruped locomotion robot. In: 2012 annual international conference of the IEEE engineering in medicine and biology society. IEEE, New York, pp 1777–1781
11. Fakhruzzaman MN, Riksakomara E, Suryotrisongko H (2015) EEG wave identifcation in human brain with emotiv epoc for motor imagery. Proc Comput Sci 72:269–276
12. Shariat S, Pavlovic V, Papathomas T, Braun A, Sinha P (2010) Sparse dictionary methods for EEG signal classification in face perception. In: 2010 IEEE international workshop on machine learning for signal processing. IEEE, New York, pp 331–336
13. Tabar YR, Halici U (2016) A novel deep learning approach for classifcation of EEG motor imagery signals. J Neural Eng 14:016003
14. Chambon S, Thorey V, Arnal PJ, Mignot E, Gramfort A (2018) A deep learning architecture to detect events in EEG signals during sleep. In: 2018 IEEE 28th international workshop on machine learning for signal processing (MLSP). IEEE, New York, pp 1–6
15. Bashivan P, Rish I, Yeasin M, Codella N (2015) Learning representations from EEG with deep recurrent-convolutional neural networks. arXiv preprint arXiv:1511.06448
16. Pion- L, Kreutz K, Makeig S (2019) ICLABEL: an automated electroencephalographic independent component classifer, dataset, and website. NeuroImage 198:181–197
17. Struck AF et al (2019) Comparison of machine learning models for seizure prediction in hospitalized patients. Ann Clin Transl Neurol 67:1239–1247
18. Li S, Feng H (2019) EEG signal classification method based on feature priority analysis and CNN, pp 403–436
19. Sharma A, Emotion recognition using deep convolutional neural network with large scale physiological data
20. George FP,Shaikat IM, Ferdawoos PS, Parvez MZ, Uddin J (2019) Recognition of emotional states using EEG signals based on time-frequency analysis and SVM classifier. Int J Electr Comput Eng (IJECE) 9(2):1012–1020
21. Doma V, Pirouz M, A comparative analysis of machine learning methods for emotion recognition using EEG and peripheral physiological signals for emotion recognition using EEG and peripheral physiological signals
22. Asghar MA, Khan MJ, Amin FY, Rizwan M, Rahman M, Badnava S, Mirjavadi SS, EEG-based multi-modal emotion recognition using bag of deep features: an optimal feature selection approach. Sensors

A Machine Learning Approach for Air Pollution Analysis

R. V. S. Lalitha, Kayiram Kavitha, Y. Vijaya Durga, K. Sowbhagya Naidu, and S. Uma Manasa

Abstract Air pollution occurs due to presence of harmful gases like dust and smoke. Inhaling these gases leads to health problem. The inhaling of dust leads to breathing problems and lung issues which are of major concern in human life. The green house gases like synthetic chemicals present due to emission of human activities. The major green house gases are carbon dioxide, chlorofluorocarbons, water vapor, ozone, methane, and nitrous oxide. Greenhouse gases absorb infrared radiation. Air pollution is monitored by Governments and various local agencies. The prime responsibility of the proposed system is to detect the concentrations of major air pollutant gases that are present in the air which cause harm to humans. Air pollution detection is developed using IoT for detecting pollutant gases using MQ2 and MQ135 sensors. The gases like carbon dioxide (CO_2), carbon monoxide (CO), ethyl alcohol, nitric oxide, nitrogen dioxide (NO_2), and sulfur dioxide (SO_2) will be detected using these sensors. The detected parameters are analyzed using machine learning (ML) algorithms to estimate air quality. The ecosystem developed helps in learning correlation among gases. This helps in estimating impact and level of air pollutants to measure air quality.

Keywords Air pollution · Internet of things · MQ2 · MQ135 and correlation

---

R. V. S. Lalitha (✉)
Department of C.S.E, Aditya College of Engineering & Technology, Surampalem, India
e-mail: rvslalitha@gmail.com

K. Kavitha
Department of C.S.E, Gokaraju Rangaraju Institute of Engineering and Technology, Hyderabad, India

Y. Vijaya Durga
TCS, Hyderabad, India

K. Sowbhagya Naidu
Aditya College of Engineering & Technology, Surampalem, India

S. Uma Manasa
Syntel, Hyderabad, India

S. Bhattacharyya et al. (eds.), *International Conference on Intelligent and Smart Computing in Data Analytics*, Advances in Intelligent Systems and Computing 1312,
https://doi.org/10.1007/978-981-33-6176-8_9

1 Introduction

In order to protect our environment, we need to monitor the pollutant gases. Several epidemiological studies have been taken up for formulation of air pollution analysis. Air pollution is one of the factors that cause deaths from lung cancer and respiratory diseases. Air pollution may have direct impact on adult deaths. World Health Organization (WHO) says that air pollution has impact on environment-related deaths. Air pollution analysis assists in reducing mortality risk of individual death rate. The prediction analysis is done using ML to take preventive measures to increase life span of individuals. IOT based air pollution detection measures presence of dangerous gases in the air. The ecosystem is developed using Raspberry PI 3, MQ2, and MQ135 sensors. WiFi module is used to upload detected parameters to ThingSpeak cloud for storing them in database. A Web server is used to deploy data from ThingSpeak for analyzing it through ML. The paper is organized into four sections. Section 1 stated the significance of air pollution detection. In Sect. 2, the previous research works are discussed. The design and implementation details are given in Sect. 3. And the machine learning-based analysis is done in Sect. 4. Conclusion states the role and impact of air pollution analysis for protecting human lives.

2 Related Work

Diffusion tubes are usually used to monitor air pollution. They are made of plastic material with a rubber stopper attached at each end. These are designed for detecting NO_2. They are large in size and are not efficient. The materials needed to perform sampling process are diffusion tubes, tube holders, survey sheet, maps, clip board, re-sealable samples bag1, and a pen. Initially, diffusion tubes are located in a specific area which is divided into grids. Then, position tubes are positioned vertically downward, and cable ties are attached if it is fixing to a pipe. Fix sample in a specific location where free circulation of air around the tube. Remove the white cap and allow it for exposure. Fill date and times in the record sheet. Note the tube condition, changes in site conditions, or anything that might affect the results. Arun Kumar presented IoT based ecosystem to estimate quality of the air using various sensors like gas, temperature, humidity, rain, and smoke. By detecting air pollution, measures can be taken to safeguard the health of people residing in that area [1]. Shah presented IoT based air pollution system using MQ135 sensor, LPG sensor, humidity sensor, and temperature sensor. The circuitry uses Arduino UNO microcontroller for connecting processing all the components data [2]. Chandana (2018) designed air pollution detection system using MQ135, MQ4, MQ5, MQ9 using Arduino UNO. The data collected by the sensors will be informed to higher authorities [3]. Setiawan and Kustiawan proposed IoT based air quality system. MQ2, MQ9 sensors, and ZH03A dust sensor are used for measuring air quality. The results are processed using ThingSpeak API [4]. El Khaili presented air quality design for urban traffic flow management for data analysis. Idrees designed IoT architecture for detecting pollution in the air. Pollution sensors and electrochemical sensors are used to detect air pollution, and IBM cloud is used for analysis. Gonçalo Marques proposed a system to using IoT for real-time monitoring in buildings. iDust sensors are used to detect dust [5]. SQL server is used to store data, and e-mail notification facility is also included. Zhao designed a smart sensor network for monitoring air quality. The information can be monitored by a Web application. PHP and nodejs are used for developing Web application, and PM2.5 is used to sense air data. MQTT protocol is used to transmit messages across IoT device and Web application [6]. Mukhopadhyay proposed design of air pollution detector and air quality meter with Arduino. Temperature sensor, humidity sensor, and gas sensors are used to sense air pollution [7]. Desai proposed a method for urban air pollution system. The system acquires CO_2 and CO levels in the air. The collected data will be stored in the Microsoft Azure services, and Power BI tool is used to transform data into information [8]. IoT based air quality monitoring and predictor systems are discussed for checking air quality in smart city applications [9, 10, 11–14].

3 Methodology

A. Circuit Analysis of IoT based Air Pollution Detection System

The Internet of Things based air pollution detection is designed using the sensors MQ2 and MQ135 sensors. The ecosystem is developed using Raspberry PI 3 B model, MQ2, MQ135 sensors, 840-point Bread board, GPIO extension board, and MCP 3008 ADC. MQ2 detects CO_2, NO_2, and NH_3. MQ135 detects CO, smoke, and LPG. ThingSpeak cloud is used to store data captured by the sensors. A Web server is used to display air pollution information and make it available over Internet. The gases sensed by the MQ2 and MQ135 are shown in Fig. 1, and circuit connections are shown in Figs. 2 and 3.

Fig. 1 Gases sensed by MQ2 and MQ135

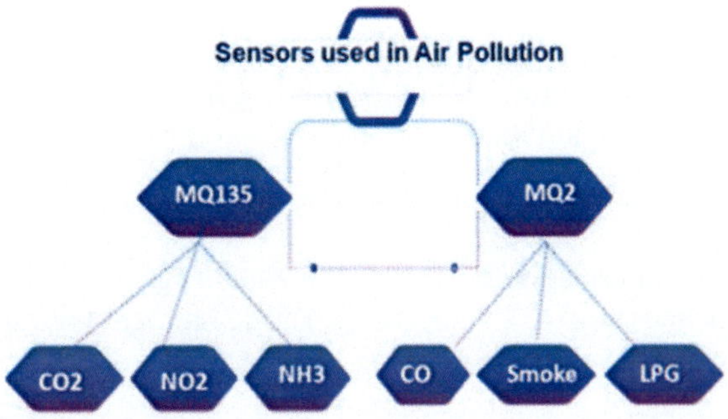

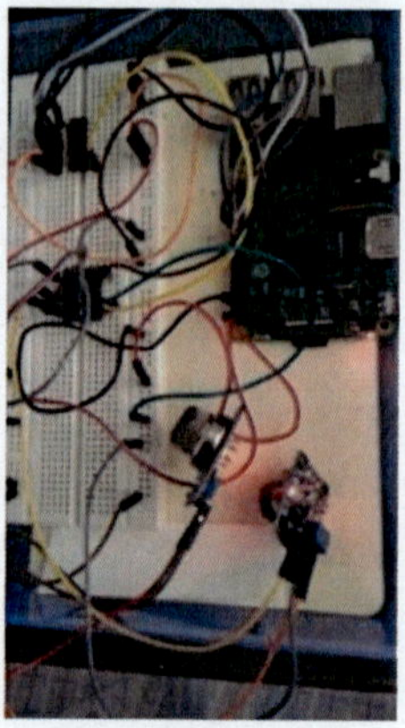

Fig. 2 Circuit connecting MQ2 and MQ135 to Raspberry PI

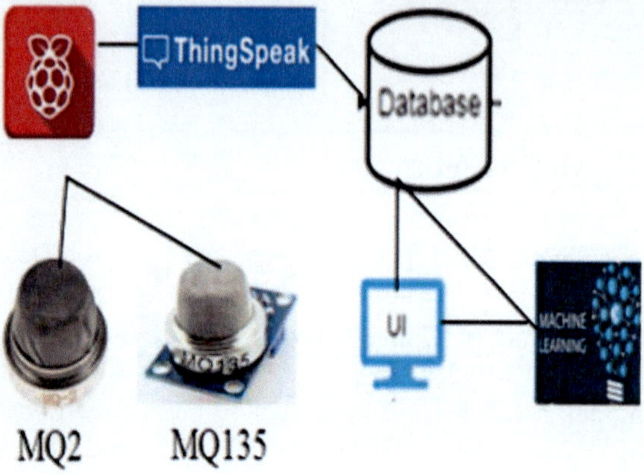

Fig. 3 Sensing and storing in cloud and data analytics using machine learning

The information sensed by MQ2 and MQ135 are uploaded in the ThingSpeak cloud instantly and stored in the database.

B. Detection of pollutants using MQ2 and MQ135 Sensors

MQ2 sensor detects gases CO_2, NO_2, and NH_3. This real-time values detected by sensor are shown in Fig. 4. And the gases CO, smoke, and LPG detected by MQ2 are shown in Fig. 5.

C. Real-time sensing of gases using MQ2 and MQ135 sensors

The information sensed by MQ2 and MQ135 in ThingSpeak cloud is depicted as below (Figs. 6, 7, 8, 9, 10, 11, and 12) for real-time statistics.

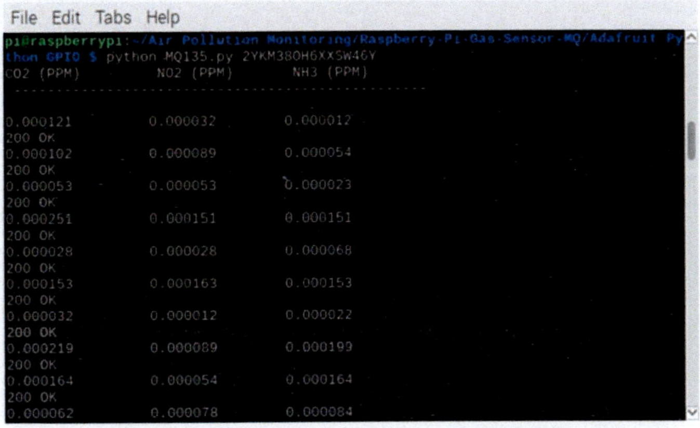

Fig. 4 Detection of gases using MQ135

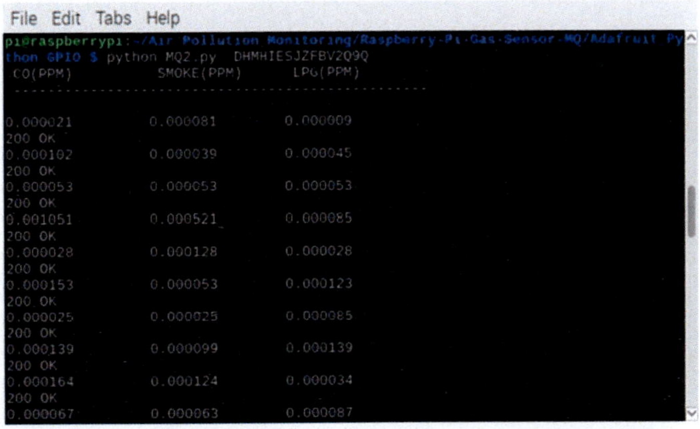

Fig. 5 Detection of gases using MQ2

4 Analysis of Linearity and Correlation Between Gases Using Machine Learning

CO, CO_2, NO_2, etc., are primary nutrients, when they are released from identifiable sources cause health risk. SO_3, H_2SO_4, and so on come under secondary air pollutants. Carbon monoxide is toxic and reduces oxygen in blood. It produces from cigarette smoke and automobiles. Sulfur dioxide produces from coal-burning power plants. It produces acids when it reacts with air. The major source of nitrogen oxide is automobiles contribute to acid rain. Ozone and H_2SO_4 are the secondary air pollutants that cause photochemical reactions in air. The correlation analysis among various pollutants are shown in Figs. 13, 14, 15, 16, 17, 18, 19, and 20.

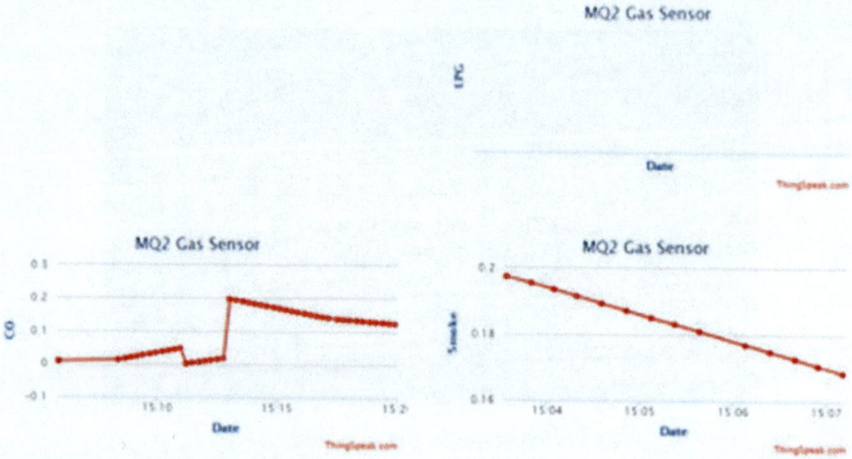

Fig. 6 Air pollution monitoring using MQ2

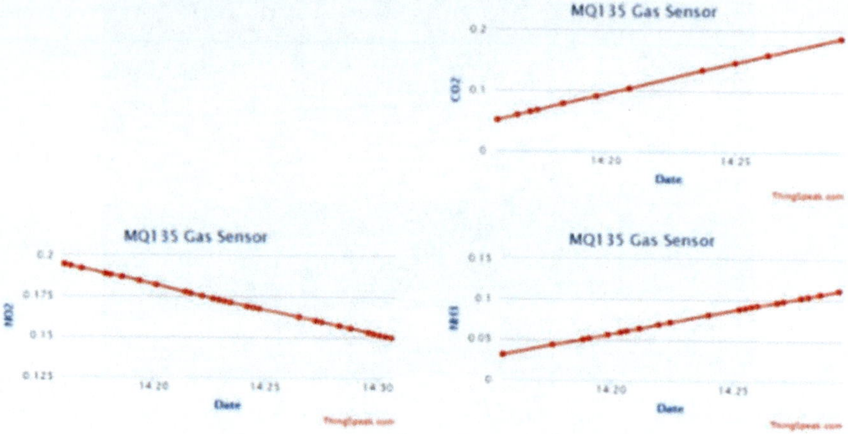

Fig. 7 Air pollution monitoring using MQ135

Fig. 8 LPG detection using MQ2

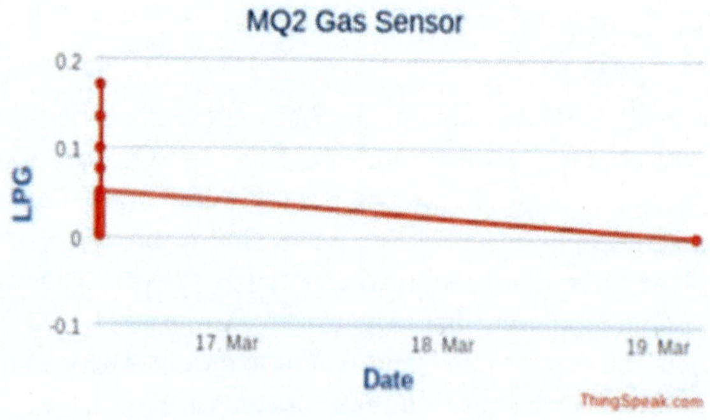

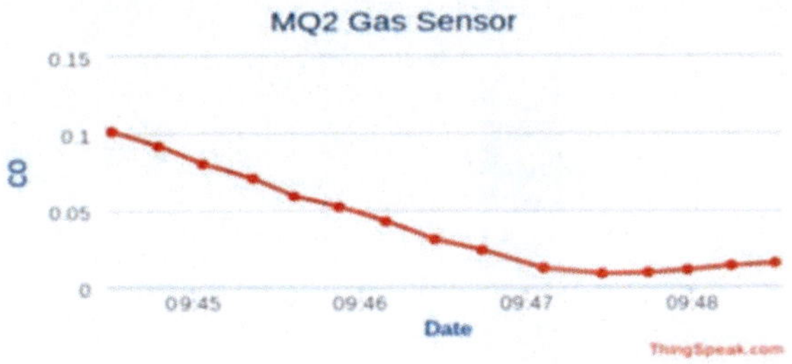

Fig. 9 CO detection using MQ2

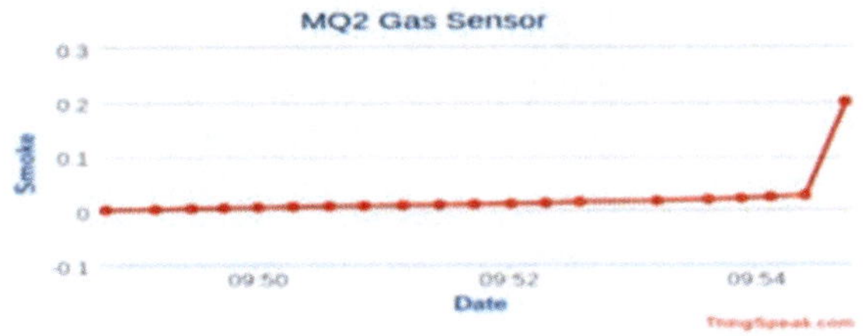

Fig. 10 Smoke detection using MQ2

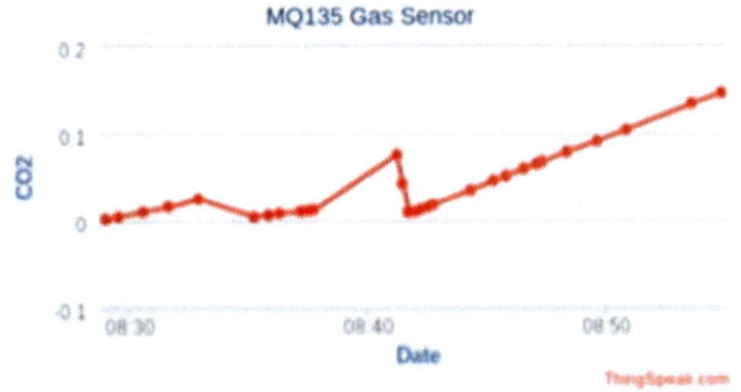

Fig. 11 CO_2 detection using MQ135

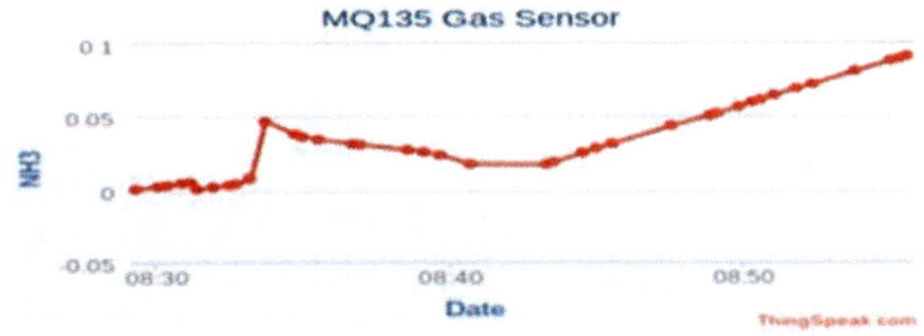

Fig. 12 NH_3 detection using MQ135

5 Conclusions

This ecosystem developed gives information of pollutants present in less amount of time. The information of air pollutants is available in the cloud; hence, the data can be analyzed from anywhere at any time. The real-time detection of air pollution levels in the environment helps government to take necessary decisions. This system is

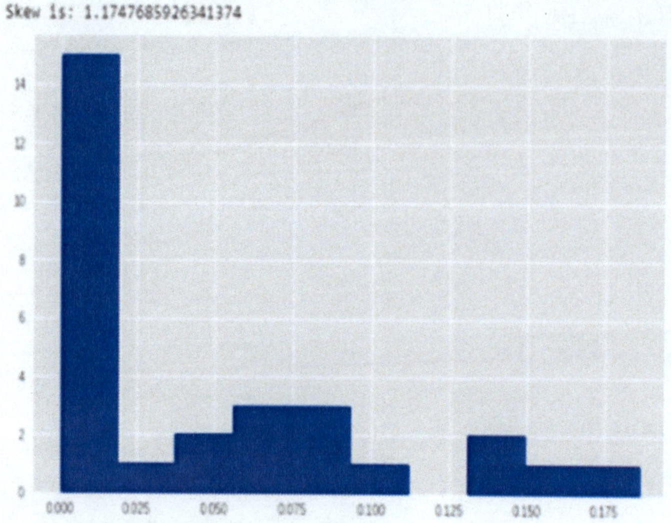

Fig. 13 Skew and histogram of CO_2

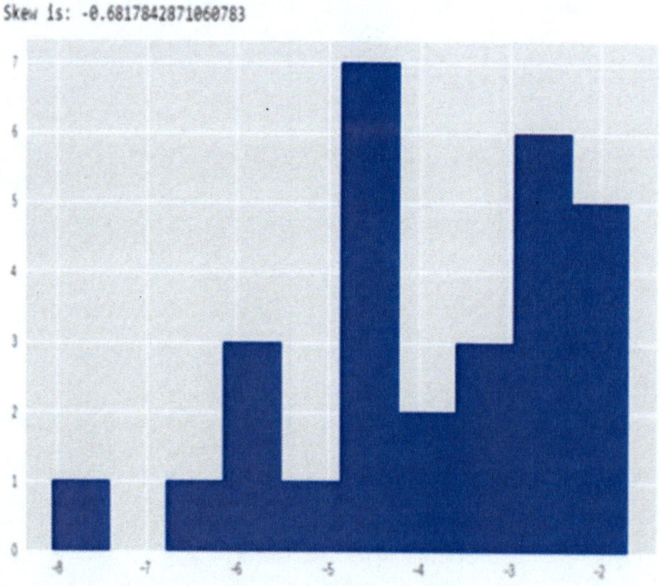

Fig. 14 Skew and histogram of CO_2

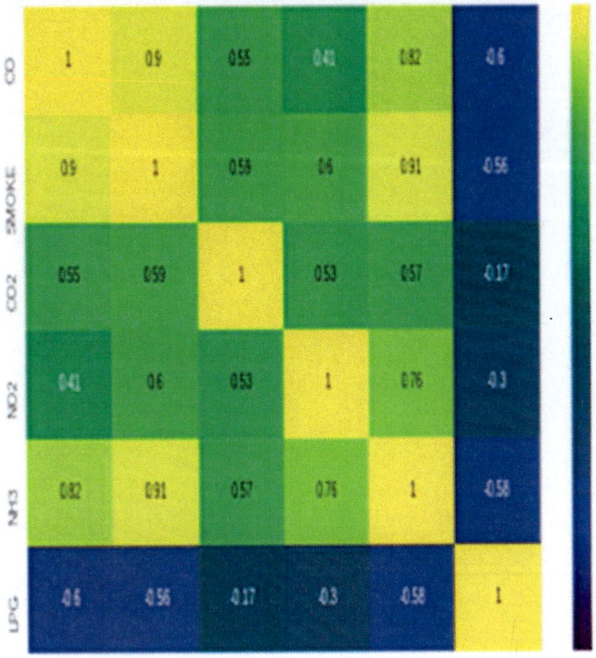

Fig. 15 Correlation between pollutants

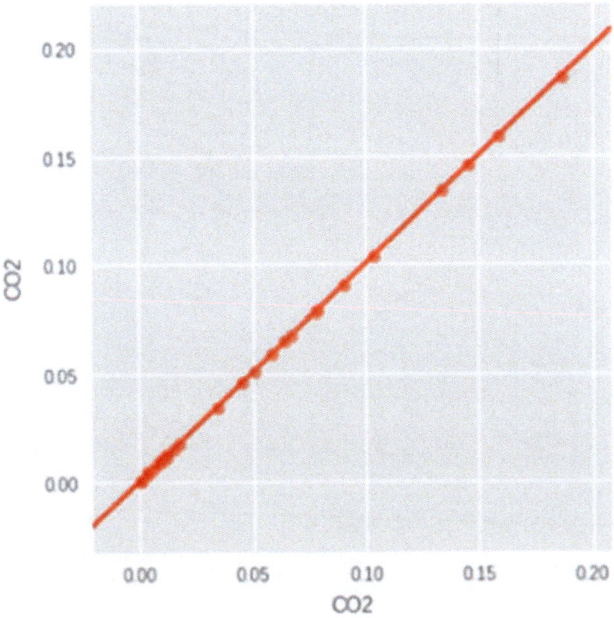

Fig. 16 Linearity of CO_2 over CO_2

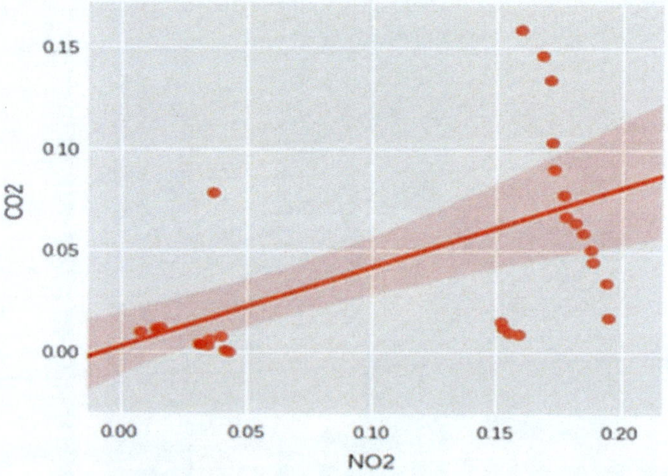

Fig. 17 Linearity between CO_2 and NO_2

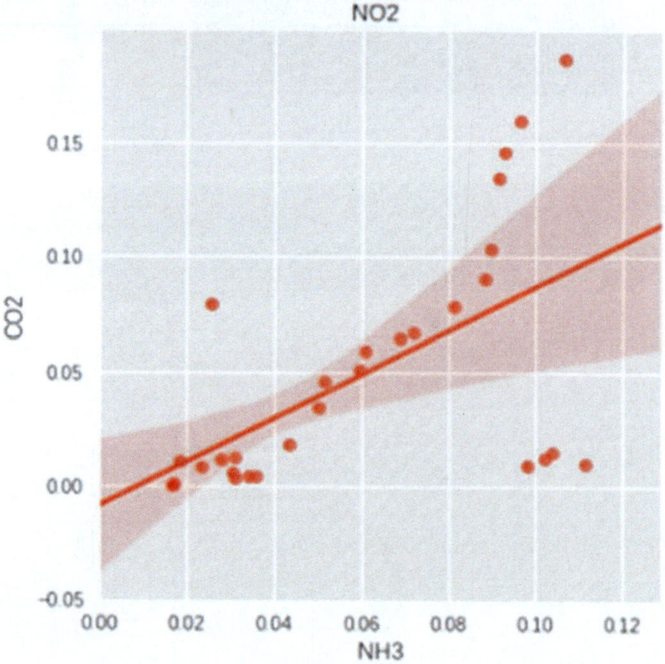

Fig. 18 Correlation between CO_2, NO_2 and NH_3

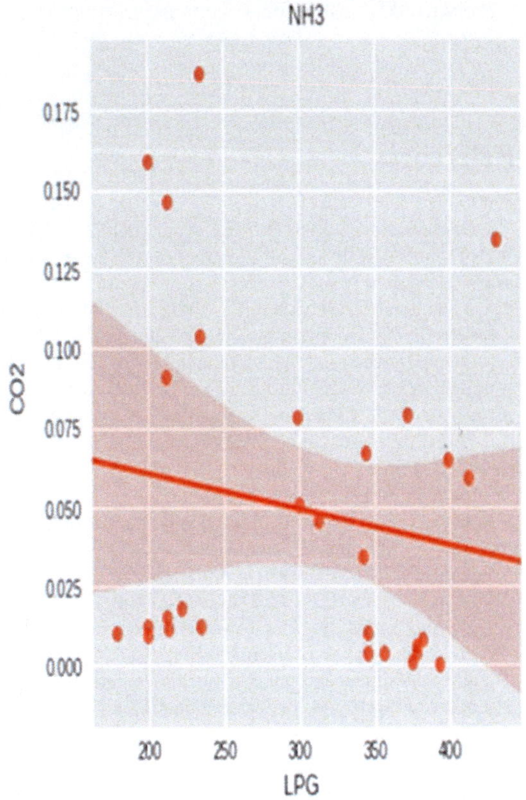

Fig. 19 Correlation between CO_2, LPG and NH_3

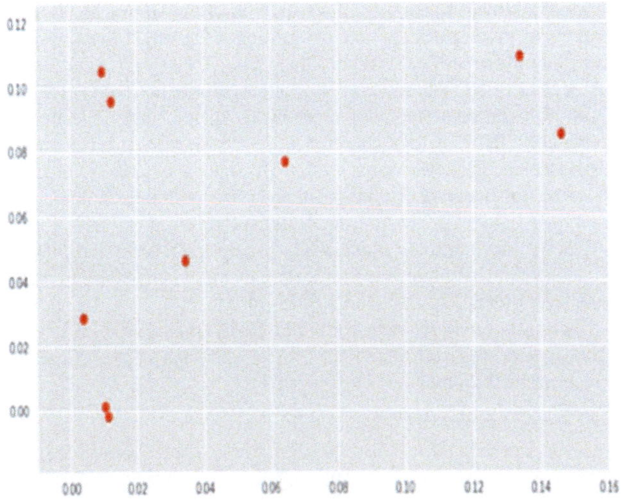

Fig. 20 Predicted value of CO_2

mainly used to researchers, because testing of gases manually takes a lot of process, time, etc.

References

1. Durga S, Raja Sekhar Babu M, Amir Gandomi H, Rizwan P, Daneshmand Md (2019) Internet of things mobile air pollution montioring system(IoT-Mobair). IEEE Internet of Things Issue 3
2. Arunkumar D, Ajaykanth K, Ajithkannan M, Sivasubramanian M (2018) Smart air pollution detection and monitoring using IoT. Int J Pure Appl Math 119(15):935–941
3. Shah HN, Khan Z, A Ali Merchant, M Moghal, A Shaikh, P Rane (2018) IOT based air pollution monitoring system. Int J Sci Eng Res 9(2)
4. Chandana B, Chandana K, Jayashree N, Anupama M, Vanamala CK (2018) Pollution monitoring using iot and sensor technology. Int Res J EngTechnol (IRJET) 05(03). e-ISSN: 2395-0056
5. Idrees Z, Zou Z, Zheng L(2018) Edge computing based iot architecture for low cost air pollution monitoring systems: a compreh syst anal des considerations and development, Sensors 18(9)
6. Gonçalo Marques ID, Roque Ferreira C, Pitarma R (2018) A system based on the internet of things for real-time particle monitoring in buildings. Int J Environ Res Public Health 15:821
7. Zhao Z, Wang J, Fu C, Liu Z, Liu D, B Li, Design of a smart sensor network system for real-time air quality monitoring on green roof, J Sens 1987931, 13
8. Mukhopadhyay A, Shuvam Paul S, Saha D, Shome K, Roy S, Ghosh S, Basu A, Sen K, R. Chatterjee, Design of air quality meter and pollution detector, In: 2017 8th annual industrial automation and electromechanical engineering conference (IEMECON), date of conference: 16–18 August 2017, Bangkok, Thailand
9. Setiawan FN, Kustiawan I (2008) IoT based air quality monitoring. In: IOP conference serial: material science engineering, pp 384 012008
10. El Khaili M, Alloubane A, Terrada L, Khiat A (2019) Urban traffic flow management based on air quality measurement by iot using LabVIEW. In: Ben Ahmed M, Boudhir A, Younes A (eds) Innovations in smart cities applications edition, SCA 2018. Lecture notes in intelligent transportation and infrastructure, Springer, Cham
11. Desai SN, Alex R (2017) IoT based air pollution monitoring and predictor system on Beagle bone black. In: 2017 International conference on nextgen electronic technologies: silicon to software (ICNETS2). IEEE, date of conference: 23–25 March 2017, Chennai, India
12. De Vito S, Massera E, Piga M, Martinotto L, Di Francia G (2008) On field calibration of an electronic nose for benzene estimation in an urban pollution monitoring scenario. Sens Actuators B: Chem 129(2):22 750–757, ISSN 0925-4005
13. De Vito S, Piga M, Martinotto L, Francia GD z(2009) CO, NO2 and NOx urban pollution monitoring with on-field calibrated electronic nose by automatic bayesian regularization. Sens Actuators B: Chem 143(1):182–191, ISSN 0925-4005
14. De Vito S, Fattoruso G, Pardo M, Tortorella F, Di Francia G (2012) Semi-supervised learning techniques in artificial olfaction: a novel approach to classification problems and drift counteraction. IEEE Sens J 12(11):3215–3224

Facial Expression Detection Model of Seven Expression Types Using Hybrid Feature Selection and Deep CNN

P. V. V. S. Srinivas and Pragnyaban Mishra

Abstract A facial expression is a natural reflection of human feelings, It is the nature of the human to reciprocate through the facial expression to the living world from where the inputs are perceived. The human science measures the emotion, feeling and sentiment by seeing the human face and face curves, but the recognition of emotion through artificial means with high accuracy and less computing resources is more challenging. In this research work, we developed a state-of-the-art procedure that recognizes the emotion of seven categories, namely Happy, Anger, Sad, Disgust, Neutral, Surprise, and Fear efficiently using deep learning. In this work, the model is trained using the fer2013 data set consists of 35887, and the CK48+ dataset consists of 3540 images. We proposed a hybrid model of feature selection that is used before feeding to the proposed computing model of CNN architecture. We claim through the use of both the models one after the other the emotions is correctly recognized with high accuracy during both training and testing phases, which the conventional method doesn't have.

Keywords Hybrid model · CNN architecture · Facial emotion · Feature selection · Fer2013 · CK48+

1 Introduction

Facial expression is a universal language through which people communicate socially, which surpasses ethnicity and cultural diversities. The information which as hard to tell can be easily conveyed through facial expressions. With the help of high-quality sensors, automatic emotion recognition has found a useful in various areas such as virtual reality applications, robotics, cyber security, psychological studies, image processing, etc. Research is being done in the areas of deep learning, machine

P. V. V. S. Srinivas (✉) · P. Mishra
Department of CSE, Koneru Lakshmaiah Education Foundation (KLEF), Guntur, India
e-mail: cnu.pvvs@kluniversity.in

P. Mishra
e-mail: pragnyaban@kluniversity.in

S. Bhattacharyya et al. (eds.), *International Conference on Intelligent and Smart Computing in Data Analytics*, Advances in Intelligent Systems and Computing 1312,
https://doi.org/10.1007/978-981-33-6176-8_10

learning and image processing for designing effective expression recognition algorithms not for ideal laboratory conditions, but also for recognition in real-time. Therefore, building a framework that is capable of detection of faces and emotions being very important in the area of research [1]. Classification done by using the visual information is not only the indicator for emotion recognition, gestures, body language, the direction of gaze and voice are some factors that contribute. Therefore, emotion recognition requires detailed knowledge of all the related factors, along with associating information to obtain better accuracy [2]. Parameterizing and recognition are the methods are used for facial emotion recognition, parameterizing methods perform segmentation on the image which assigns a binary label to each pixel to obtain a boundary to the face located in the given image [3], recognition methods are applied on the data after applying parameterizing methods to recognize emotions. Feature selection, classification, extraction and classification are the steps in deep learning and machine learning approaches for recognizing expressions in faces [4]. Image standardization, Face detection and component detection, Decision function are the steps in Geometric Feature-Based Process [4].

1.1 Edge Detection and CNN

Edge detection is one of the image processing method for locating the bounds of objects in images. It really works by means of detecting discontinuities in brightness, it is used in areas such as machine vision, computer vision, and image processing for data extraction and segmentation [5]. Edge detection models are classified into sketch models, edge features, and gradient filters. Segmentation and region identification, object searching and tracking, medical image segmentation are some application areas of edge detection [6]. In recent studies Convolutional neural network (CNN) is a class of deep learning networks has attained much attention, from the raw input high-level features are automatically extracted, and the extracted features are more powerful than the features human-designed [7]. CNN based methods are categorized based on the properties of network used and are classified as Basic CNN's, Scale-aware models, Context-aware models, and Multi-task frameworks [8]. Image recognition and OCR, Object detection for self-driving cars, Face recognition on social media, and Image analysis in healthcare are some real-time application areas where CNN's are used.

2 Related Work

Matsugu et al. [9] designed a CNN based on rule-based algorithm for detecting expressions in faces, resulted in an accuracy of 96.7% while detecting smiles in still images. Mohammed et al. [10] proposed a technique which uses curve let features, the features are reduced dimensionally by using bidirectional weighted modular PCA and these features are given as input to Extreme Learning Machine (ELM) resulted in recognition faster than existing systems and is independent of number of hidden neurons and size of the training data. Rivera et al. [11] proposed a method which encodes directional information of the face's textures (i.e., the texture's shape) in a compact manner, the image is divided into several regions, and the distributed features are mined and concatenated into a feature vector which is used as a face descriptor. Ebrahimi et al. [12] provided a RNN for modeling Spatio-temporal evolution through the aggregation of facial features to carry out emotion recognition in video which outperformed all the sophisticated methods used by challenge winners of 2013.

Yu et al. [13] proposed a method which consists of a face detection module and classification module with the ensemble of more than one convolutional neural networks where each model is separately trained on FER2013 and SFEW 2.0 datasets which resulted in a validation accuracies of 61.29% and 55.96%. Zhang et al.[14] proposed a detector that deals with occlusions and pose variations to estimate the intensities of 18 selected action units neural networks and support vector regression techniques are used and Fuzzy c-means clustering technique is used identify the emotions. Mollahosseini et al. [15] collected facial expression images from the World Wide Web by using three search engines and trained the model in in various scenarios and resulted in an accuracy of 82.12%. Guo et al. [16] released a dataset named iCV-MEFED dataset that contains labels and compound emotions belongs to 50 classes.

Le et al. [17] proposed a Recursive Encoder and Decoder Network that adds the connections that skipped during encoding and decoding stages and used the resulted information in evaluation metrics such as ODS F-measure, OIS F-measure, and Average precision when applied on BSDS500 and NYUD datasets. Liu et al.[18] designed an integrated module that permits to choose features at different levels dynamically depending on the characteristics allocates information for different tasks, Experimentation was done on multiple databases and performed better than some existing methods. Liu et al. [19], proposed a versatile and hearty edge fragment finder where images were characterized into three classes, based on consistency with the gradient, percentage value attached with the reference. Using the predictive curvature method the anchors were joined into non-identical edge segments, each of them is a pixel of a wide chain of 1-pixel, clean, and connective. Resulted in better accuracy.

Zhang et al. [20] proposed a model that learns saliency by labeling data using scribbles. An edge detection task that localizes the edges of the object was proposed to recursively consolidate all scribble annotations which are useful for supervising high-quality saliency maps training that outperformed many of the existing weakly supervised and unsupervised methods. Wang et al. [21] developed a monitoring system that monitors the growth of an apple in its growth period using edge detection deep learning network. Experiments showed that an F1 score of 53.1% on the test set, mean absolute error was found to be 0.90 mm which was reduced by 67.9% compared to the circle fitting based method and resulted in an accurate and effective system to monitor the growth of apples. Lo et al. [22] proposed micro-expression recognition based graph classification network(MER-GCN) extracts features to Action

Units(AU) using 3D Conventional Networks and is applied to Graph Convolutional Network (GCN) layers to identify the dependency between Micro Expression categorization and action unit nodes. Experimentation showed that it outperformed CNN based MER networks.

3 Proposed Model

3.1 About the Model

In the present work we constructed a hybrid edge detection model that selects the features and a CNN model that recognizes facial expressions. Initially, all the images are resized and normalized for consistency in the image features.

The resulted images are applied to hybrid edge detection feature selection model to extract the informative edges. Perwitt, Canny, Sobel, and Laplacian edge detection techniques are used in this model, and the resultant folder which consists of images obtained by applying various edge detection techniques is given as input to the CNN model proposed for training and validation. CNN model used here consists of 3 convolutional, 3 max-pooling, 2 dense, 1 dropout and 1 flatten layers.

3.2 Data Flow of the Model

The data flow of the model proposed is given in the Fig. 1. Initially the image is preprocessed using resize and normalization techniques after this the input is given to convert into the hybrid image set by applying multiple edge detection techniques, then the resulted image set is given to the CNN Architecture that was proposed for training and testing. The training using TrDf (Train Set) is done. After training the architecture the model will classify the images into any of the Happy, Sad, Fear, Disgust, Neutral, Surprise, and Anger based on the input given.

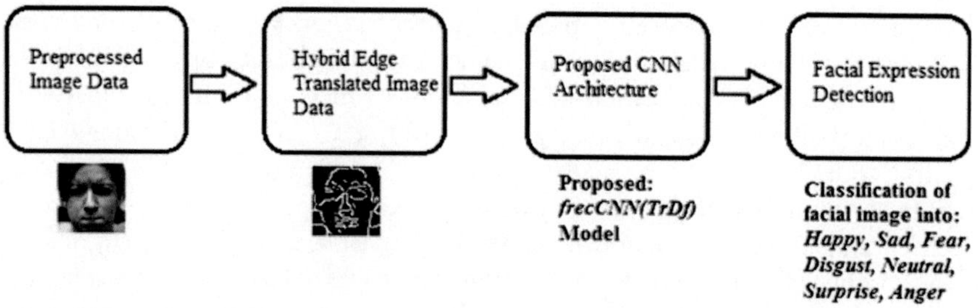

Fig. 1 Data flow of the model

3.3 Proposed Algorithm and Model

3.3.1 Algorithm of the Hybrid Model

```
Input: Fer Image S_i
ImageS_i = {im_1, im_2, ..., im_n} //Set of All The Images
Output: Facial Expression
FacImgRecogAdv(ImageS_i) //Algorithm For Facial Emotion Recognition
Begin
  if len(ImageS_i) = ∅ then //Image set Is empty
    return Exit //Exits from the Block as image set is empty
  else
  Begin
      for i in 1 to n do //Loop to read images
        Begin
          im_i ← resize(im_i, 128, 128) //Image is converted to sizeof 128X128
          im_ni ← (N max − N min) * 1/(1 + e^(−(im_i − β)/α)) + N min //Normalization of image using min−max
          imgset[] ← ⋃ im_ni //All resized and Normalized images are stored in imageset
        end
      end for
  end
  df ← EdgeDetecAlg(imgset[]) //Filters the images by applying edge detection technique
  Ldf ← lab(df) //Assigns Labels to imagesAssigns Labels to images
  (TrDf, TsDf) ← Split(Ldf, m, n − m) //Splits images to Training and Testing sets
  FrecCNN ← FrecCNN(TrDf) //Model for Traing the data
  Evaluation ← FrecCNN(TsDf) //Evaluation of Model by Test set
 end else
end
```

```
Input: Ldf //Dataframe with Labels Assigned
Output: TrDf and TsDf //Seperate Train and Test Dataframes
Split(Ldf, m, n − m) //Algorithm to Split Dataframe to Train and Test Dataframes
   Begin
    for i in 1 to m do //Loop to create Train dataset by selecting random images
      Begin
        TrDfim ← rand(Ldf(img_i)) //Selects random image from Ldf and Assign to Train dataframe
        Ldf ← Ldf ⌈ img_i //removes selected dataframe from input dataframe
        TrDf ← ⋃ TrDfim //Selected images are assigned to Train dataframe
      end
    end for
    for j in m − n to n do //Loop to create Test dataset by selecting random images
      Begin
        TsDfim ← rand(Ldf(img_j)) //Selects random image from Ldf and Assign to Test dataframe
        Ldf ← Ldf ⌈ img_j //removes selected dataframe from input dataframe
        TsDf ← ⋃ TsDfim //Selected images are assigned to Test dataframe
      end
    end for
  end
```

```
Input: imgset[] //Contains resized and normalized images of ImageS_i
Output: Hybrid Filtered images after applying Edge detection techniques
EdgeDetecAlg(imgset[]) //Algorithm for Hybrid Edge images Creation
   Begin
      l ← len(imgset[]) //Total number of input images
      n_1 ← rand(l) //Random number to select the number of images from input set
      for i in 1 to n_1 do //Loop to filter selected images by canny technique
        Begin
          im_ei ← imread(im_ni) //To read image
          Edim_i ← Canny(im_ei) //Filters imags by Canny Edge Detection Technique
          df ← ⋃ Edim_i //Filtered image is assigned to a dataframe
          imgset[] ← imgset[] − im_ni //Filtered image is removed from input set
        end
      end for
      l ← l − n_1 / Number of images left after applying Canny
      n_2 ← rand(l) //Random number to select the number of images from input set
      for i in 1 to n_2 do //Loop to filter images by Sobel technique
       Begin
        im_ei ← imread(im_ni) //To read image
        Edim_i ← Sobel(im_ei) //Filters imags by Sobel Edge Detection Technique
        df ← ⋃ Edim_i //Filtered image is assigned to a dataframe
        imgset[] ← imgset[] − im_ni //Filtered image is removed from input set
       end
     end for
     l ← l − n_2 //Number of images left after applying Canny and Sobel
     n_3 ← rand(l) //Random number to select the number of images from input set
     for i in 1 to n_3 do //Loop to filter images by Perwitt technique
      Begin
        im_ei ← imread(im_ni) //To read image
        Edim_i ← Perwitt(im_ei) //Filters imags by Perwitt Edge Detection Technique
        df ← ⋃ Edim_i //Filtered image is assigned to a dataframe
        imgset[] ← imgset[] − im_ni //Filtered image is removed from input set
      end
    end for
    n_4 ← l − n_3 //Number of images left after applying Canny and Sobel
    for i in 1 to n_4 do //Loop to filter images by Laplacian technique
      Begin
        im_ei ← imread(im_ni) //To read image
        Edim_i ← Laplacian(im_ei) //Filters imags by Laplacian Edge Detection Technique
        df ← ⋃ Edim_i //Filtered image is assigned to a dataframe
        imgset[] ← imgset[] − im_ni //Filtered image is removed from input set
      end
    end for
   return df //returns the resulted Hybrid dataframe of filtered images
end
```

3.3.2 Description of CNN Architecture

```
Model: "sequential_1"
_________________________________________________________________
Layer (type)                 Output Shape              Param #
=================================================================
conv2d_1 (Conv2D)            (None, 48, 48, 6)         456
_________________________________________________________________
max_pooling2d_1 (MaxPooling2 (None, 24, 24, 6)         0
_________________________________________________________________
conv2d_2 (Conv2D)            (None, 24, 24, 16)        2416
_________________________________________________________________
activation_1 (Activation)    (None, 24, 24, 16)        0
_________________________________________________________________
max_pooling2d_2 (MaxPooling2 (None, 12, 12, 16)        0
_________________________________________________________________
conv2d_3 (Conv2D)            (None, 10, 10, 64)        9280
_________________________________________________________________
max_pooling2d_3 (MaxPooling2 (None, 5, 5, 64)          0
_________________________________________________________________
flatten_1 (Flatten)          (None, 1600)              0
_________________________________________________________________
dense_1 (Dense)              (None, 128)               204928
_________________________________________________________________
dropout_1 (Dropout)          (None, 128)               0
_________________________________________________________________
dense_2 (Dense)              (None, 7)                 903
=================================================================
Total params: 217,983
Trainable params: 217,983
Non-trainable params: 0
```

3.4 *FaceImgRecog Advanced*

FaceImgRecogAdv model takes input images from an ImageSt and classifies the images based on their emotions. In the proposed model Happy, Sad, Fear, Disgust, Neutral, Surprise, and Anger are the seven emotions that taken into consideration. If the ImageSt is empty the model exists without performing any operation or else the images are read one after the other and resized into 128 × 128 using resizes function, and then normalized using min-max normalization and the resulted images are given to EdgeDetecAlg as input. The EdgeDetecAlg extracts the features of the images by applying edge detection techniques and the resulted images are placed in a data frame df. The resulted data frame df is returned to the model on which the labels are added using the label encoding technique, and the resulted data frame be named as Ldf, Ldf is then split into two different sets TrDf and TsDf by using the Split function. These sets are used for training and testing the FrecCNN model. FrecCNN model is trained by using TrDf data frame, and then validated using TsDf data frame and finally the model classifies the input image into any of the seven emotions that are being matched.

3.4.1 EdgeDetecAlg

EdgeDetecAlg function takes resized and normalized images as inputs, the features of the images are extracted by using edge detection techniques, and the resulted feature extracted images are given to FaceImgRecogAdv model in the form of a data frame. Canny, Laplacian, Sobel, and Perwitt are the edge detection techniques used here. Out of all the images obtained as input here some of them are selected randomly, on the randomly selected images canny edge filtering is applied, and the resulted images are stored in a data frame df. The images which were selected randomly are removed from the input dataset to avoid duplication. After applying Canny filtering again images are selected randomly and Sobel edge filtering is applied, resulted images are stored in data frame df and input images selected are removed from the image dataset. The same process is followed while applying Laplacian and Perwit edge filtering techniques. Finally, the resultant data frame df is returned to FaceImgRecogAdv.

3.4.2 Split

Split function will split the image data frame into TrDf and TsDf into m, n-m where m is the number of training images to be selected from the labelled data frame Ldf, n is the total number of images in the Ldf. In general the split is done 80:20 ratio, i.e. 80% for training and 20% for testing, m number of images are selected randomly from the labelled data frame df and assigned to a new label TrDf which is used for training the FrecCNN model. Randomly selected images are removed from Ldf to avoid duplication of data and the remaining images left in Ldf are assigned to another label TsDf that is used for validating the FrecCNN model.

4 Experiment and Results

Hybrid feature extraction edge detection methods data frame obtained by applying fer2013 dataset resulted in better accuracy when compared to existing edge detection techniques data frames, It has also been observed that execution time reduced to more than 50% by using edge detection algorithms. Also observed that our model performed well on larger dataset fer2013 when compared to CK48+. The proposed model resulted in a testing accuracy of 86.01% on fer2013 dataset whereas Sobel, Laplacian, Perwitt, Canny and original data frame (Data frame without applying edge detection techniques) resulted in accuracies of 83.48, 84.30, 84.74, 83.57, and 84.19% respectively and also observed that our model test accuracy becomes consistent after few epochs and other techniques test accuracy is reduced as the number of epochs increases. Experimentation is done for 50 epochs with a batch size of 64 and observed that the proposed method took 5 s for each epoch, whereas, the average time taken on the original data set is 11 s. The same Experimentation is done by using CK48+ dataset and resulted in accuracy of 91.92% which outperformed Sobel and Laplacian, and avg time taken for each epoch is 1 s for all.

Table 1 Data set details

Data set	Name and No. of images in each emotion							Total images
	Happy	Sad	Angry	Disgust	Sad	Surprise	Neutral	
CK48+	621	336	540	531	336	996	216	3540
Fer2013	8989	6077	4954	547	6077	4033	6197	35,887

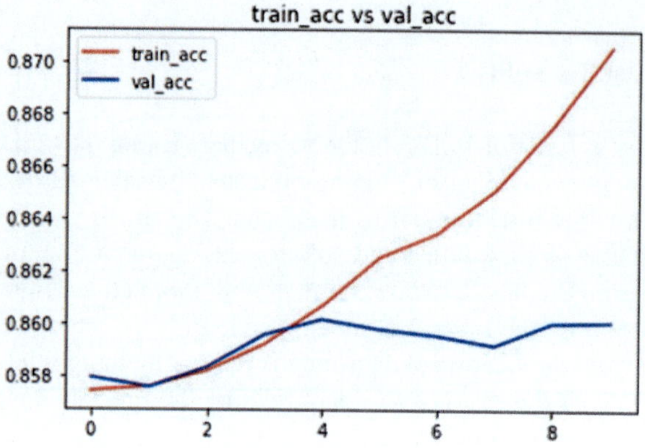

Fig. 2 Hybrid feature selection on Fer2013

4.1 Dataset and Execution

Fer2013 and CK48+ are the datasets used in this model for experimentation. Fer2013 consists of 35887 images of seven different emotions (Happy, Anger, Sad, Disgust, Neutral, Surprise and Fear) with image dimension's 128 × 128 × 3. And CK48+ dataset consists of 3540 images with same dimensions and emotion categories of fer2013. Execution of the model is done on the Google cloud platform called as goggle research colabs Which Provides 12 GB NVIDIA Tesla K80 GPU, CPU: 1xsingle core hyper threaded Xeon Processors @2.3Ghz i.e. (1 core, 2 threads) and a disk space of 68.40 GB (Table 1).

4.2 Graphical Representation of Results

See Figs. 2, 3, 4, 5, 6, 7.

4.3 Comparison Table

See Tables 2, 3 and Figs. 8, 9.

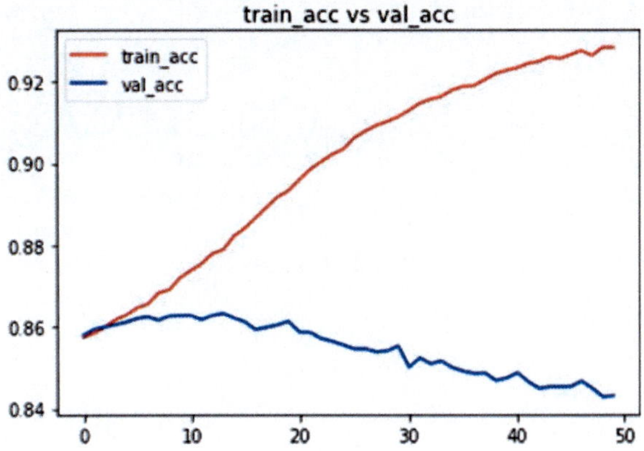

Fig. 3 Laplacian on Fer2013

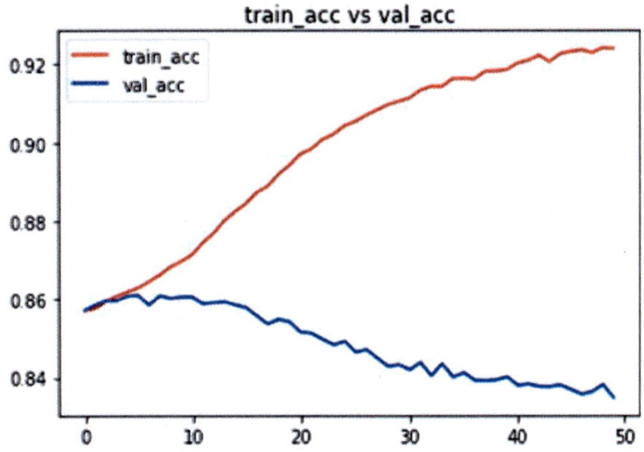

Fig. 4 Sobel Fer2013

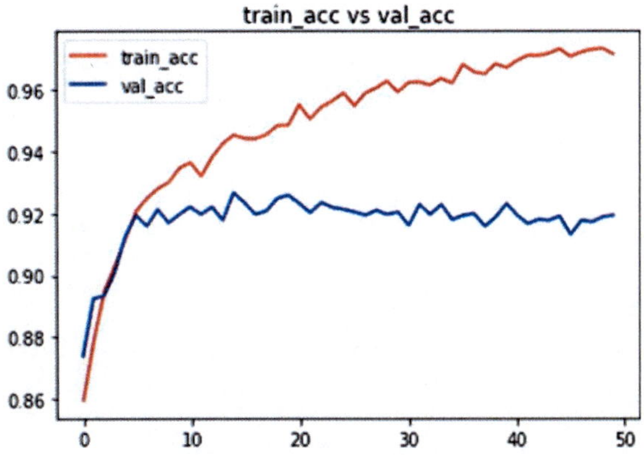

Fig. 5 Hybrid feature selection on CK48+

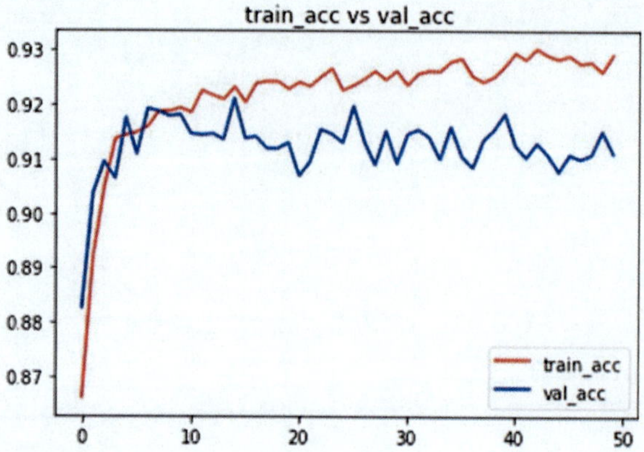

Fig. 6 Laplacian on CK48+

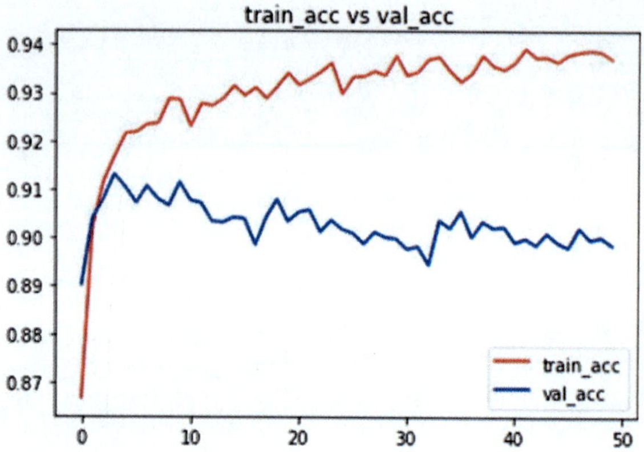

Fig. 7 Sobel CK48+

Table 2 Comparison table on fer2013 and CK48+ datasets

Tech Used	Train Acc	Test Acc	Train loss	Test loss	Epoch time (s)
Hyb Fet Sel Meth	0.8784	0.860	0.288	0.353	5
Sobel	0.967	0.834	0.0911	0.588	4
Laplacian	0.965	0.843	0.0916	0.536	2
Canny	0.961	0.835	0.103	0.562	4
Perwitt	0.966	0.847	0.0952	0.535	3
Org dataset	0.963	0.841	0.099	0.54	11

5 Conclusion and Future Work

In the proposed model here we designed an hybrid feature selection model which constructs a data frame of images by applying Canny, Sobel, Perwitt and Laplacian edge detection techniques on the images randomly and the resulted image data

Table 3 Comparison table on fer2013 and CK48+ datasets

Tech used	Train Acc	Test Acc	Train loss	Test loss	Epoch time (s)
Hyb Fet Sel Meth	0.991	0.919	0.026	0.418	2
Sobel	0.941	0.892	0.0803	0.138	1
Laplacian	0.952	0.907	0.094	0.180	1
Canny	0.948	0.928	0.096	0.260	1
Perwitt	0.942	0.921	0.110	0.152	1
Org dataset	0.934	0.912	0.137	0.191	2

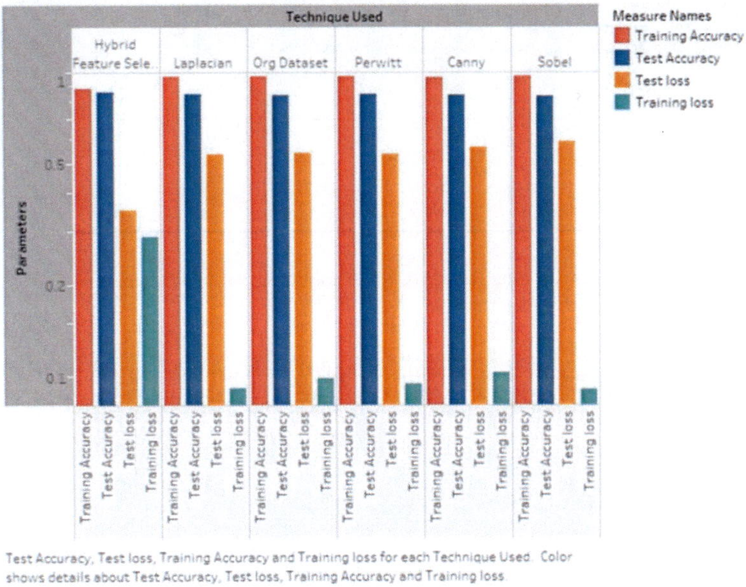

Fig. 8 Graphical representation of Table 2 (Fer 2013 dataset on various parameters

frame is given as an input the CNN Model (FrecCNN Model). Fer2013 and CK48+ datasets are taken as inputs. The datasets are converted into data frames by applying edge detection techniques along with our hybrid feature selection technique and are given for FrecCNN Model for training and validation. It is observed that our model resulted in efficient test accuracy when compared to others on Fer2013. And also our model outperformed Sobel and Laplacian techniques. Our model resulted in 86% Test and 87.8% Training accuracy on Fer2013 Dataset and 91.9% Test Accuracy and 99.1% Training Accuracy on CK48+ dataset. The proposed model performed more efficiently on larger image dataset fer2013 which contains more than 37,500 images. A better hybrid model which can improve the training and testing accuracy

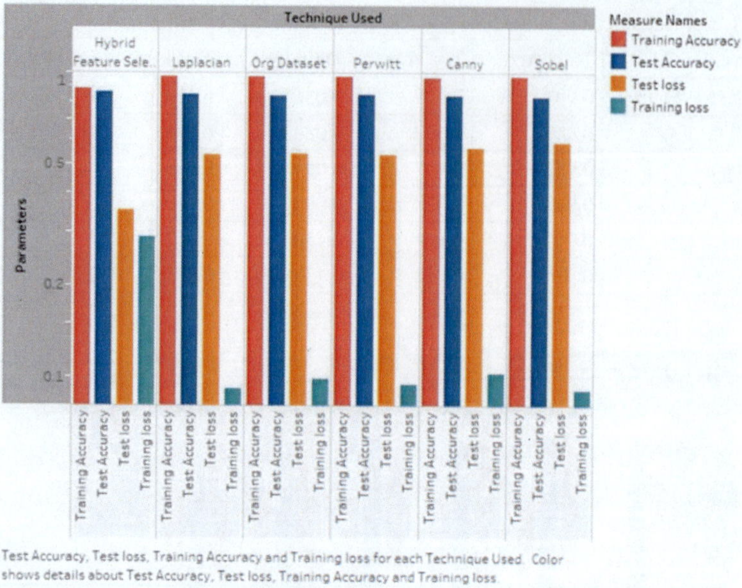

Fig. 9 Graphical representation of Table 3 (CK48+ dataset on various parameters)

and other performance measures applied on any dataset, increasing the test accuracy by compromising model over fitting on training dataset are the scope for future extension of this work.

References

1. Mehta D, Siddiqui MFH, Javaid AY (2018) Facial emotion recognition: a survey and real-world user experiences in mixed reality. Sensors 18(2):416
2. Ekman P (1977) Facial action coding system
3. Zhang C, Zhang Z (2010) A survey of recent advances in face detection, TechReport, No. MSR-T201066, Microsoft Corporation, Albuquerque, NM, USA
4. Kumari J, Rajesh R, Pooja K (2015) Facial expression recognition: a survey. Procedia Comput Sci 58:486–491
5. Muthukrishnan R, Miyilsamy R (2011) Edge detection techniques for image segmentation. Int J Comput Sci Info Technol 3(6):259
6. James Alex Pappachen (2016) Edge detection for pattern recognition: a survey. Int J Appl Pattern Recogn 3(1):1–21
7. He K, Xiangyu Z, Shaoqing R, Jian S (2016) Deep residual learning for image recognition. In: Proceedings of the IEEE conference on computer vision and pattern recognition, pp 770–778
8. Sindagi Vishwanath A, Patel Vishal M (2018) A survey of recent advances in cnn-based single image crowd counting and density estimation. Pattern Recogn Lett 107:3–16
9. Masakazu M, Katsuhiko M, Yusuke M, Yuji K (2003) Subject independent facial expression recognition with robust face detection using a convolutional neural network. Neural Netw 16(5–6):555–559

10. Mohammed AA, Rashid M, Wu QMJ, Sid-Ahmed MA (2011) Human face recognition based on multidimensional PCA and extreme learning machine. Pattern Recogn 44(10–11):2588-2597
11. Rivera AR, Jorge RC, Chae OO (2012) Local directional number pattern for face analysis: face and expression recognition. IEEE Trans Image Process 22(5): 1740–1752
12. Ebrahimi Kahou S, Michalski V, Konda K, Memisevic R, Pal C (2015) Recurrent neural networks for emotion recognition in video. In: Proceedings of the 2015 ACM on international conference on multimodal interaction, pp 467–474
13. Yu Z, Zhang C (2015) Image based static facial expression recognition with multiple deep network learning. In: Proceedings of the 2015 ACM on international conference on multimodal interaction, pp 435–442
14. Zhang L, Mistry K, Jiang M, Neoh SC, Hossain MA (2015) Adaptive facial point detection and emotion recognition for a humanoid robot. Comput Vis Image Underst 140:93–114
15. Mollahosseini A, Hassani B, Salvador MJ, Abdollahi H, Chan D, Mahoor MH (2016) Facial expression recognition from world wild web. In: 2016 IEEE Conference on computer vision and pattern recognition workshops (CVPRW) (June 2016) https://doi.org/10.1109/cvprw.2016.188
16. Guo J, Lei Z, Wan J, Avots E, Hajarolasvadi N, Knyazev B, Anbarjafari G (2018) Dominant and complementary emotion recognition from still images of faces. IEEE Access 6:26391–26403. https://doi.org/10.1109/access.2018.2831927
17. Le Truc, Duan Ye (2020) REDN: a recursive encoder-decoder network for edge detection. IEEE Access 8:90153–90164. https://doi.org/10.1109/access.2020.2994160
18. Liu J-J, Hou Q, Cheng M-M (2020) Dynamic feature integration for simultaneous detection of salient object, edge and skeleton. arXiv preprint arXiv:2004.08595(2020)
19. Liu Y, Xie Z, Liu H (2020) An adaptive and robust edge detection method based on edge proportion statistics. IEEE Trans Image Process 29:5206–5215. https://doi.org/10.1109/tip.2020.2980170
20. Zhang J, Yu X, Li A, Song P, Liu B, Dai Y (2020) Weakly-supervised salient object detection via scribble annotations. In: Proceedings of the IEEE/CVF conference on computer vision and pattern recognition, pp 12546–12555
21. Dandan W, Li C, Song H, Xiong H, Liu C, He D (2020) Deep learning approach for apple edge detection to remotely monitor apple growth in orchards. IEEE Access 8:26911–26925. https://doi.org/10.1109/access.2020.2971524
22. Lo L Xie H-X, Shuai H-H, Cheng W-H (2020) In: MER-GCN: micro expression recognition based on relation modeling with graph convolutional network. arXiv preprint arXiv:2004.08915(2020)

A Fuzzy Approach for Handling Relationship Between Security and Usability Requirements

V. Prema Latha, Nikhat Parveen, and Y. Prasanth

Abstract Security is an essential part of the improvement for value programming, so as Usability is natural and significant factor for creating quality system. The discrepancy among Usability and protection be generally perceived examine issue in diligence as well as for scholarly community. Disappointment to plan frameworks, which are at the same time usable as well as secure, may perhaps cause incident anywhere individual mistakes show the way towards safety breaks. Scholarly study distinguishes to facilitate usability vs. safety struggle can be real best handle by requirement along with design phase of the framework improvement. The principle target of the security is to give restricted access to the security concentrated data though the goal of usability is to give simple access of the verified application. Usable security can be more interesting because of the expanding use of PCs with upgraded usability and protection criteria in it. While recovering the usability through security of system, fundamental securities as well as usability qualities assume a significant work. Thus, usable security assessment utilizes security and usability credits towards accomplish ideal security actions through usability. In this paper a Fuzzy approach system is assess to identify the needs and overall usable—secure and the effect of safety on the Usability and vice versa assessed by quantitatively. The outcomes got with ends helpful for professionals to get better usable–secure of the system.

Keywords Safety · Usability · Fuzzy · Secure system and usable system

1 Introduction

With rapid increase during Internet usage, cybercrimes have become more and more popular. In addition, protection measures are used to protect against misuse users and device resources. Such frameworks decide the set of the rules to define the abuse among the stop users and device resources from having any adverse effects. Some studies had been cited to develop the security services of software to recognize

V. Prema Latha (✉) · N. Parveen · Y. Prasanth
Department of C.S.E, Koneru Lakshmaiah Education Foundation, Vaddeswaram, 522502 Guntur, AP, India
e-mail: premawilliams@gmail.com

S. Bhattacharyya et al. (eds.), *International Conference on Intelligent and Smart Computing in Data Analytics*, Advances in Intelligent Systems and Computing 1312,
https://doi.org/10.1007/978-981-33-6176-8_11

and identify ways to estimate security. Occasionally, however, a person who uses the program can turn into weakest link himself, and inadvertently attract attacks. Avoidance of non-authorization [1] is the main objective of the protection at the same time as usability focus on easiness of 'holding easy' formula for users. Organizations should therefore concentrate on safeguarding security with usability together.

According to the researcher [2] the inherent conflict exists among usability along with protection. Here, an e.g. featuring the authentication password to highly structured the tension among usability and protection. The secure aspect indicates passwords are long enough, must be changed normally, must contain case adjust with the special characters etc. Nevertheless, these passwords are hard to memorize from user's aim of vision. When we enforce the safety strategy, they include an unfavorable effect on system usability and if we don't introduce them, we risk doing so compromise system security. The area that considers human aspects relating to safety [3] and usability combination with protection is recognized as usable–secure. It should be remembered to facilitate all [4] modern information system implements password-based verification today. Sometimes password specifications be multipart, which leads in the direction of cases anywhere user use strategies such as pre-texting or reprocess of the similar password on different location to make sure reputation.

Usability be defined [2] as point to a result may be use by particular user to get individual objectives by quality, adequacy as well as fulfillment in predetermined setting of utilization. As this meaning focus mostly on client goal, speed essential to reach goal along with user approval; [5] additional definition given by the researcher focal point on further usability mechanism such the same as understanding, reputation, error. Security concepts [6] generally turn around attackers as valid users mainly of point in time concession system. This was generally due to the question so as to innovator usually view usability and safety as attach type towards a completed product and the variance of importance among device holder along with its user [7].

Secure software systems usability assessments model [2] involve procedures which deviate from standard Human Computer Interaction techniques [8]. Whitten discusses the distinctions among security software and some other applications, along with why secure software usable assessment is difficult to assess. In addition to addressing aspects of educational software (such as learning skills), safe-ware, and common end user software discusses properties to compose safety hard. These contain the less important intent things, concealed fault things, reflection things and the most vulnerable connection things. The usability assessment [2] of safe software's should not concentrate on usability to keeping out of protection: in some situations, it has important to include complex behavior, for security purposes. In comparison, it is achievable towards decline the safety of method through simplifies or automating assured essentials which classically get better usability.

There is lots of work accessible in study field; it is not included in literature to determine the characteristics of protection along with usability through applicability to actual world efforts. Furthermore, the client is the one approving the security setting. Utilizable and reliable [9] infrastructure is therefore the necessitate of creation of today. The safety along with usability characteristics together participate a significant role in maintaining software safety. According to the researcher Usability [2] along with safety attributes like CIA i.e. Confidentiality [10], Integrity, Availability and EEU i.e. Effectiveness [6], Efficiency, User satisfaction can affect usability and security [6] of software services. The role of these attributes in ensuring protection is special, but significant. Therefore, evaluation has not been achieved through ignoring attributes of usability or else protection. Reflection of together protection and usability attributes can result in other efficient and accurate evaluation [11]. Therefore, evaluation of the functional protection was a question of decision building, since each company adopts its individual policy along with method. The evaluation helps decision buildings understand the expectations as maintaining usable–secure.

In this paper Fuzzy assessment approach [9] the evaluation, a hierarchy is required to identify the artificial attribute by usability protection. Thereafter, a hierarchy of usable–secure attributes is specified after that section to discuss and analyze the usable–secure of the program [12]. Using the Fuzzy Inference System [9] procedure, Computer Usability-Security was assessed. The results obtained through the consideration can help safety designers improve usable–secure through software improvement.

2 Relationship Between Usability and Security

The result for Usability and security are therefore attributes that can trade off against each other. For instance, expecting clients to change their passwords occasionally may improve security yet puts a more important influence on clients [2, 6, 13]. throughout safety architecture, compromise among usability. In addition, theoretic protection is usually not acknowledged like a basic standard. Some authors argue that while usability is within center of attention during software growth, security is not compromise. CIA's evaluation and maintenance during software development proves in the direction of on its own greatest traditions to get safe apps. Hence, this is why every person needs towards put together a high-secure design as well as the safety design makes the applications less usable due to the composite processes involved. This problem triggers worries for end users [14].

Usable–secure seems to exist the ideal result to all problems of usability and security that were there [5] Usable–secure and its evaluation concentrate on top of the compensations and disadvantages of together approaches, as well as a result is build by means of a suitable method to make sure usability by means of protection. Therefore, security [6] has three big usability factors that have an indirect impact. The three factors are: effectiveness [15], performance, satisfaction and the security of user errors. Therefore, CIAAN is the defense foundation. Confidentiality [10] refers to authorizing permitted way into responsive as well as secure information in the sense of protection. Integrity is an attractive quality that the right assertion and declaration establishes. In situation of a PC, availability refers to a user's facility towards way in sequence or else assets for a particular period. Usable–secure possibly improved by focus on CIA with EEU together. The relation between usability and security requirements by using security attributes like confidentiality [10], integrity, availability and usability [2] attributes like effectiveness [15], efficiency, and user satisfaction.

2.1 Usability

Effectiveness—According to the researcher [15] a program is only effective if its users are in a position to accomplish expected objectives. It is possible that an unsuccessful program is neglected. The Effectiveness was calculated in the way of whether or not the user can complete a specific task. For most research, this method is acceptable; anywhere a method consists of a only one stage to facilitate can be completed throughout a distinct pathway. Composite and multi-stage projects, however, can involve a additional definition of completion or collapse that might contain rates like partial collapse/ performance.

- Efficiency—As clients may utilize a framework to accomplish a explicit objective, accomplishment in itself isn't adequate. The objective must be accomplished inside an adequate measure of time and exertion. What is the worthy measure of time or on the other hand exertion in one framework or setting may not be in another [16]. To this respect, a framework is appraised as productive corresponding to other comparable frameworks or built up benchmarks. Productivity is caught by estimating an opportunity to finish a task or the quantity of snaps/catches squeezed to accomplish required objectives.
- User Satisfaction—while target investigation of convenience examination of frameworks is normal, clients' abstract evaluation is pivotal to a framework's achievement. For instance, a framework might be usable (by ease of use guidelines) however clients may mark it unhygienic. As it were, a framework will undoubtedly flop in any event, when it is usable on the off chance that it isn't satisfactory to clients. Client fulfillment can be surveyed through meetings and rating scales.

2.2 Security

- Confidentiality—According to several researchers [10] Confidentiality is referred to as privacy and defense of access by unauthorized persons to information. This restricts access as a security policy that guarantees that until permission is granted no one can access the data or information. Confidentiality acts as a privacy that restricts access to personal information that requires a trusted, binding requirement mechanism. And its comprehensiveness, comprehensibility and allied elements. Security requests that secret data ought not to be revealed freely.
- Availability—Setting target for accessibility is a complex process. The details must be accessible whenever it is necessary for any software system to provide its services. These actions demonstrate accuracy and efficiency in the processing of

information. This solid data must be ensured by giving least benefit benefits so as to maintain a strategic distance from uncertainty with the goal that the accessible data can be verified. This is the fact that the security is reluctantly decreasing when information is available at the highest priority. However, service securities need adequate protection in the form of physical security that acts as fundamental precautionary security, and it is essential for the system to meet the availability requirements of the user.

- Integrity—According to the researcher Integrity process protect data from unapproved modification and give affirmation within the precision as well as completion of an information and towards secure data incorporates the two in sequence i.e., put away going on frameworks as well as information to facilitate transmit among frameworks, for e.g., electronic post. In looking after honesty, it isn't immediately significant towards be in charge of right to use next to the support level, however to additionally assurance to structure consumers be presently ready to modify data to facilitate they are really approved towards change.

3 Fuzzy Approach to Develop Usable-Secure System

According to LotfiZadeh, a university lecturer at UC Berkeley in California, first used the name fuzzy logic in the midst of 1965. He noticed that traditional machine logic could not manipulate data that reflected individual or undefined human being facts. Unclear logic was extended to different field, from the direct hypothesis to AI. Numerous researchers have done usability and safety related research work [13]. MCDA plays a significant position in the success of different competing assessment objects, together with multi attribute usefulness hypothesis and analytical chain of command method as well as blurred analytical chain of command process. Therefore, all decision analysis methods are characterized by the identification of targets and alternative weights. A method of evaluation for usable–secure on behalf of completion and simplicity of use was proposed with the aid of the MCDA system, since usable–secure evaluation be a multicriteria crisis. The current input aims at evaluating the usable–secure by the aid of Fuzzy towards break down of a multi criteria problem [9]. Usable-safety is typically a qualitative indicator. It is a dispute to quantitatively evaluate the usable–secure [17]. Furthermore, usable–secure attributes play an important role for software secure usability (Fig. 1).

Here, FIS (The Fuzzy Inference System) is used for handling relation between security and usability requirements by Mamdani FIS. FI Unit be the most important part of a fuzzy logic unit with management while its main function. This use "IF...... THEN" set of laws beside among "OR"//"AND" connectors to represent basic rules used for decisions. A fuzzification machine [9] allows various fuzzification methods to be implemented and transforms crisp data into fuzzy information. After translating crisp input into fuzzy input, understanding base gathering of the set of laws base and record is created. The fuzzy contribution Defuzzification unit is gradually converted to crisp output.

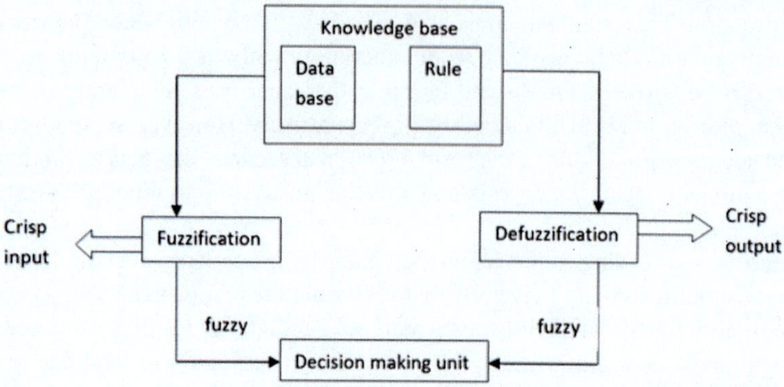

Fig. 1 FIS

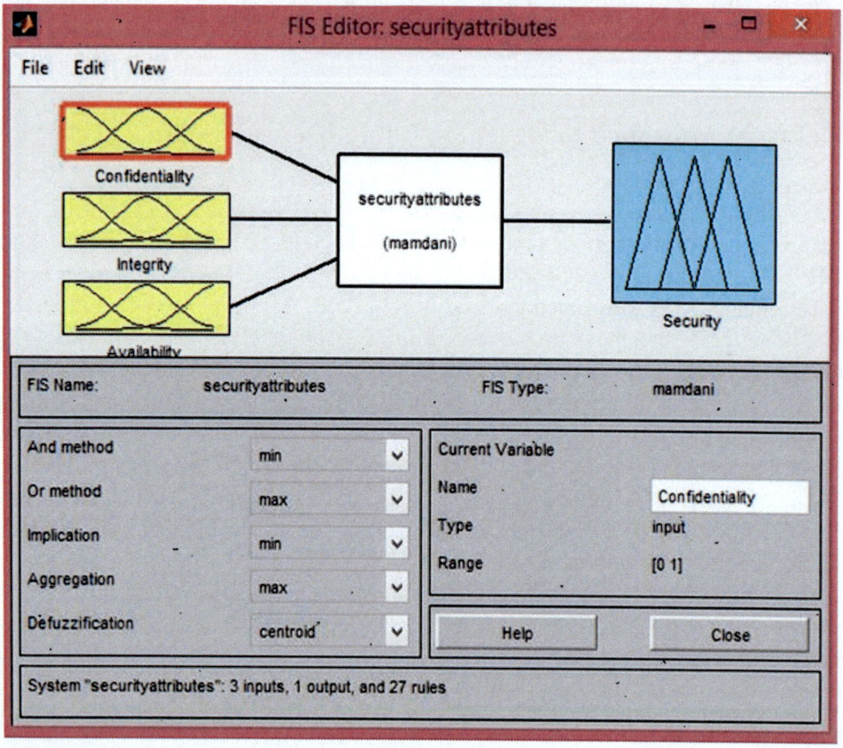

Fig. 2 Security attributes FIS with 3 inputs and 1 outputs

4 Implementation and Results

Figure 2 gives the snap of MATLAB window while using FIS editor in support of 3 inputs and 1 output, of FIS-1(Securityattributes_fis). Here we contain 3 input variables as: Confidentiality, Integrity, Availability and 1 output variables as: Security. The next step is to set membership function for every variable input and output. There are various membership features but we used the Triangular membership feature and Trapezoidal membership feature as they are better suited for this method.

After establishing the membership functions the next step is to create the rules. Figure 3 is the Rule-editor in the fuzzy system Securityattributes_Fis

Figure 4 is the Rule-editor in the fuzzy system Usabilityattributes_Fis. These rules can also be customized through interface of Rule-Editor. The program includes a total of 27 rules. Total number of rules = $3^3 = 27$ Rules.

Figure 5 is the Rule-editor in the fuzzy system SU_Fis. These rules can also be customized through interface of Rule-Editor. The program includes a total of 9 rules. Total number of rules = $3^2 = 9$ Rules (Fig. 6).

Once the rules are generated, they are used through the fuzzy inference engine to compute the respective output. Based on the rules triggered in the database the

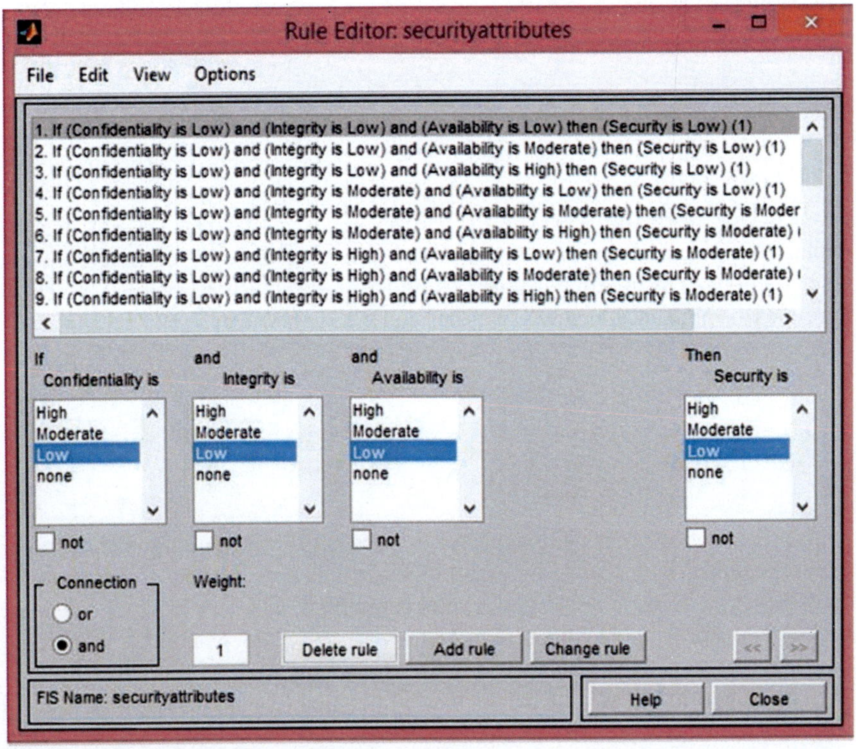

Fig. 3 Rule–Editor window for securityattributes_FIS

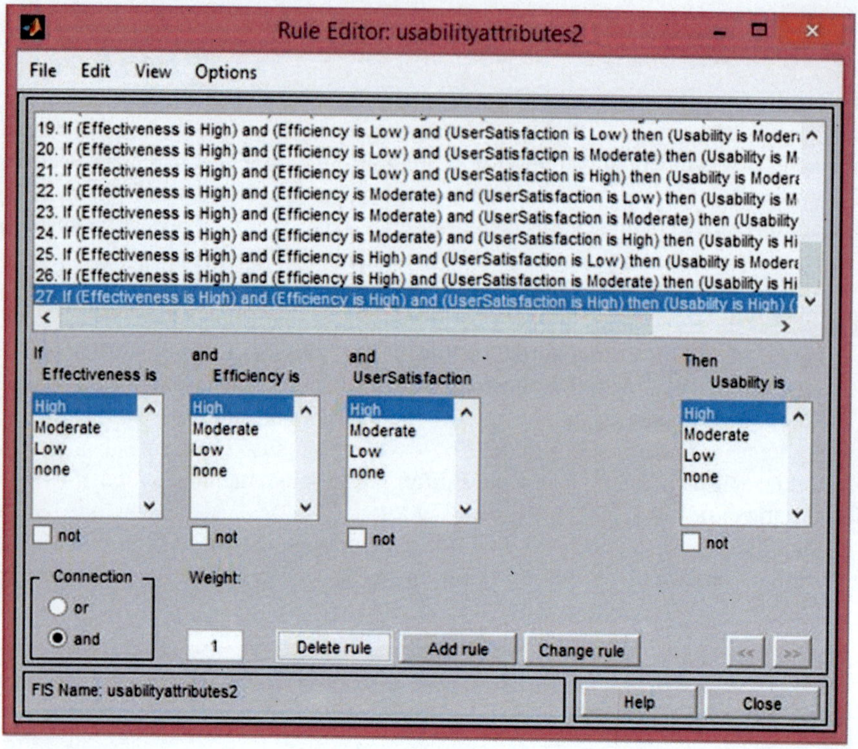

Fig. 4 Rule–Editor window for usabilityattributes_FIS

output is calculated and is shown to the user as the defuzzified value. Once the output is evaluated, the surface viewer can be generated. Secuable of surface viewer which is obtained by the combination of security and usability attributes. The yellow represents the high, the blue represents low and the sea green represents the moderate values.

5 Conclusion

In this present system of paper is expected to assess attributes of usability and protection are established, and software usability-security is examined. Usability-security assessment Is a decision issue with several parameters, and This is why Fuzzy was used in this paper approach to determine the usable–secure. Using the fuzzy logic move towards to calculate conquests between usability and security attributes has two advantages: first, since the data is inaccurate, the FI is competent of measuring these data kind to decide the correct ideals. Second, by decoupling variables, fuzzy inference be capable of grip system dependency between changeable. The most

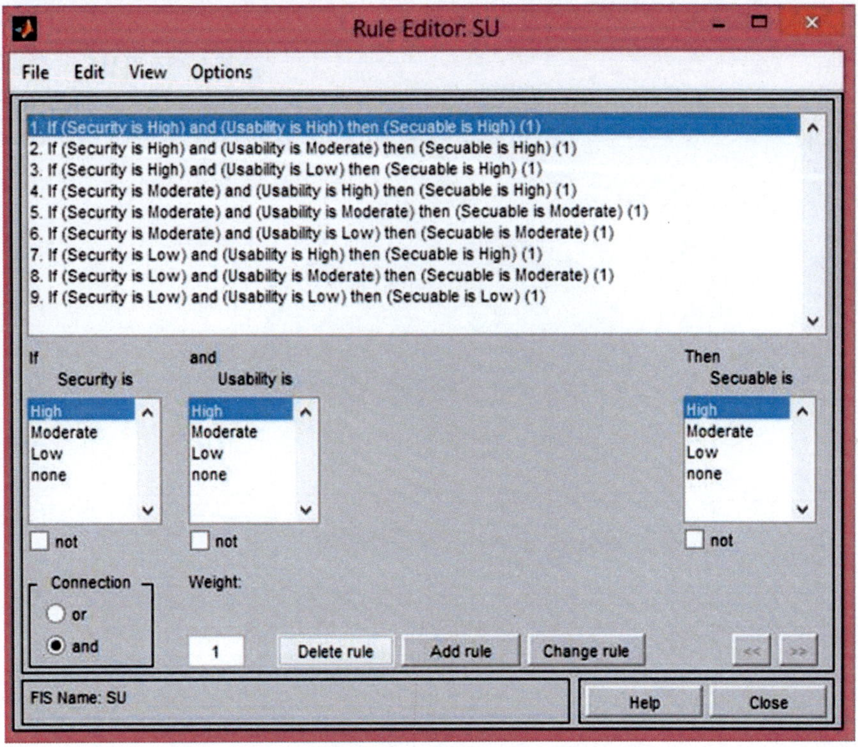

Fig. 5 Rule–Editor window for usabilityattributes_FIS

important weight attributes were evaluated. To ensure usable-secure, The developers want to concentrate initially on the protection of client errors, and secondly on the productivity to ensure usability-security and web services.

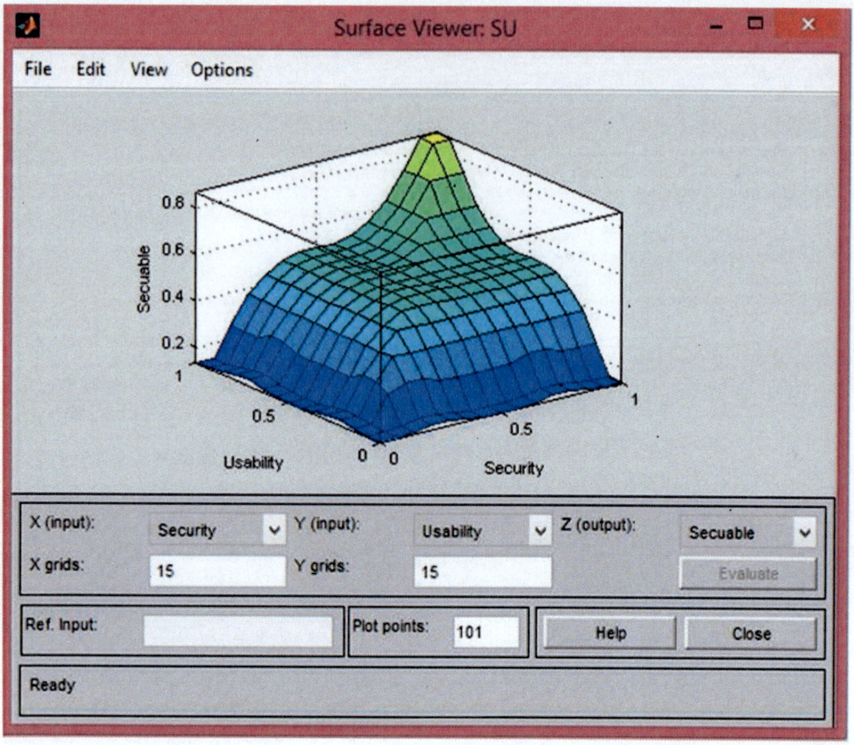

Fig. 6 Surface viewer of SU_FIS

References

1. Kainda R et al (2010) Security and usability: analysis and evaluation. In: International conference on availability, IEEE
2. Saxena S, Agarwal D (2017) A systematic literature review and implementation of software usability estimation model for measuring the effectiveness (IJETAE) 7(7)
3. Wijayarathna C et al (2018) A methodology to evaluate the usability of security APIs. IEEE, ICIAfS, pp 1–6
4. Merdanoğl N et al (2018) In: A systematic mapping study of usability versus security, IEEE, pp 1–6
5. Javed Y et al (2011) In: Captchæcker: reconfigurable CAPTCHAs based on automated security and usability analysis, IEEE
6. Saxena S, Agarwal D (2018) Model to quantify security for adoption of effective e-procurement process. J Emerg Technol Innov Res (JETIR) 5(5):792 –796
7. Alsuhibany SA et al (2018) A proposed approach for handling the tradeoff between security, usability, and cost. ICCIS, IEEE, pp 1–6
8. Parveen N, Roy et al (2020) Human computer interaction through hand gesture recognition technology. Int J Sci Technol Res 9(4):505–513 ISSN: 2277-8616
9. Saxena S, Agarwal D (2019) Towards a fuzzy logic rule based prediction for effective adoption of e-procurement system on cloud environment (IJEAT). 8(5) ISSN: 2249–8958
10. Surabhi S, Devendra A (2018) Confidentiality assessment model to estimate security during effective E-procurement process. Int J Comput Sci Eng 6(1):361–365

11. Nikhat P et al (2014) In: Integrating security and usability at requirement specification process, IJCTT
12. Riaz M et al (2016) In: Systematically developing prevention, detection and response patterns for security requirements, IEEE
13. Kumar SA, Vidyullatha P (2019) A comparative analysis of parallel and distributed FSM approaches on large-scale graph data. Int J Recent Technol Eng Open Access 7(6):103–109
14. Pellakuri V, Rao DR (2016) Training and development of artificial neural network models: single layer feed forward and multilayer feed forward neural network. J Theor Appl Inf Technol Open Access 84(2):150–156
15. Surabhi S, Devendra A (2019) A model to quantify effectiveness assessment model through security and correctness assessment for adoption of the e-procurement (February 24, 2019). In: Proceedings of international conference on sustainable computing in science, technology and management (SUSCOM), Amity University Rajasthan, Jaipur, India, February 26–28. Available at SSRN https://ssrn.com/abstract=3358745 or https://doi.org/10.2139/ssrn.3358745
16. Jammalamadaka K, Parveen N (2019) Holistic research of software testing and challenges . Int J Innov Technol Exploring Eng (IJITEE) 8(6S4):1506–152.1 ISSN: 2278-3075
17. Parveen N et al (2015) Model to quantify confidentiality at requirement phase. In: ACM International conference on advanced research in computer science engineering and technology (ACM ICARCSET)
18. Wang Y et al (2017) Usability and security go together: a case study on database. In: ICRTCCM, IEEE, pp 49–54
19. Vidyullatha P, Rajeswara Rao D (2016) Knowledge based information mining on unemployed graduates data using statistical approaches. Int J Pharm Technol 8(4):21961–21966

Naive Bayes Approach for Retrieval of Video Object Using Trajectories

C. A. Ghuge, V. Chandra Prakash, and S. D. Ruikar

Abstract The popularity of video recordings either on mobile devices or video surveillance has contributed to the demand for video data applications. As a result, the management of video has become significant in the object retrieval process. Video object retrieval is seen as a major issue in the management of video objects. Object tracking is therefore a significant step in detecting and tracking video objects. Hence, object tracking is a major step, which detects and tracks the video objects using a hybrid model named Nearest Search Algorithm–Nonlinear Autoregressive Exogenous Neural Network. The tracked events are further employed for training, and the recognized events interrelated to the query is processed by proposed Naïve Bayes classifier for retrieving the highly relevant object trajectories and the events associated with it. The performance of the proposed Naïve Bayes classifier is greater when compared with other existing techniques with maximal precision of 81.985%, recall of 85.451%, and F-measure of 86.847%, respectively.

Keywords Video surveillance · Naive bayes classifier · Video retrieval · Neural network

1 Introduction

The rapidly increasing technological developments in the field of video capture have increased the accessibility of an enormous mass of videos thereby attracting the

C. A. Ghuge (✉) · V. Chandra Prakash
Department of Computer Science and Engineering, Koneru Lakshmaiah Education Foundation, Vaddeswaram, Guntur, AP, India
e-mail: caghugeklu@gmail.com

V. Chandra Prakash
e-mail: vchandrap@kluniversity.in

S. D. Ruikar
Department of Electronics Engineering, Walchand College of Engineering, Sangli, Maharashtra, India
e-mail: ruikarsachin@gmail.com

S. Bhattacharyya et al. (eds.), *International Conference on Intelligent and Smart Computing in Data Analytics*, Advances in Intelligent Systems and Computing 1312,
https://doi.org/10.1007/978-981-33-6176-8_12

researchers by its wide application like video archives, entertainment and news broadcasting [1]. Video object retrieval is a significant area of research in image processing [2, 3]. Due to the complex training method and the dynamic model appearance and position of objects in each frame, weakly supervised object detection is considered a major challenge. The conventional approaches to tackling issues are to consider the location of objects, which are of great interest to static images [4]. In video object retrieval, most of the existing techniques cannot detect using crowded videos due to occlusions [5]. A huge amount of video cameras are installed entirely over the place for security. Due to this, there is an imperative need for developing techniques using videos, which can substitute the human operators for monitoring the area under observation. Recognizing and tracking systems, different multi-object tracking techniques are examined for tracking the objects. The tracking issues are modelled as a dynamic system that is represented using the states of the discrete domain [6, 7]. Object tracking is the method of determining the location of moving objects and other relevant details in image sequence [8]. However, the improper matching of the trajectories corresponds to an appropriate matching scheme, resulting in an error.

The purpose is to propose a method of tracking and retrieving video objects from the videos. The proposed technique is devised in two stages, namely tracking and retrieving objects. The main contribution is given below:

Proposed Naïve Bayes classifier for video object retrieval: The major contribution is Naïve Bayes classifier for retrieving the relevant objects from video. The Naïve Bayes classifier is to retrieve the related objects given by the user query.

In paper, introduction section relevant to video retrieval is given in Sect. 1. Section 2 elaborates on various video-retrieval techniques. Section 3 deliberates the proposed technique for training the NB classifier. Section 4 determines the outcomes of the methods for the video object retrieval, and finally, Sect. 5 provides the summary.

2 Motivations

This section discusses latest approaches, their benefits and drawbacks and addresses the paper's research gaps.

2.1 Literature Review

Lai [1] suggested a method of trajectory and its appearance. However, the outcomes stand reasonable, some learning approaches might be improve the accuracy. Sihao Ding et al. [9] suggested a SurfvSurf video-retrieval system that experiments on huge amount of video surveillance data and considerably minimize data volume. Lin et al. [10] the method was seen as a weakly supervised approach, requiring important and irrelevant frames of the input videos to obtain suitable results for retrieval. Nguyen et al. [11] developed a fusion used for boosting the accuracy of instance for search systems. Initially, the object detectors were utilized based on a denser feature to determine the similarity score and object bounding box. Query scheme was devised based on three weighting functions for evaluating the final similarity score-based object detector and bag-of-visual-words; the method was flexible. Durand et al. [12], developed a method for video retrieval based on video segmentation, which helped to shorten the time taken for retrieval. The long videos were detected using a spatio-temporal interest points (STIPs) detection algorithm. For selecting the key frames, the region of interest (ROI) was created based on STIP, and the saliency detection of the ROI was used for screening out the video key frames. Then, the captions of the videos were generated by adding the vectors to the conventional LSTM's. Garcia et al. [13] developed a feature fusion method using multimodal graph learning for retrieving the 3D objects. However, the method failed to use different types of features and distance functions for generating geo-location-based applications.

2.2 *Research Gaps*

The challenges faced by conventional video object retrieval methodologies are described below:

- The main challenge is that most of the existing video-retrieval approaches face is the effectiveness and accuracy of the videos from the databases [14].
- While dealing continuously monitoring systems, there are many factors such as distance, dissimilarity, and obstruction. Furthermore, the retrieval of highly specific structures object and the trajectory of the object's path is a major concern [15, 16].

3 Proposed Method

Need for video object retrieval is to track the video objects from the frames. The main drawback associated with detecting the objects are the video cameras and occlusions. The proposed model uses the training phase for learning the indexed database and testing phase for retrieving the relevant objects based on a user query. In the training phase, the key frames in the video are chosen considering the frames, for which initially the object detection of the individual frames is determined using a hybrid model named NSA-NARX.

In the testing phase, the query is given as an input for extracting the object location. After positioning the object, the events tracked by the tracking method and the input must be matched according to the NB classifier is used for retrieving correct video frames.

3.1 Object Tracking Based on Hybrid NSA-NARX Model

The Nearest Search Algorithm is to determine position of object in video and tracking object using Nonlinear Autoregressive Exogenous Neural Network used in nonlinear time series, and it has considerable significance compared to other models. This systems key benefit is the efficient learning rate, which meets easily to the desired solution. Finally, NSA-NARX neural network uses the merits of both NSA and NARX thereby attains object tracking is given as,

$$H_k^u = \frac{o_k^u(\text{NSA}) + o_k^u(\text{NARX})}{2} \tag{1}$$

3.2 Retrieval of Objects Using the Naive Bayes Classifier

The NB classifier is well known for its speed, as it poses the ability to make predictions in real time. The NB classifier is described as a probabilistic classifier which is derived using specific features based on the Bayes theorem. It is used to find the mean and variance for each sample and then determines the posterior function. The Naive Bayes classifier is utilized for retrieving the events. The equivalent class label κ for each event can be generated using the Naive Bayes classifier. The relevant objects from the classified events is given as,

$$\kappa = \arg\max_{Z=1}^{T} \text{post}\left(E_Z \middle| N\right) \tag{2}$$

4 Results and Discussion

The proposed technique is evaluated with respect to the existing methods based on precision, F-measure and recall parameter. The analysis is done on video taken from the CAVIAR database [17].

4.1 Performance Metrics

The method used different performance measures adapted to analyze the performance and is briefed below.

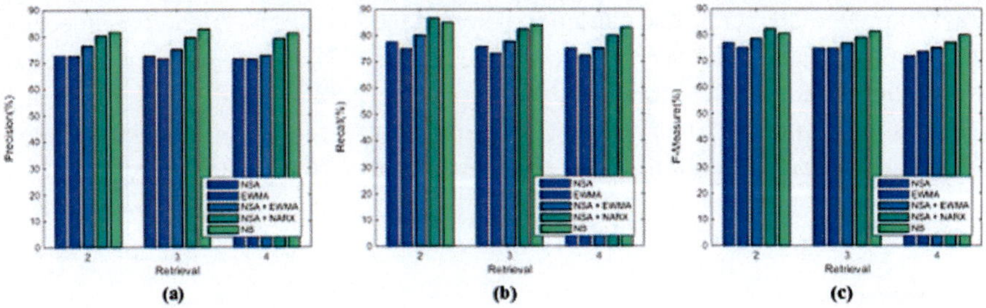

Fig. 1 Analysis of video using **a** Precision, **b** Recall, **c** F-measure

- ***Precision***: The precision is the most pertinent objects amongst the retrieved objects.
- ***Recall***: The recall determining the complete set of relevant videos.
- ***F-measure***: Defined as harmonic mean of precision and recall.

4.2 *Comparative Analysis*

The analysis is made using the comparative method like NSA + EWMA, Nearest Search Algorithm-based non-autoregressive neural machine (NSA + NARX), and Nearest Search Algorithm [18].

The comparison between proposed NB and existing techniques is done using recall, F-measure, and precision. In Fig. 1a, the retrieval objects is 2; the precision calculated by existing NSA is 72.681%; EWMA is 72.468%; NSA + EWMA is 76.422%; NSA + NARX is 80.220%, and proposed NB is 81.508%. The analysis of recall shows in Fig. 1b. The retrieval objects are 2; the recall values calculated by existing NSA is 77.377%; EWMA is 74.894%; NSA + EWMA is 80.121%,;NSA + NARX is 86.574%, and proposed NB is 84.793%. The analysis of F-measure shows in Fig. 1c. The retrieval objects are 2, the f-measure values computed by NSA is 76.879%; EWMA is 75.231%; NSA + EWMA is 78.568%; NSA + NARX is 82.277%, and proposed NBis 80.475%.

5 Conclusion

A video object retrieval strategy is proposed for tracking the objects from the videos. The proposed technique is devised in two phases, namely object tracking and retrieval. At first, the location of the objects is tracked by finding the object location by employing a hybrid model named NSA-NARX. Here, the spatial tracking is done using NARX, whereas visual tracking is done by the NSA model. The Naive Bayes classifier is trained using the indexed database. In retrieval, the query of the tracked object is given to the classifier, wherein the matching is done for retrieving the relevant objects. The performance of the proposed NB is grater when compared with other existing techniques with precision of 81.985%, recall of 85.451%, and F-measure of 86.847%, respectively. In future, this research work can be extended further by utilizing the optimization method to improve the performance.

References

1. Lai Y, Yang C (2015) Video object retrieval by trajectory and appearance. IEEE Trans Circuits Syst Video Technol 25(6):1026–1037
2. Pande SD, Chetty MSR (2019) Position invariant spline curve based image retrieval using control points. Int J Intell Eng Syst 12(4):177–191
3. Awate G, Bangare S, Pradeepini G, Patil S (2019) Detection of alzheimers disease from mri using convolutional neural network with tensorflow arXiv:1806.10170
4. Bilen H, Pedersoli M, Tuytelaars T (2015) Weakly supervised object detection with convex clustering. In: Proceedings of the IEEE conference on computer vision and pattern recognition, pp 1081–1089
5. Ghuge CA, Ruikar SD, Chandra Prakash V (2018) Query-specific Distance and hybrid Tracking model for video object retrieval. J Intell Syst 27(2):195–212
6. Cheng HY, Hwang JN (2011) Integrated video object tracking with applications in trajectory-based event detection. J Visual Commun Image Represent 22(7):673–685
7. Wagdarikar AMU, Senapati RK (2019) Optimization based interesting region identification for video watermarking. J Info Secur Appl 49:102393
8. Ghuge CA, Ruikar SD, Prakash VC (2018) Support vector regression and extended nearest neighbor for video object retrieval. Evol, Intel
9. Ding S, Li G, Li Y, Li X, Zhai Q, Champion AC, Zhu J, Xuan D, Zheng YF (2016) SurvSurf: human retrieval on large surveillance video data. Multimedia Tools and Appl 1–29
10. Lin TC, Yang MC, Tsai CY, Wang YCF (2015) Query-adaptive multiple instance learning for video instance retrieval. IEEE Trans Image Process 24(4):1330–1340
11. Nguyen VT, Le DD, Tran MT, Nguyen TV, Ngo TD, Satoh SI, Duong DA (2019) Video instance search via spatial fusion of visual words and object proposals. Int J Multimedia Info Retrieval 1–12
12. Durand T, He X, Pop I, Robinault L (2019) Utilizing deep object detector for video surveillance indexing and retrieval In: Proceedings of international conference on multimedia modeling, Springer, pp 506–518
13. Garcia N (2018) Temporal aggregation of visual features for large-scale image-to-video retrieval. In: Proceedings of the 2018 ACM on international conference on multimedia retrieval, pp 489–492
14. Dyana A, Das S (2010) MST-CSS (Multi-Spectro-Temporal Curvature Scale Space), a novel spatio-temporal representation for content-based video retrieval. IEEE Trans Circuits Syst Video Technol 20(8)
15. Castañón G, Elgharib M, Saligrama V, Jodoin P (2016) Retrieval in long-surveillance videos using user-described motion and object attributes. IEEE Trans Circuits Syst Video Technol 26(12):2313–2327
16. Hsieh J, Yu S, Chen Y (2006) Motion-based video retrieval by trajectory matching. IEEE Trans Circuits Syst Video Technol 16(3):396–409
17. CAVIAR database.https://homepages.inf.ed.ac.uk/rbf/CAVIARDATA1/
18. Ghuge CA, Chandra Prakash V, Ruikar SD (2020) Weighed query-specific distance and hybrid NARX neural network for video object retrieval. Comput J 63(11):1738–1755

Mobility-Aware Clustering Routing (MACRON) Algorithm for Lifetime Improvement of Extensive Dynamic Wireless Sensor Network

Rajiv Ramesh Bhandari and K. Raja Sekhar

Abstract Wireless sensor network is growing rapidly in recent era. The scalability and mobility impose remarkable challenges and degrade overall lifetime of network. The versatile topology with evolving parameters such as location and coverage needs to be modified for extensively dynamic network. The flat sensor network degrades the network's total lifespan, because it absorbs a lot of resources. Clustering with one-hop distance in sensor network is the best way to elongate network lifespan. Clustering along with adaptive sleep scheduling using reinforcement algorithm produces better results by eliminating the issue of idle listening. The proposed mobility-aware clustering routing algorithm (MACRON) along with self-healing scheduling for extensively dynamic network to handle network communication with one-hop distance and probability distribution function will give better results as compared to RI-MAC, A-TDMA, AODV and MEMAC. The experimental analysis shows that MACRON gives better results in terms of throughput, delay, packet delivery, hop and mean deviation.

Keywords Sleep scheduling · Clustering · Wireless sensor network

1 Related Work

In fastest-growing wireless sensor network, mobility of node is one of the most important parameters that need to be considered while deploying the network. Mobility of any node among the network depends on coverage and location. Most of the conventional protocols were not able to handle the extensively dynamic networks. The mobility of code can be classified into three patterns like sensor mobility, base station mobility and cluster head mobility [1]. Flat wireless sensor network is aggregating data at each individual level and degrading overall network lifetime, whereas hierarchical networks are more powerful and elongating lifetime of network through clustering. For extensively dynamic network, hierarchical- or cluster-based routing

R. R. Bhandari (✉) · K. Raja Sekhar
Department of Computer Science and Engineering, Koneru Lakshmaiah Education Foundation, Vaddeswaram, Andhra Pradesh, India
e-mail: rajivrbhandari@gmail.com

S. Bhattacharyya et al. (eds.), *International Conference on Intelligent and Smart Computing in Data Analytics*, Advances in Intelligent Systems and Computing 1312,
https://doi.org/10.1007/978-981-33-6176-8_13

are the best suitable solutions in terms of scalability, effective communication and coverage. Some of the best possible solutions over traditional clustering algorithms are machine learning, artificial intelligence and fuzzy logics. There are multiple ways to predict mobility like location-based and prediction-based; out of these, global positioning system and coverage give us better results. Depending on the location and coverage, nodes are taking decision of joining and leaving. In most of the deployment, nodes are connected to cluster head through multihop connectivity and degrade the performance of overall network [2–4].

1.1 Need of Scheduling in Wireless Sensor Network

Energy is one of the most important parameters in wireless sensor network. Simple approach to meet coverage objective is to keep all nodes alive all time, but keeping all nodes alive will drain the energy of all members fastly and not all nodes are taking active participation in communication at same time. Making all nodes alive will create huge collision in media access control layer, and gradually, whole network will get down. Minimal subset of deployed sensors kept alive to extend the lifespan of the network, and remaining sensors should be retained in sleep mode. This kind of strategy will rise new overheads in the system like need to alternatively keep subset alive/sleep until no more subset will remain, and then, there is problem of scheduling them. This approach would not work well for large sensor network. Lots of research have been carried out to handle the large sensor network through centralize scheduling and distributed scheduling [5]. Centralized approach can suffer from scalability problem, central failure point and lack of stability. The problem with distributed approach is that decision-making is based on a simplistic greedy approach and hence does not solve the scheduling problem [6, 7].

The proposed framework focuses on incorporating hybrid scheduling methods to produce better scheduling performance. There are several ways to boost sensor network lifespan like placement of nodes, sleep/wakeup scheduling and optimization of coverage. This paper focuses on sleep/wakeup scheduling approach. Several sleep/wakeup approaches have recently been developed, such as on-demand, synchronous and asynchronous approach. This paper proposes self-adaptive sleep/wakeup approach which is asynchronous one [8].

The following points show the main contribution of this paper

1. The problem of node mobility with cluster head in wireless sensor network is dealt with by modifying mobility-conscious media access control (MEMAC).
2. The dynamic sleep/wakeup scheduling using machine learning approach with modified MEMAC improves overall lifetime of network.

The need of clustering and scheduling algorithm is described in Sect. 1. The latest problems in design are discussed in the Sect. 2; here, the background knowledge of novel approach for MACRON algorithm is elaborated.

2 Proposed Work

The proposed mobility-aware clustering routing protocol (MACRON) mainly focuses on clustering for widely dynamic environment. In addition to that, paper also proposes self-adaptive sleep scheduling using reinforcement learning algorithm [1, 2].

The base station broadcasts its location with all sensor nodes in the network. Sensor node sends its IP address and energy level along with its location to base station. The base station calculates unit area and average number of cluster nodes in the network. The cluster heads are calculated based on iterative probability distribution. The probability is calculated by considering the distance and energy level of cluster head [9, 10].

If more than one node has the max probability, then base station will find the average probability value to decide the cluster head. All cluster heads are connected at one-hop distance with sensor nodes. The base station initiates the clustering process same as LEACH protocol [11–13].

Once the clustering is done in wireless sensor network, then cluster chooses the tentative CH based on the shortest reachability. If the cluster member belongs to the other cluster, then it sends the leave message to the old CH and sends the join message to the newly selected CH based on the minimum distance. Cluster member belongs to the other cluster and receives the message from the shortest reachable CH; then, it performs the cluster shifting by joining in the new CH. If CH received the CH announcement from the other overlapping CH, then it checks the cluster probability [14, 15]. The Fig. 1 shows basic architecture of MACRON algorithm and Fig. 2 shows reinforcement algorithm with self-adaptive sleep scheduling.

The node with the greater probability retains the head position, so the lower probability CH performs the cluster shifting process by sending the shifting message to both CM and overlapping CH.

1. The shifted CM nodes are joined to the overlapping CH if it is in reachable distance.
2. Cluster head assigns unique slot to all cluster member for data transmission.

Sleep scheduling approach for traditional sensor network consumes huge energy as idle state affects and consumes energy. The new scheduling approach uses machine learning algorithm to predict the next state of execution based on reinforcement learning. This learning approach avoids idle state and making network self-adaptive to decide when to transmit the packet [16, 17].

2.1 Proposed Algorithm

The proposed mobility-aware clustering routing algorithm is mainly classified into three main parts like network and cluster head formation, leave, join and shift algorithm and adaptive sleep scheduling using reinforcement algorithm.

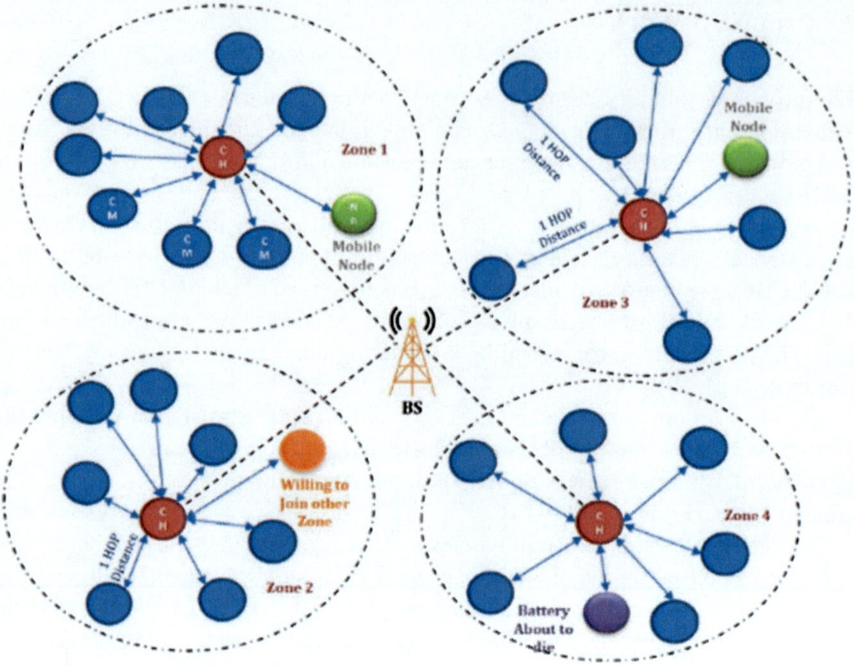

Fig. 1 WSN architecture

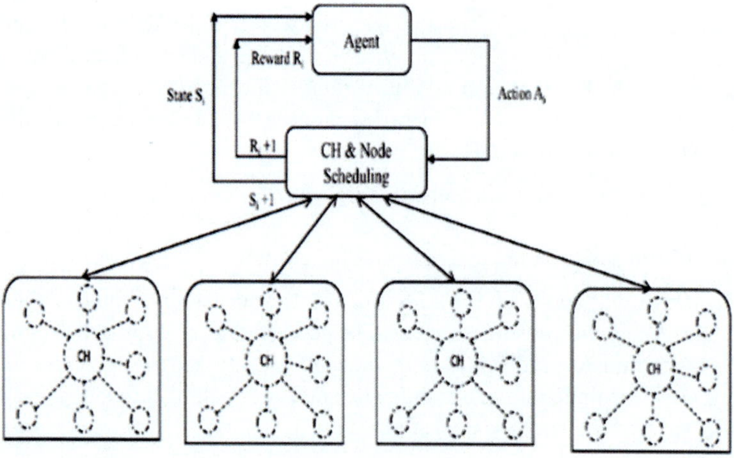

Fig. 2 Wireless sensor network: self-adaptive sleep scheduling

2.1.1 Network and Cluster Head Formation Algorithm

```
Step 1: Node 0 < - Base Station (BS) with X, Y and B_Add
Step 2: rh - > X = node_ - > X( );rh - > Y = node_- > Y( );
ih - > daddr( ) = IP_BROADCAST;
Step 3: Node send its location and energy to base station.
Step 4: Base station creates location table
{add (ih - > saddr (), rh - > X, rh - > Y, rh- > E)};
Step 5: Cluster table is maintained by Each Node
Step 6: Calculate unit area = nodes (nn)/ upper_X * upper_Y
Step 7: Calculate Average cluster nodes
Avg_c_n = unit_area*M_PI*n_- > coverage*n_- > coverage
Step 8: Calculate Number of Clusters
n_cluster = nodes (nn)/avg_c_n
Step 9: Initially clusters are formed by one hop distance
     While(cluster_cnt !=0)
For every distinct pair of nodes (i, j)
        P1<-location-table[i]; P2<-location-table[j];
        If (d1<node_coverage)
    _1_hop[i][_1_count[i]+++ = cluster_nodeid[j]
Step 10: Calculate probability distribution
Step 11: Calculate CH based on Max Prob & Average Prob Value
Step 12: Cluster Formationmax_ = prob[i];
    cluster_->add(nid); &Cluster_.remove(nid);
```

2.1.2 Algorithm for Leave, Join & Shift Algorithm

```
Step 1: CM chooses the tentative CH based on the shortest
     reachability.
Step 2: if(status == MEM)
     S_Leave(head_id)- > old_CH; S_Join(head_id)- > new_CH;
Step 3: CM receives new CH announcement
     sendLeave(head_id)- > o_CH;sendShift(head_id)- > n_CH
Step 4:
   If (prob[currCH] > prob[overlapCH])
   for all CM ∈ overlapCH
   S_Leave(head_id)- > overlapCH; S_Join(head_id)- > currCH
Step 5: CH assigns uniform slot to all CM ∈ CH
Step 6: CH sends time slot to all CM ∈ CH
Step 7: while ( slot ! = CM_Slot); Mode(CM) = Sleep;
```

2.1.3 Algorithm and Scheduling

Step 1: A is set of n available action $\{aa_1, aa_2, \ldots, aa_n\}$,
$a_i \in \{trans, sleep, idle\}$, s_{curr} is current_state_action,

s_{next} is next state_of_action.
Step 2: each action $aa_i \in A$
define value function $Q_i := 0$; define rule $\gamma \cdot \frac{1}{n}$
according to the rule γ (s_{curr}, aa_i) select an action
aa_i of s_{curr}
Step 3: if the selected rule $a_i := trans$
Time slot selected by node to transmit packet.
detect payoff ∂ and s_{next}; update Q_i
$Q_i(s_{curr}, a_i) \leftarrow (1 - nr_1)Q_i(s_{curr}, a_i) + nr_1(\partial + nr_2 \max(s_{next}, a_{i+1}))$
Step 4: if the selected action $a_i \neq sleep$
update policy $\gamma(s_{curr}, a_i)$ based on approx.rule $\forall a_i \in A$
Step 5: calculate the average payoff ∂_{avg}

3 Results

The proposed MACRON protocol is compared with receiver-initiated MAC, source-initiated MAC, AODV and MEMAC. Simulation in NS2 with node size varies from 10 to 40 nodes. The proposed MACRON protocol shows better performance in terms of delay, packet delivery ratio, throughput, hop count and mean deviation. Tables 1, 2, 3, 4 and 5 shows MACRON yields better results as comparied to RI-MAC,A-TDMA, AODV and MEMAC.

Table 1 Results for delay calculations

Number of nodes	Receiver initiated MAC	Advertisement-based TDMA	Adhoc on-demand distance vector	Mobility-aware MAC	MACRON
Node 10	5.5	4.2	0.4	0.15	0.2
Node 20	7.6	5.9	1	0.21	0.1
Node 30	8.6	5.5	2.5	0.25	0.21
Node 40	10.5	5.3	3.5	0.28	0.32

Table 2 Results for packet delivery ratio

Number of nodes	RIMAC	Advertisement-based TDMA	AODV	MEMAC	MACRON
Node 10	97.085	99.87	99.58	99.84	98.93
Node 20	97.33	99.87	98.42	99.77	99.91
Node 30	96.53	99.7	97.37	99.73	99.86
Node 40	95.03	99.38	96.32	99.7	101.72

Table 3 Results for throughput

Number of nodes	RIMAC	Advertisement-based TDMA	Adhoc on-demand distance vector	Mobility-aware MAC	MACRON
Node 10	0.78	0.97	9	6.15	10.93
Node 20	2.06	1.96	8	5.79	11.91
Node 30	2.93	2.94	9	7.27	10.86
Node 40	3.87	4.23	7	7.69	11.72

Table 4 Results for average energy consumption

Number of nodes	RIMAC	Advertisement-based TDMA	MACRON
Node 10	71	114	60.52
Node 20	180	112	58.66
Node 30	309	118	34.79
Node 40	405	135	18.92

Table 5 Results for hop count

Number of nodes	RIMAC	MEMAC	MACRON
Node 10	3	6	2
Node 20	19	7.4	2
Node 30	28	5	2
Node 40	38	5	2

4 Conclusion

The fame of wireless sensor network has grown swiftly in coming years. Movement of nodes and energy efficiency in cluster sensor network have imposed significant challenges for design of MAC protocol with scheduling of nodes in heterogeneous environment. The MACRON comprises modification in mobility-aware media access control (MEMAC) [1] with dynamic sleep/wakeup scheduling using reinforcement learning algorithm which does not use traditional duty cycling method. This machine learning approach enables each cluster head and nodes to dynamically decide its own schedule to enhance lifetime of networks. The proposed algorithm shows significant improvement in end-to-end delay, throughput, packet delivery ration and hop count in extensive dynamic network over traditional static network. Figures 3, 4 and 5 shows significant improvement in end to end delay, Packet delivery Ratio, Throughput and average energy consumption.

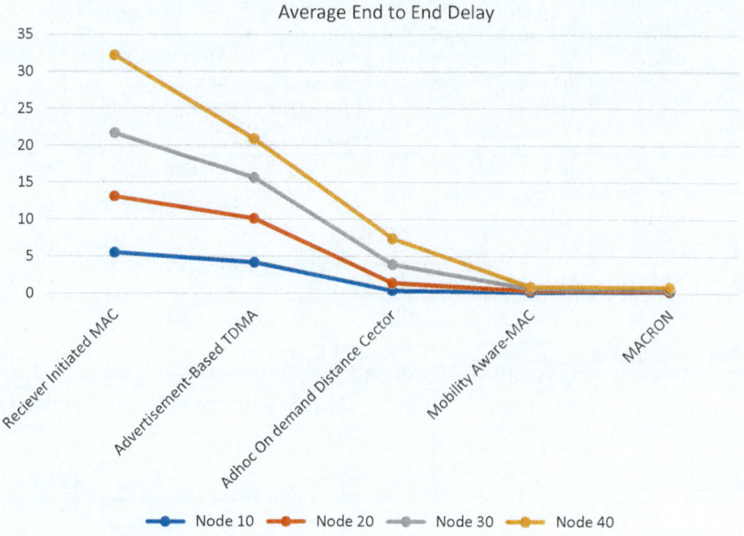

Fig. 3 Results for end-to-end delay

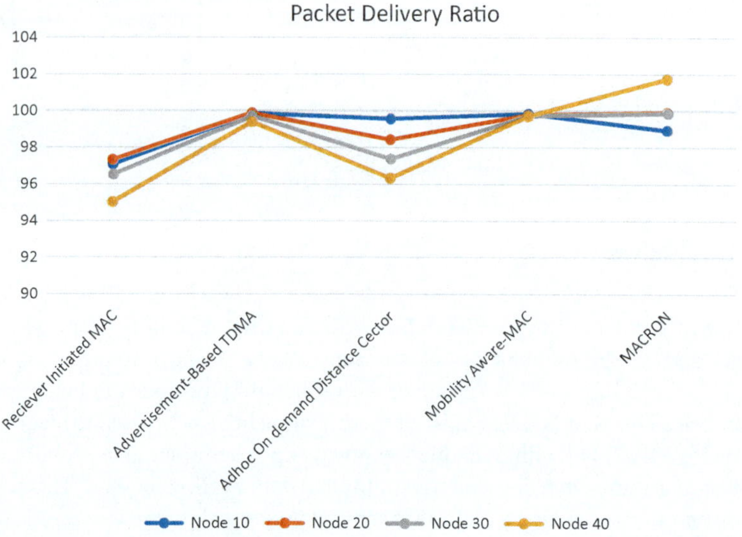

Fig. 4 Results for delivery of packet

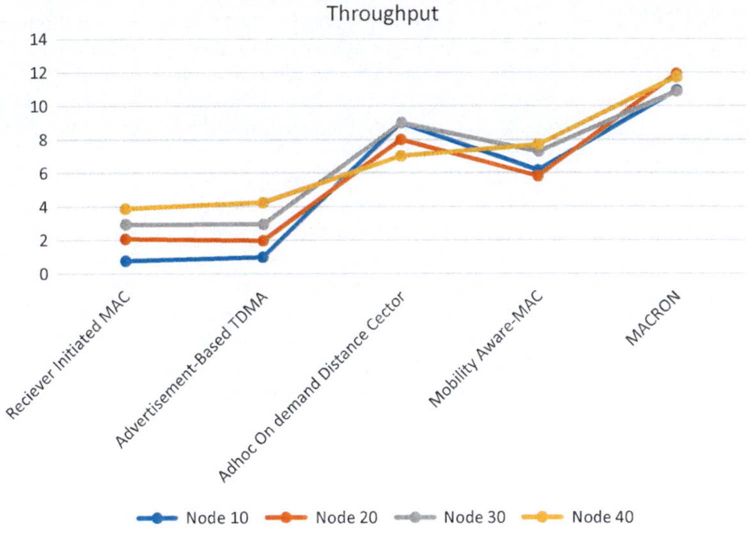

Fig. 5 Results for throughput

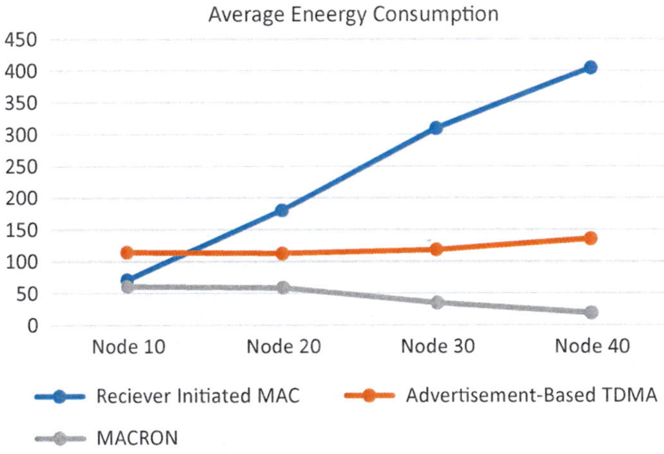

Fig. 6 Results of average energy consumption

References

1. Yahya B, Ben-Othman J (2009) An adaptive mobility aware and energy efficient MAC protocol for wireless sensor networks. In: 2009 IEEE symposium on computers and communications, Sousse, pp 15–21. https://doi.org/10.1109/ISCC.2009.5202382
2. Srie Vidhya Janani E, Ganesh Kumar P (2015) Energy efficient cluster based scheduling scheme for wireless sensor networks. Sci World J. https://doi.org/10.1155/2015/185198

3. Kathavate PN, Amudhavel (2018) Energy aware routing protocol with Qos constraint in wireless multimedia sensor networks. J Adv Res Dynam Control Syst. ISSN 1943–023X
4. Anusha M, Vemuru S (2018) Cognitive radio networks: state of research domain in next-generation wireless networks—an analytical analysis. In: Mishra D, Nayak M, Joshi A (eds) Information and communication technology for sustainable development. Lecture notes in networks and systems, vol 9. Springer, Singapore. https://doi.org/10.1007/978-981-10-3932-4_30
5. Ye D, Zhang M (2018) A self-adaptive sleep/wake-up scheduling approach for wireless sensor networks. IEEE Trans Cybernet 48(3):979–992. https://doi.org/10.1109/TCYB.2017.2669996
6. Zhang Z, Shu L, Zhu C, Mukherjee M (2018) A short review on sleep scheduling mechanism in wireless sensor networks. In: Wang L, Qiu T, Zhao W (eds) Quality, reliability, security and robustness in heterogeneous systems QShine 2017. Lecture notes of the institute for computer sciences, social informatics and telecommunications engineering, vol 234. Springer, Cham
7. Zareei M, Islam AKM, Vargas-Rosales C, Mansoor N, Goudarzi S, Rehmani MH (2017) Mobility-aware medium access control protocols for wireless sensor networks: a survey. J Netw Comput Appl 104. https://doi.org/10.1016/j.jnca.2017.12.009
8. Wan R, Xiong N, Loc NT (2018) An energy-efficient sleep scheduling mechanism with similarity measure for wireless sensor networks. Hum Cent Comput Inf Sci 8:18
9. Anant RM, Prasad MSG, Wankhede Vishal A (2019) Optimized throughput and minimized energy consumption through clustering techniques for cognitive radio network, Int J Innov Technol Explor Eng (IJITEE) 8(4S2). ISSN: 2278-3075
10. Shaik S, Ratnam DV, Bhandari BN (2018) An efficient cross layer routing protocol for safety message dissemination in VANETS with reduced routing cost and delay using IEEE 802.11p. Wireless personal communications, June 2018. https://doi.org/10.1007/s11277-018-5671-z
11. Bhandari RR, Rajasekhar K (2016) Study on improving the network life time maximization for wireless sensor network using cross layer approach. Int J Electr Comput Eng 6(6):3080. http://doi.org/10.11591/ijece.v6i6.pp3080–3086
12. Mohammad H, Chandrasekhara S, Sastry A ACNM: advance coupling network model sleep/awake mechanism for wireless sensor networks. Int J Eng Technol [S.l.] 7(1.1):350–354. ISSN: 2227-524X
13. Ayushree M, Arora S (2017) Comparative analysis of AODV and DSDV using machine learning approach in MANET. J Eng Sci Technol 12:3315–3328
14. Bhandari RR, Rajasekhar K (2020) Energy-efficient routing-based clustering approaches and sleep scheduling algorithm for network lifetime maximization in sensor network: a survey. In: Ranganathan G, Chen J, Rocha Á (eds) Inventive communication and computational technologies. Lecture notes in networks and systems, vol 89. Springer, Singapore
15. Rao YM, Subramanyam MV, Prasad KS (2018) Cluster-based mobility management algorithms for wireless mesh networks. Int J Commun Syst. https://doi.org/10.1002/dac.3595
16. Amiripalli SS, Bobba V (2019) An optimal TGO topology method for a scalable and survivable network in IOT communication technology. Wireless Pers Commun 107:1019–1040
17. Kumar KH, Srinivas VYS, Moulali S (2019) Design of wireless power transfer converter systems for EV applications using MATLAB/ simulink. Int J Innov Technol Explor Eng 8(5):406

An Extensive Survey on IOT Protocols and Applications

K. V. Sowmya, V. Teju, and T. Pavan Kumar

Abstract The most buzzed word in the modern era is internet of things which connects almost all devices and humans in the world in the coming future. IOT has made lives of humans comfortable by reducing the man efforts where the work to be by done humans will be done by machines. This paper presents an extensive survey on the communication protocols that are used in internet of things (IOT). The protocols used in IOT are different in a way that they are light in weight compared to the protocols used by the conventional networking devices.

Keywords IOT · Communication protocols · MQTT · CoAP · HTTP · AMQP · DDS

1 Introduction

Internet of things can be defined as a system which consists of objects, machines, animals, people, etc., interconnected to each other where the data can be transferred between anyone and anything. With minimal or sometimes, no human intervention the system could work thereby making the whole system intelligent. The things in IOT can be generally categorized into three groups viz.

1. Objects that collect the information and send it
2. Objects that receive the information and act on it
3. Objects that can do both

K. V. Sowmya (✉) · V. Teju · T. Pavan Kumar
Koneru Lakshmaiah Education Foundation, Vaddeswaram, Guntur, India
e-mail: sowmyakambhampati@kluniversity.in

V. Teju
e-mail: teju@kluniversity.in

T. Pavan Kumar
e-mail: pavankumar_ist@kluniversity.in

S. Bhattacharyya et al. (eds.), *International Conference on Intelligent and Smart Computing in Data Analytics*, Advances in Intelligent Systems and Computing 1312,
https://doi.org/10.1007/978-981-33-6176-8_14

Objects that collect the information could be sensors which measure the physical parameters of the environment like temperature, humidity, pressure, etc., and send the information to the top layer devices.

Objects that receive the information could be controllers, gateways, restful servers or cloud servers where they process the information that is received from the lower level devices and act upon the data that may lead to taking a decision according to the current situation of the system.

Objects that can do both the things could both collect the information and receive the information. Upon the received information, necessary action is taken on the data

Internet of things has made the human life easier in the way of reducing the human efforts. Imagine a refrigerator connected through IOT, where it tracks the amount of vegetables in the tray and places the order by itself if the vegetables are running out of stock which reduces the human effort. Internet of things has been extended in almost all fields of engineering, medicine, manufacturing, etc. IOT can be sandwiched with other technologies like AI, ML, HPC, etc., which furthermore increases the scalability and importance of IOT.

2 Related Work

For any device or server to communicate with another device or server certain protocols need to be followed. Protocols define the way of communication between the devices. In IOT each layer uses a different protocol. When the data is to be traversed from one layer to another it must undergo protocol conversion.

In [2–6] authors mentioned about the basic issues in an IOT system and algorithms and protocols used in IOT are also proposed

3 Block Diagram of IOT

The basic block diagram of IOT is as shown in Fig. 1 where it consists of the following layers

1. Device Level
2. Controller Level
3. Restful Server Level
4. Gateway Level
5. Cloud Level

Device Level: This level consists of sensors which are able to collect the information from surroundings that can be sent to the higher levels.

Controller Level: This level receives the data from the devices and then processes it. Controller is the device which acts as the main unit where it does all the processing of the data.

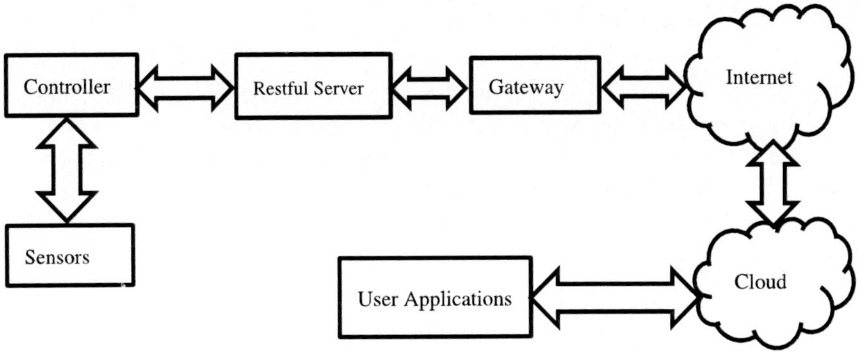

Fig. 1 Block diagram of IOT representing different levels

Restful Server Level: This level services the requests that are sent by the users to know the status of the devices that are situated remotely from them.

Gateway Level: This level is used to route the data from the devices to cloud level and then carries the request sent by the users to Restful server layer.

Cloud Level: This level stores the data generated and processed through the whole IOT network.

4 Applications of IOT

We can understand the beauty of IOT by considering some of the application areas. The applications considered here will be known to everyone in general but the role of IOT played in these systems is unique of its kind.

1. Smart Home: Smart home is a system where all the appliances in home are connected to each other and they are controlled by the user remotely. User can switch on or off the appliances using some app or through voice control even..
2. Smart Cites: This is a system where the livelihood of humans is enhanced through making the applications related to customers smart. One such area could be road traffic where in some large metropolitan cities, there is a huge demand to regulate the traffic to avoid congestions at many junctions.
3. Smart Irrigation System: This is a system which has made the irrigation to be done in a smarter way by informing the farmer about the amount of water to be sprinkled to the crops everyday by deploying a soil moisture sensor in the field.
4. Smart Industry: This is a system where all the machines in an industry are connected through M2M communication. Apart from connecting, the machines together if IOT is made part of the system it can reduce almost all the human efforts.

5 IOT Protocols at Different Layers

As IOT involves many layers and the data transmission from layer to layer follow different set of protocols. As shown in Fig. 1, it consists of device level, controller level, restful server level, gateway level, and cloud level. All these levels can be mapped to different layers of the TCP/IP model. The four major layers where the whole communication in IOT happens are as shown in Fig. 2 proposed by the author in [1].

1. Link Layer

Link layer is responsible for routing the data over the physical medium. Some of the link layer protocols from the context of IOT are:

802.3 Ethernet: The data link layer consists of two layers viz. physical and medium access control (MAC) whose standards are defined by IEEE 802.3. There are many standards defined under 802.3 like 802.3 is the standard for 10BASE5 Ethernet where a coaxial cable is used as a medium,

802.11 Wi-Fi: A set of physical and MAC layer protocols for local area networks (LANS) are defined by IEEE 802.11.

802.16 Wi-Max: The Wi-Max is family of wireless broadband communication standards where they define multiple physical layers and MAC layer.

802.15.4 LR-WPAN: LR-WPAN is a standard defined for low rates wireless personal area networks. Physical and MAC layer controls are specified by this standard.

2G/3G/4G- Mobile communication: These mobile communication standards starting from 2G form the basis for data mobility from the source to destination. 2G includes GSM and CDMA, 3G includes UMTS and CDMA2000, 4G includes LTE.

2. Network/Internet Layer

This layer routes the data packets from the source to destination.. The protocols included in this layer are:

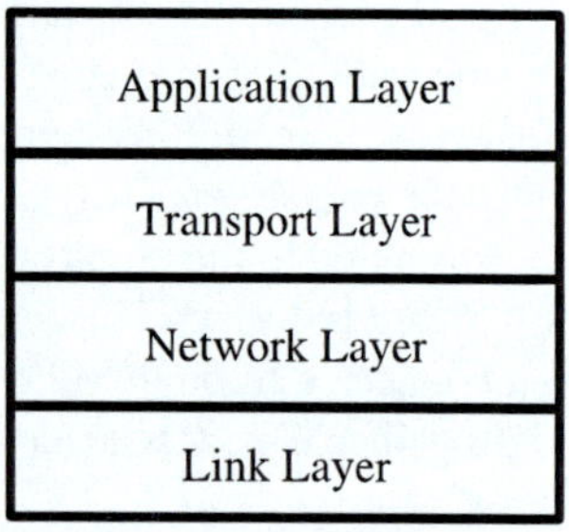

Fig. 2 Layers in IOT architecture

IPv4: IPv4 is an internet protocol that assigns unique addresses to the devices using the internet. It uses a 32 bit addressing scheme which allows assigning 2^{32} addresses to the devices.

IPv6: With the increasing demand of addresses that need to be assigned to the devices connected to the internet IPv6 was invented which uses a 128 bit addressing scheme that can accommodate 2^{128} devices with unique identity.

6LOWPAN: With the idea that low power devices also must be able to participate in IOT system 6LOWPAN was invented. As the name suggests, IPv6 over low power wireless personal area networks it is used for the devices that consumes less power.

3. Transport Layer

Message transfer from one end to other end is ensured by this layer, i.e., it sees to it that the message is transferred from the source to destination correctly the protocols involved in this layer are:

TCP: Transmission control protocol is one of the famous transport layer protocols that are used along with HTTP, HTTPS, SMTP, and FTP. This TCP protocol is connection oriented where it ensures that data packets has reached the correct destination and in order.

UDP: User datagram protocol is unlike TCP which requires an initial setup before transmitting the data. It is a connectionless protocol which is used to send small amounts of data.

4. Application Layer

This layer defines how the applications talk with the lower layers and coordinate to send data over the network. The protocols that fall under this category are:

HTTP: Hyper text transfer protocol (HTTP) is an application layer protocol which is used to transfer documents over the web. This protocol forms the foundation for World Wide Web (WWW).

CoAP: Constrained application protocol (CoAP) is used for constrained nodes and networks which is also a specialized web transfer protocol like HTTP as shown in Fig. 3. This is one of the lightweight protocols that is used in IOT as it allows the constrained devices and constrained networks to join the system with low bandwidth.

Web Socket: Web socket protocol allows bi-directional communication between the user's browser and server.

MQTT: Message queuing telemetry transport (MQTT) protocol is a light weight protocol in internet of things which uses publish-subscribe model.. The client publishes messages to the topics on server where the messages are forwarded by the broker to the clients subscribed to those topics as shown in Fig. 4.

XMPP: Extensible messaging and presence protocol, as the name implies is a protocol that enables the communication between two systems in real time, i.e., the data packets from sender to receiver does not introduce any network load unlike the traditional web-based mechanisms as shown in Fig. 5.

DDS: Data distribution service protocol allows device to device or machine to machine communication. This protocol follows publish-subscribe model where

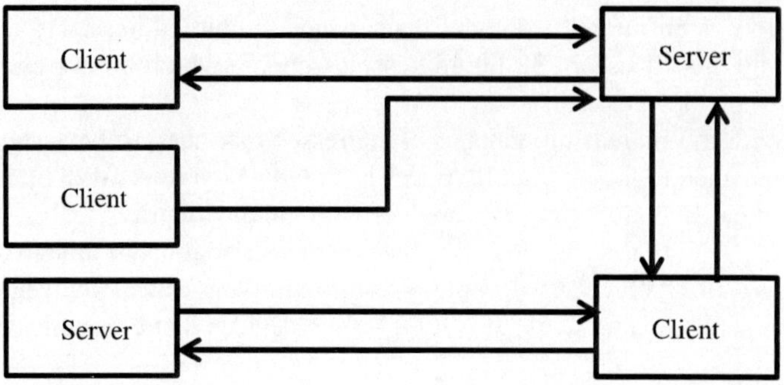

Fig. 3 CoAP protocol

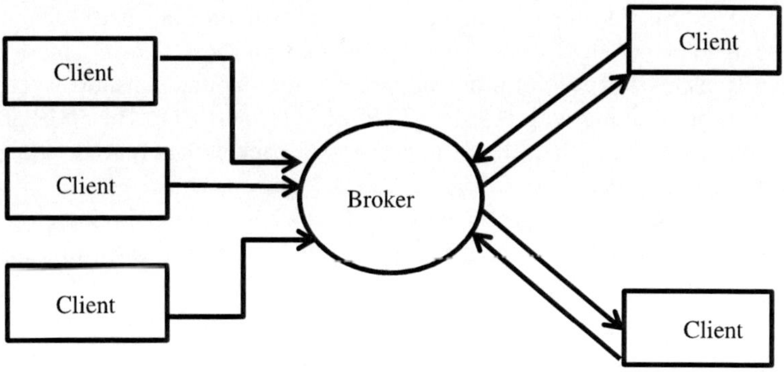

Fig. 4 MQTT Protocol

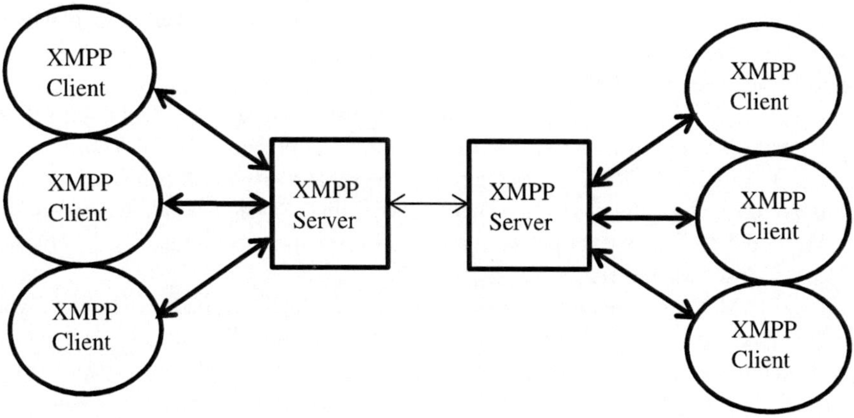

Fig. 5 XMPP protocol

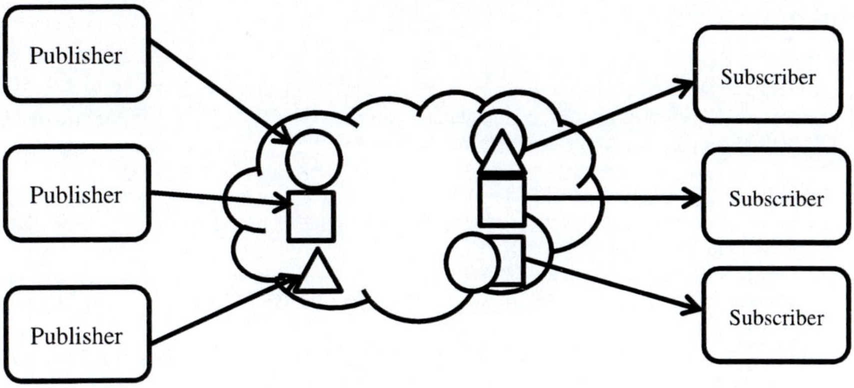

Fig. 6 DDS protocol

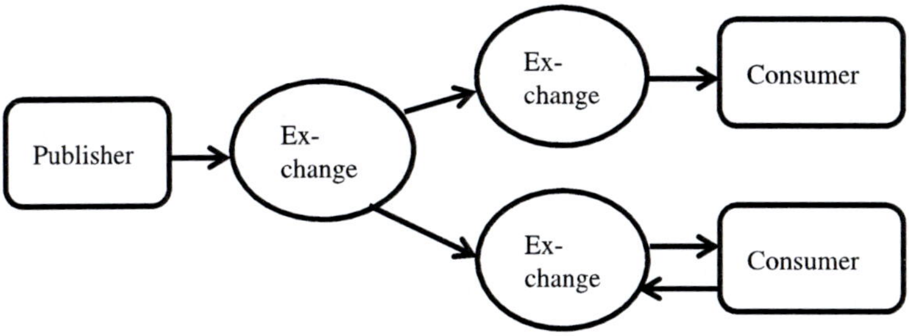

Fig. 7 AMQP protocol

the publishers (devices that generate data) publishes the messages and subscribers (devices that want to take the data) subscribe to that message as shown in Fig. 6.

AMQP: Advanced message queuing protocol allows the systems to exchange data between them mostly business exchanges as shown in Fig. 7.

6 Conclusion

In this paper, a survey was done on the protocols used in IOT systems. According to the literature survey done, it was found that the most widely used protocols in IOT are MQTT, CoAP, AMQP, HTTP. As IOT is finding widespread use in every field, lightweight protocols are of utmost demand. Among the above said protocols, MQTT and CoAP are lightweight. Also, a survey on the some of the IOT applications is presented.

References

1. Arshdeep B, Vijay M (2014) In: Internet of things: a hands-on approach
2. Sowmya K, Chandu A, Nagasai A, Preetham C, Supreeth K (2020) Smart home system using clustering based on internet of things. J Comput Theoretical Nanosci 17:2369–2374. https://doi.org/10.1166/jctn.2020.8897
3. Sowmya KV, Harshavardhan J, Pradeep G (2020) Remote monitoring system of robotic car based on internet of things using raspberyy Pi. J Compu Theoretical Nanosci 17:2288–2295. https://doi.org/10.1166/jctn.2020.8886
4. Teju V, Sai K, Swamy, Bharath K (2020) Mining environment monitoring based on laser communication with internet of things. J Comput Theor Nanosci 17:2375–2378. https://doi.org/10.1166/jctn.2020.8898
5. Teju V, Krishna N, Reddy K (2020) Authentication process in smart card using Sha-256. J Comput Theoretical Nanosci 17:2379–2382. https://doi.org/10.1166/jctn.2020.8899
6. Sowmya K , Sastry Dr (2018) Performance evaluation of IOT systems–basic issues. Int J Eng Technol 7:131. https://doi.org/10.14419/ijet.v7i2.7.10279

Review on Cardiac Arrhythmia Through Segmentation Approaches in Deep Learning

P. Jyothi and G. Pradeepini

Abstract Identifying the precise Heart Sounds (HS) positions inside a Phonocardiogram (PCG); otherwise, Heart Sounds Segmentation (HSS) is a vital phase for the automatic examination of recordings of HS, permitting for the categorization of pathological proceedings. Analysis of HS signals (explicitly, PCG) in the last some decades, particularly for automated HSS and also classification, was largely learned and also stated to encompass the possible value for detecting pathology precisely in medical applications since the bad outcomes in these stages will ruin or shatter the HS detection system's efficiency. Therefore, the PCG detection issues to implement a new efficient algorithm are required to be discussed. Here, the recently published pre-processing, segmentation, Feature Extractions (FE), and also classification techniques along with their top-notch of PCG signal examination were reviewed. Associated studies are contrasted with their datasets, FE, and the classifiers that they utilized. This effort aims to analyze all the research directions in PCG detection techniques. At the last of this appraisal, several directions for future researches toward PCG signal analysis are rendered.

Keywords Phonocardiogram (PCG) · Cardiac auscultation · Feature extraction · Heart sound segmentation · Classification

1 Introduction

The primary reason for demise athwart the globe will be on account of Cardiovascular Diseases (CVD). In 2008, around 17.3 million populaces died because of heart-related issues, which represent almost 30 (%) of all worldwide deaths. A basic screening tool that is utilized in the prime healthcare for examining the heart's proper

P. Jyothi (✉) · G. Pradeepini
CSE Department, Koneru Lakshmaiah Education Foundation, Vaddeswaram, Vijayawada, AP, India
e-mail: jyophani.reddy@gmail.com

G. Pradeepini
e-mail: pradeepini_cse@kluniversity.in

S. Bhattacharyya et al. (eds.), *International Conference on Intelligent and Smart Computing in Data Analytics*, Advances in Intelligent Systems and Computing 1312,
https://doi.org/10.1007/978-981-33-6176-8_15

functioning is the cardiac auscultation. However, the requirement of trained physicians stands as a major con for this method. In the traditional auscultation technique, there is a chance that the human ears might overlook the lower-frequency elements, such as a murmur, which could be obviously recognized during the spectrogram illustration of the HS. For this, a graphical illustration of the HS has been generated, i.e., PCG, for enhanced elucidation along with the heart-linked disease diagnoses, which serves a means to register the auscultation findings precisely.

Usually, the PCG comprises events, such as S1, S2 —HS for adults (healthy). The S3 as well as S4—associated sounds could be heard in fit elder populace along with kids. These HS elements are the changes that happen in the blood flow's direction inside the heart, which is exhibited in Fig. 1. These HS are formed by the heart valves' vibration as closure as well as opening take place, by means of moves which takes place through mechanical of complete myocardium along with structures of association. Every heartbeat is activated through impulse electrically within the heart that brings about the ventricles and atrium make contract as well as relax alternatively. These HS signals hold the heart's physiological together with pathological traits. Thus, heart diseases are visually emerged in the equivalent PCG signals.

The "4" locations: (a) Aortic, (b) Pulmonic, (c) Tricuspid, and (d) Mitral areas are utmost frequently utilized to listen as well as transduce the HS that are labeled as per the positions through the valves could efficiently will heard. The location of these heart valves along with arteries related to auscultation is exhibited in Fig. 2.

The integration of an assortment of signals pre-processing operations, say signals denoising, signals segmentation FE, together with classification, is vital to make a system for HS signals analysis. The segmentation is utilized for detecting the basic HS, which are the vital physical traits of the heart. The classification's performance [1] is usually centered on the FE and HSS results; thus, the HSS plays a chief part on the automated HS classification.

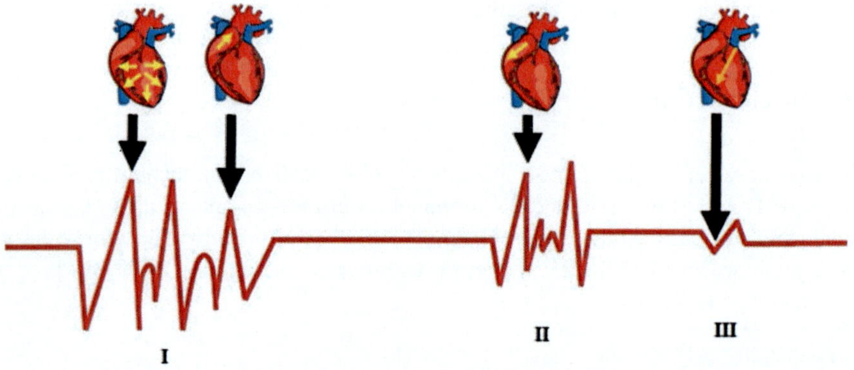

Fig. 1 HS Components representation graphically and changes in corresponding blood flow in the heart

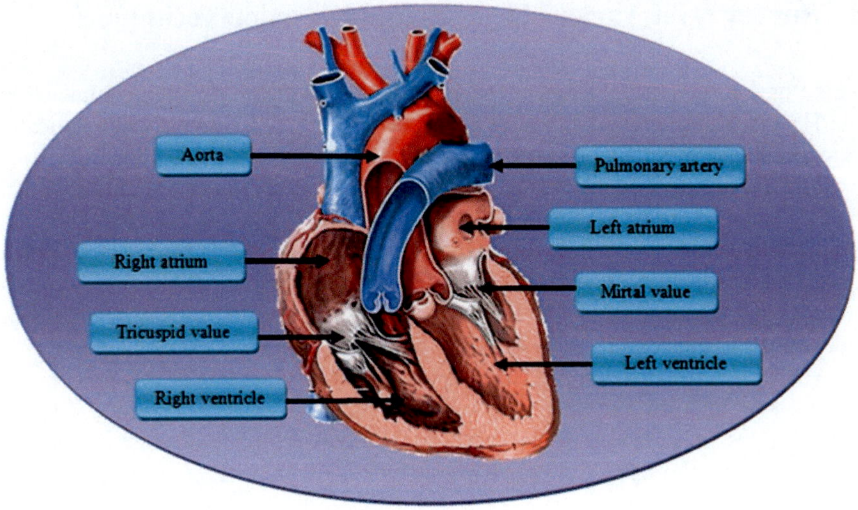

Fig. 2 A view of heart

General structure:

Figure 3 implies the HS detection system's general flow. Figure 3 encompasses "4" phases: (a) pre-processing, (b) segmentation, (c) FE, and the (d) classification model. Primarily, the signal is preprocessed that cleans the signal by means of eradicating the undesirable

frequency together with unwanted noises. The second step of pre-processing is segmentation, which ascertains the boundaries of cardiac cycles as of contiguous HS signals. After that, the FE technique is implemented for dimension reduction. Next, classification is executed to detect the HS.

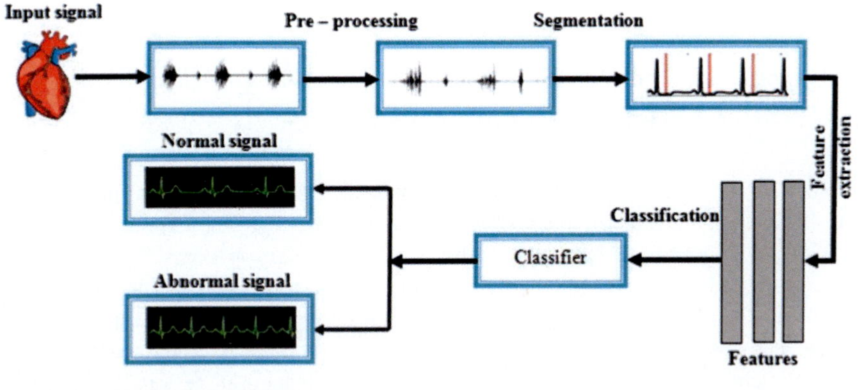

Fig. 3 General structure of HS detection

2 Survey Over Various Heart Sound Detection Techniques

This stage discusses the distinctive research works, which have been completed in the HS detection field. A technique aimed at filtering in addition to automatically categorizing ventricular beats. The implemented Switching Kalmans Filter (SKF) [2] approach facilitated the automated assortment of the utmost possible form, whilst concurrently filtering the signal utilizing suitable preceding knowledge. HS was presented via wavelet packets decomposition trees. Information gauges were stated on the basis of HOC's Wavelet Packet (WP) co-efficients. The propitious outcomes implied that the competency of HOC of WP co-efficients for capturing HS's non-linear traits to be utilized for fundamental assortment.

Analyzing PCG done through technique called digital processing of signal. Information of diagnostic provided through Phonocardiogram (PCG) which evaluates heart failures and defects related to the heart. Normal and abnormal conditions of the heart measured through PCG signals which are unable to hear through human ear.

2.1 Heart Sound Detection Using Empirical Mode Decomposition

An automatic segmentation [3] algorithm aimed at the discovery of the first (diastole-S1) and second (systole-S2) of HS and also the systole period together with diastole period devoid of utilizing the electro-cardiogram references. This work utilized Empirical Modes Decomposition (EMD) [4] for generating intensity envelopes of the principal HS on the time domain. The detection method's sensitivity was 88.3 (%) aimed at S1 in addition to S2; in addition, the precision was 95.8 (%) aimed at S1 as well as S2. The chief cons that the algorithm encompassed were that it concentrated only on detecting HS and not on distinguishing their timing

2.2 Heart Sound Detection Through Tunable Quality Wavelet Transform (TQWT)

Puneet Kumar and Anil Kumar Tiwari rendered a stronger algorithm intended for the PCG segmentation utilizing a Wavelet Transform (WT) termed Tunable Qualities WT (TQWT). In the technique, initially, the PCG was pre-processed to lessen the dimension, and next, the signal was decomposed utilizing TQWT. Then, the Fanos factor was employed to efficiently choose an adaptive level having a low level of noise. The employed adaptive thresholding technique suppressed the level of noise as of the chosen level that enhanced the segmentation accurateness in the presence of noise.

2.3 Heart Sound Detection Using Feature Extraction

Amir Mohammad Amiri and Giuliano Armanowe offered a technique to execute segmentation as well as FE, for separating HS signals in "2" sets: (i) innocent along with (ii) pathological murmurs. The HS's segmentation on single cardiac cycles (i.e,. S1 as well as S2 murmurs) utilized WT along with k-mean clustering approach. Two FE techniques recommended for HS classification. In the primary one, curve fitting was utilized for accomplishing the data embraced in the series of the HS signal. The K-Nearest Neighbor (KNN) classifiers with Euclidean distance were utilized during classification. The recommended FE techniques had high-quality performance contrasted to earlier techniques, for example, Filter banks along with WT. Chiefly, the fractal dimension's performance was considerably improved than the curve fitting technique.

3 Comparative Analysis of Various Segmentation Approaches Used in HS Detection

The HSS aims to recognize the starting and ending of HS. It also targets to segment the S1, diastole, S2, as well as systole for the succeeding FE. Some segmentation technique Hidden Markov Model (HSMM) [5] recommended for addressing issues of accurate initial and secondary HSS within real-world and noisy PCG recordings with performance of 98.28% sensitivity and 98.36% F1-score. Continuous Density—Hidden Morkov Model (**CD-HMM**) based on MSAR, this suggested Markov switching autoregressive model (MSAR) was proffered, which utilized the integration of SKF, the fusion of refined SKF, SKF, and also the SKF-Viterbi (duration-depended Viterbi algorithm) for HS estimation with 90.19% F1 score and 84.2% Accuracy.

HMM—Mel Frequency Cepstrum Co-efficients (**MFCC**) model. Fusion of **HMM** as well as Adaptive Neuro Fuzzy Inference System (**ANFIS**), These suggested classifiers were well-trained utilizing the pre-extracted traits for exactly identifying abnormal and normal heart murmurs with 97.9% acuuracy.

3.1 Heart Sound Detection Based on S-Transform

Ali Moukadem et al. proffered a methodology for HSS centered on S-transform approach. The proffered segmentation strategy has three blocks. In the initial block, the scheme termed SSE computed the local spectrum associated Shannon Energy (SE). S-transform computes this SE for all samples of HS signal. The SE content of such an S-transform of local sounds was optimized by utilizing the windows width optimization algorithm. The S-matrix's single value decomposition was implemented to categorize S1 and also S2. The frequency of HSs made the detection task of higher-frequency signatures extremely difficult.

A scheme for HSs classification utilizing a discrete TF energy trait centered on the approach of S-transform. Initially, the HS signal was denoised utilizing a wavelet threshold denoising strategy with the optimum parameters. The presentation of extra HSs culling operation ameliorated the double threshold (DT) approach. Then, the HS signal containing an extra or murmur HSs was localized and also segmented utilizing the enhanced DT approach.

3.2 Classification Techniques for Heart Sound Detection

The ML usage "Classification" is utilized to effectually classify the inputted patterns onto particular classes. Numerous parameters, namely (a) accuracy of classification, (b) performance of algorithm's, and (c) computational resource are considered for selecting relevant classifiers.

Classification methods of HS detection SVM and KNN classifiers whose features are Total Standard Deviation of signal (ST) having drawback of Complex on account of countless features, Total Variance of signal (VR), and MFCC and AdaBoost [6] whose features are Springer features and Custom features (MFCC, HSMM-QF, etc.) and having drawback of it does not pay attention to long-term recordings. Non-linear **SVM** via Radial Base Function (**RBF)** whose features are time feature and frequency feature having drawback of frequency and spectral features continually alter in respect of time, which makes HSS a hard task.

4 Heart Sound Detection Using Deep Learning Approaches

A 1D CNN [7] framework, which has bifurcated HS signals into abnormal and normal most directly independent ECG. The HS's deep features were well-extracted utilizing the denoising auto-encoder algorithm and sent to the1D CNN as the input feature. The experiential outcomes evinced that the framework utilizing deep traits has the strongest anti-interference competency on considering MFCC. The 1D-CNN framework had top-level accuracy during classification, higher precision, maximal F-score, and even classification ability when contrasted to backpropagation (BP) NN scheme (Table 1).

Discussion: The performance rendered by several HS classification approaches in respect of specificity along with sensitivity is evinced in Fig. 4. For HS classification utilizes the Multi-Level Basis Selection (MLBS) [7] of WP decomposition (WPD), which acquired the sensitivity rate and also specificity rate up to 97.830% and 97.460%, respectively. Subsequently, for HS classification utilize the SKF model, Caffe framework [8] (i.e., convolutional architecture for fast feature embedding), and one dimensional CNN, respectively. The sensitivity rates of are 94.740, 93.120,

Table 1 Comparative analysis of deep learning approaches on HS classification

Author name	Database	Features	Deep learning techniques	Experimental results
Das et al. [9]	PhysioNet/CinCchallenge 2016	MFCC, STFT and Cochleagram	Artificial NN (**NN**)	Accuracy: 95%
Demiret al. [10]	HSs Challenge (CHSC)	Short-time fourier transform (STFT)	Convolutional NN (**CNN**)	Precision: 76% Specificity: 95%
Messner et al. [11]	PhysioNet/CinC challenge 2016	Spectrogram, MFCC and envelope features	Deep recurrent NN (**DRNN**)	F1- score: 96%
Acharya et al. [12]	open-source PhysioBank MIT-BIH Arrhythmia database	Daubechies wavelet	9-layer deep CNN (**DCNN**)	Sensitivity: 96.01% Accuracy: 93.470% Specificity: 91.64%

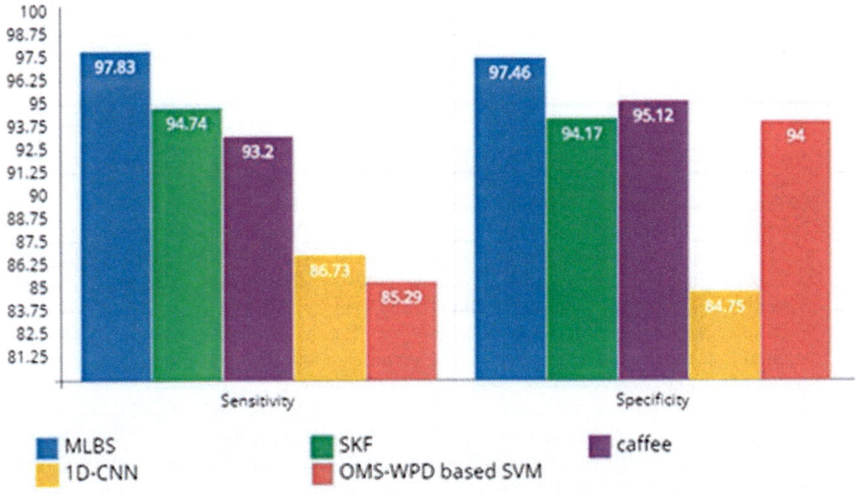

Fig. 4 Performance comparison of various heart sound classification techniques regarding sensitivity and specificity

and 86.730%, respectively, and their specificity rates are 94.17, 95.120, and 84.75%, respectively. OMS-WPD (optimal multi-scale WPD) centric SVM classifier for HS detection, which has the least sensitivity along with specificity values contrasted to other approaches. Heart sound signals recorded through various electrical devices are motivated for efficiency in detecting

1. Various heart-related diseases identified at earlier stage through efficient techniques with CNN
2. Efficient algorithms used for detecting the cause of specific heart-related disease identified through objective 1

5 Conclusion

Auscultation is the utmost utilized technique for recognizing CVDs, which is the chief cause of death all through the globe. This paper renders a literature survey on disparate segmentation and classification approaches related to HS detection; the importance of HS detection is also detailed and as well the various sorts of heart detection process and their limitations are briefly discussed. This literature work enlightens disparate existing approaches of HS detection suggested by diverse researchers, which assists the researchers for the forthcoming effort in this specific area. On examining the survey, deep learning-centric HS detection approaches are more accurate when contrasted to other algorithms. But, the requisite of high training time is the major demerit of deep learning approaches. Hence, the future directions grounded in this survey are the investigation of optimized deep learning methodologies with reduced training time to enhance system efficiency.

References

1. Bangare SL, Pradeepini G, Patil ST (2017) Brain tumor classification using mixed approach. In: 2017 International conference on information communication and embedded systems, ICICES
2. Ghahjaverestan NM, Ge D, Hernández AI, Shamsollahi MB (2015) Switching kalman filter based methods for apnea bradycardia detection from ECG signals. Physiol Meas 36(9):1763
3. Inthiyaz S, Madhav BTP, Kishore PVV (2018) Flower image segmentation with PCA fused colored covariance and gabor texture features based level sets. Ain Shams Eng J 9(4):3277–3291
4. Bajelani K, Navidbakhsh M, Behnam H, Doyle JD, Hassani K (2013) Detection and identification of first and second heart sounds using empirical mode decomposition. Proc Inst Mech Eng Part H: J Eng Med 227(9):976–987
5. Kamson AP, Sharma LN, Dandapat S (2019) Multi-centroid diastolic duration distribution based HSMM for heart sound segmentation. Biomed Signal Process Control 48:265–272
6. Shi K, Schellenberger S, Michler F, Steigleder T, Malessa A, Lurz F, Koelpin A (2019) Automatic signal quality index determination of radar-recorded heart sound signals using ensemble classification. IEEE Trans Biomed Eng 67(3):773–785
7. Fatemeh S, Shyamala D, Azreen A, Azrul J, Ramaiah ARA (2013) Multi-level basis selection of wavelet packet decomposition tree for heart sound classification. Comput Biol Med 43(10):1407–1414
8. Dominguez-Morales JP, Jimenez-Moreno MJG, Jimenez-Fernandez AF (2017) Deep neural networks for the recognition and classification of heart murmurs using neuromorphic auditory sensors. IEEE Trans Biomed Circuits Syst 12(1):24–34
9. Das S, Pal S, Mitra M (2019) Supervised model for Cochleagram feature based fundamental heart sound identification. Biomed Signal Process Control 52:32–40
10. Demir F, Şengür A, Bajaj V, Polat K (2019) Towards the classification of heart sounds based on convolutional deep neural network. Health Info Sci Syst 7(1):16

11. Messner E, Zöhrer M, Pernkopf F (2018) Heart sound segmentation—an event detection approach using deep recurrent neural networks. IEEE Trans Biomed Eng 65(9):1964–1974
12. Acharya UR, Oh SL, Hagiwara Y, Tan JH, Adam M, Gertych A, San Tan R (2017) A deep convolutional neural network model to classify heartbeats. Comput Biol Med 89:389–396

Fast Medicinal Leaf Retrieval Using CapsNet

Sandeep Dwarkanath Pande and Manna Sheela Rani Chetty

Abstract Geometrical feature descriptors that describes the shape of the object are efficiently used for image feature delineation in several image recognition applications. The proposed approach implements a medicinal leaf classification system using a Bezier curve and CapsNet. A new feature vector consisting of control points (CP) of a Bezier curve and discrete fourier transform (DFT) is proposed. It also proposes a novel approach for the CP detection for feature representation. The extracted CPs are further used to find out the DFT. CPs and DFTs are further used to train the CapsNet for image classification. The CapsNet is trained to classify the input image to a particular class within a desired range of similarity. The proposed system is compared with other classification systems and the comparison reveals that the proposed system outperforms other classification systems in many parameters.

Keywords Bezier curve · CapsNet · Control point extraction · Leaf retrieval · Discrete fourier transform

1 Introduction

Plants plays a crucial role in our environment. Huge number of plant species are found in the universe. Plants are an integral part of our life. India is one of the countries having largest biodiversity. Thousands of plant species found in India are having medicinal properties. Currently, numerous plant species are at the threat of their extinguishment. An effective and efficient leaf retrieval and classification system is always crucial to recognize the plants species of user's interest based on query. Essentially, leaf retrieval is playing a crucial role in gaining visual information and imparting

S. D. Pande (✉) · M. S. R. Chetty
Department of Computer Science and Engineering, Koneru Lakshmaiah Education Foundation, Vaddeswaram, AP, India
e-mail: sandeep7887pande@gmail.com

M. S. R. Chetty
e-mail: sheelarani_cse@kluniversity.in

S. Bhattacharyya et al. (eds.), *International Conference on Intelligent and Smart Computing in Data Analytics*, Advances in Intelligent Systems and Computing 1312,
https://doi.org/10.1007/978-981-33-6176-8_16

knowledge through it. Representation of image feature has a vital role in the accuracy of image retrieval application. Feature representation is established based on the content of an image where, color, texture, or shape descriptions are employed for its representation. The accuracy of the approaches depends on the retrieval algorithm and the representative features. Shape representation has an advantage of low complexity coding effort for image representation. These features are dominantly been used in current image retrieval system. Various methods were developed to achieve the objective of faster retrieval with better accuracy in topological representation. Shape, color, and texture features are employed in most of the preceding re-searches for plant breed classification by making use of images of a leaf. In [1], the combination of geometrics features, color moments, vein features are used to generate FD as a feature vector and lacunarity-based texture features. Further, it feeds these features to the PNN classifier for leaf classification. An approach using multiscale triangles describing local features of the shape contour points of the leaf; multiscale triangular representation (MTR) is presented in [2]. CNN and machine learning are used in [3] for medicinal leaf classification. It uses leaf area, diameter, length, perimeter, and width, as a feature for CNN and SVM, Naïve Bayes, K-NN, discrimination for classification. In [4], the leaf classification is attained by employing a k-NN classifier. The method considers a vast number of features; hence, it is an older and complex approach. In [5], various components are combined hierarchically to form a robust and strong classifier for spectral information. The authors of [6] have proposed NN method and combined thresholding for extraction of vein patterns from leaf images. In [7], Beziers curves are used to represent the tip and base as a representative feature. It involves many trigonometric and approximation computations to obtain the feature vector. The shape descriptors used as a feature large in count which takes large memory storage and higher search overhead. The larger descriptive feature also leads to higher probable misclassification in recognition. The constraint of feature representation is focused, and a new feature extraction method based on CP representation is developed. This paper outlines a linear coding approach in CP extraction for high variant feature description.

2 Proposed Approach

The shapes considered in research work are outlines of leaf images which are open or closed curves in a single plane. Here, dataset of images of leaves of hundred species is used. There are total 1600 images for 100 species. Many of species which are listed here are having medicinal applications.

2.1 Pre-processing

The pre-processing stage outputs the boundary co-ordinates of shape present in the input image. The first step is binarization of the shape image that converts the gray level image to binary. The shapes obtained are sometimes corrupted; hence, a denoising step is applied. To get boundary, latest marching squares algorithm is used [8, 9]. Further, 10 segments are generated, and CPs for each segment are extracted using the contour co-ordinates ($x(u)$, $y(u)$). The curvature coding is applied to extract the shape features, defining dominant curve regions. The curvature, C, for a given contour co-ordinates (x, y) defined by [10] is given by,

$$C(i) = \frac{x'(i)y''(i) - y'(i)x''(i)}{\left[x'(i)^2 + y'(i)^2\right]^{3/2}} \tag{1}$$

Here, (x', y') and (x'', y'') represents first and second derivative of x, y contour co-ordinates, respectively. This curvature represents the curvature pattern for the extracted contour. A smoothening of the contour reveals in the dominant curvature patterns. The curvature C with the Gaussian factor is defined by [9],

$$C(i,\sigma) = \frac{\left(G'_x(i,\sigma)G''_y(i,\sigma)\right) - \left(G''_x(i,\sigma)G'_y(i,\sigma)\right)}{\left(G'_x(i,\sigma)^2 + G''_y(i,\sigma)^2\right)^{3/2}} \tag{2}$$

Wherein, the CPs are developed over the fitting curvature. An iterative process was carried out to derive the tangential variation points over the boundary regions. The process is, however, iterative and results in large overhead, as well leads to selection of over biased or under biased edge regions. To overcome the selection issue, a linear interpolation of the boundary region is developed. This approach transforms the extracted curvature to a linear plane and performs a CP extraction based on a max-peak threshold. The CPs are extracted as a max-peak (Mp) threshold, where the point is derived based on the maximum curvature limit obtained for an image. A threshold based on the max-peak level is derived as a 50% of the derived value to declare the peak as CP. The peak limits above the threshold margin are taken as the CPs. Here, the selection achieves two main objectives, (1) The iteration overhead of tangential search is eliminated, (2) the misclassification of dominant curvatures in image representation was overcome by thresholding over the max-peak value. This process leads to more accurate CP selection and, hence, the representative feature [9]. The CPs of Bezier and extreme points of each segment of the leaf image are used as shape signature to compute the DFTs. A fast fourier transform algorithm is used to compute the DFTs efficiently. DFT converts a signal from time or space band to frequency band and conversely. These shape descriptors store the local shape features in time and frequency band and are capable to differentiate small variations in patterns [11].

2.2 *CapsNet Design and Training Process*

Sequence of multiple convolutional kernels bundled together is known as a capsule. Capsule networks consists of large number of these capsules. Each capsule operates at local level of features. Global understanding of features is done by communication between various capsules using routing paths [12]. In this experiment, input size is kept as 10 by 10. As the input size is small, first layer kernel size is set to 3 by 3. Also, reduction in input is not required, so stride is kept as 1. Number of outputs from first layer are set to 256. In second layer, 24 primary capsules are used together. Again, kernel size is kept to be 3 by 3. 256 outputs from previous layer act as input to this layer. There can be three stages of routing possible. Output layer has capsules same to the number of classes in input data. Training dataset of all images converted in forms of DFTs is used as input to CapsNet. Each image is pre-processed and its CPs along with DFTs are extracted. The DFT values in a matrix form act as a single input. So, training set of all such matrices extracted from all training images is used.

3 Experimental Setup and Results

The pre-processing gives set of curve points which represents boundary of a shape or object. It is further divided into 10 segments. The pin pointed approach detects CPs in lesser iterations. The generated CPs are used to derive Bezier whose curve points considered to compute the DFTs as an optimal feature vector. For each segment, 10 such 100 DFTs are calculated. Then, these DFTs are used to train the CapsNet to classify the images. All steps of proposed work are shown in Fig. 1. The proposed approach is implemented in Python 3.7 with the help of Tensorflow GPU [13] library and Keras software. Simulations are performed on three laptops as given in Table 2.

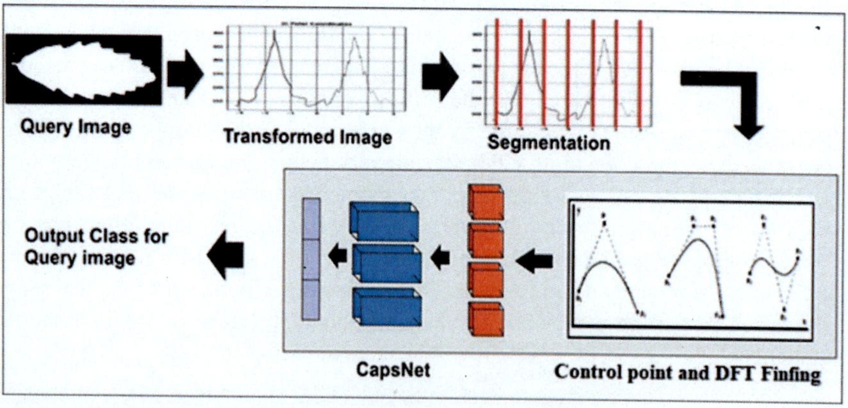

Fig. 1 Algorithm flow

The performance is evaluated and compared. It is noticed that the image processing techniques works better on GPUs [14].

3.1 Evaluation Parameters

The proposed approach's performance is assessed in terms widely used evaluation parameter for CBLC systems termed as accuracy. It can be defined mathematically as:

$$\text{Accuracy} = \frac{\text{Number of correctly classified images}}{\text{Total number of testing images}} * 100 \tag{3}$$

The proposed approach is compared in the regard of performance with those of various pioneer shape-based image retrieval methods, identified as MTR [2], and hierarchical approach using multiple descriptors [5]. Multiple iterations are performed on dataset with different samples. Then, results are averaged out as mean results. These results are compared with existing techniques and are shown in Table 1. Proposed method has high accuracy. The proposed method outperforms in processing time due to the efficient method used for CP generation and also reduced processing time in feature matching due to the use of DFTs in CapsNet. Table 2 shows the training time

Table 1 Results from leaf dataset

Plant Species Names	Images classified correctly	Images classified incorrectly	Accuracy		
			MTR [2]	Hierarchical [5]	Proposed
Acer Opalus	33	02	93.4	93.8	97.7
Magnolia Salicifolia	32	03	90.6	90.2	97.5
Acer Palmatum	34	01	96	95.1	95.1
Betula Austrosinensis	31	04	86.6	90.6	97.5
Quercus Afares	32	03	89.2	88.2	95.5

Table 2 Training time for CPU and GPGPU

Sr. No.	System configuration	Training time (Seconds)
1	Core i5 Processor, 8 GB RAM	1272.1479
2	Core i7 Processor, 8 GB RAM	1141.2731
3	Core i7 Processor, Nvidia GeForce GTX 860 m 4 GB GPU, 8 GB RAM	140.6436

required to execute the proposed approach. The proposed approach gives superior results on GPGPU than CPU.

4 Conclusion

This research work has designed a framework that implements a linear coding of Bezier curve CP computation for image retrieval, a linear transformation and a feature selection approach for geometrical feature representation. Here, novel way of using CPs as shape signature of an object is proposed. To detect the CPs, new and efficient approach are used. This approach minimizes the processing overhead and search delay by reducing feature vector size. The proposed approach has an advantage of distortion suppression and dominant feature extraction. Generated CPs are further transformed into optimal feature vector DFT. In this approach, from image, only DFTs are selected as input for the CapsNet so it takes less time for training. This approach is position and orientation invariant. Due to all these reasons proposed method outperforms others in terms of computation complexity and memory efficiency. Results prove that proposed method achieves feature selection accuracy. The research work obtains better results, performance, and acceptable accuracy compared to other CBLC systems.

References

1. Kadir A, Nugroho L, Susanto A, Santosa P (2011) Leaf classification using shape, color, and texture features. Int J Comput Trends Technol 1(3):306–311
2. Moune S, Yahiaoui I, Verroust A (2013) A shape-based approach for leaf classification using multiscale triangular representation. In: Proceedings of the 3rd ACM conference on International conference on multimedia retrieval (ICMR'13), New York, USA, pp 127–134
3. Caoa J, Wanga B, Brown D (2016) Similarity based Leaf Image retrieval using multiscale R-Angle sescription. Inf Sci 374:51–64
4. Mallah C, Cope J, Orwell J (2013) Plant leaf classification using probabilistic integration of shape, texture and margin features. In: Proceedings of the international conference on signal processing, pattern recognition and applications, Innsbruck, Austria, pp 279–286
5. Chaki J, Parekh R, Bhattacharya S (2018) Plant leaf classification using multiple descriptors: a hierarchical approach. J King Saud Univer-Comput Info Sci
6. Fu H, Chi Z (2006) Combined thresholding and neural network approach for vein pattern extraction from leaf images. IEEE Proceed Visual Image and Signal Process 153(6):881–892, IEEE
7. Cerutti G, Tougne L, Mille J, Vacavant A, Coquin D (2013) Understanding leaves in natural images—a model-based approach for tree species identification. Comput Vis Image Understand 117(10):1482–1501
8. Pande SD, Chetty MSR (2019) Position invariant spline curve based image retrieval using control points. Int J Intell Eng Syst 12(4):177–191
9. Pande SD, Chetty MSR (2020) Linear bezier curve geometrical feature descriptor for image recognition. Recent Adv Comput Sci Commun 13(5):1–12

10. Abbasi S, Mokhtarian F, Kittler J (1999) Curvature scale space image in shape similarity retrieval. Multimedia Syst 7(6):467–476
11. Winograd S (1978) On computing the discrete fourier transform. Math Comput 32(141):175–199
12. Pande SD, Chetty MSR (2018) Analysis of capsule network (Capsnet) architectures and applications. J Adv Res Dynam Control Syst 10(10):2765–2771
13. Abadi M, Barham P, Chen J, Chen Z, Davis A, Dean J (2016) Tensorflow: a system for large-scale machine learning. In: Proceedings of 12th the USENIX symposium on OS design and Implementation, Savannah, GA, USA, pp 265–283
14. Kulkarni JB, Chetty MSR (2017) Depth map generation from stereoscopic images using stereo matching on GPGPU. J Adv Res Dynam Control Syst 9(18):736–747

Risk Analysis in Movie Recommendation System Based on Collaborative Filtering

Subham Gupta, Koduganti Venkata Rao, Nagamalleswari Dubba, and Kodukula Subrahmanyam

Abstract The main aim of any project or software is to provide customer satisfaction at the end. The problem in Movie Recommendation System is unusual recommendation of movies to users, i.e., liking and disliking of recommended movie. This problem or risk impacts customer satisfaction, as a result of which the software will not be used much by the end users, and the company will be in huge loss. So, this paper provides you a detail description of recommendation system, steps of how to analyze risks and how to tackle or mitigate them using genetic algorithm based on collaborative filtering approach. Single and multiobjectives were implemented.

Keywords Recommendation system (RS) · Collaborative filtering (CF) · Risk management · Genetic algorithm (GA)

1 Recommendation System

The recommender framework is a brilliant separating apparatus for producing a rundown of potential of most loved things for the client to diminish the time required by client to pick among countless decisions in sites and encourage the procedure recommendations for books on Amazon or motion pictures on Netflix are certifiable instances of the activity of industries quality recommender frameworks, and the structure of such proposal motors relies upon the area of the information accessible [1].

In this paper, we propose a recommendation system that enables the user to watch a movie among many movies that are available by providing him a list of movies as per the interest of the user [2]. The recommendation system is a tool for generating a list of potential favorite items for the user to reduce time and also reduce the

S. Gupta · N. Dubba (✉) · K. Subrahmanyam
Koneru Lakshmaiah Education Foundation, Vaddeswaram, AP, India
e-mail: nagamalleswary@kluniversity.in

K. V. Rao
Vignan's Institute of Information Technology, Visakhapatnam, AP, India

S. Bhattacharyya et al. (eds.), *International Conference on Intelligent and Smart Computing in Data Analytics*, Advances in Intelligent Systems and Computing 1312,
https://doi.org/10.1007/978-981-33-6176-8_17

ambiguity of the user [3]. It reduces the time needed by the user to choose among a huge number of choices in Web sites and facilitate the process.

There are many algorithms proposed for the development of a recommendation system [4, 5]. For our project, we are using the adaptive genetic algorithm and collaborative filtering for the development of a recommendation system. Genetic algorithm uses biologically inspired techniques such as genetic inheritance, natural selection, mutation and reproduction to give the best possible solution of the given problem [6].

1.1 Types of Recommendation System

The below diagram shows types of recommendation system (Fig. 1):

2 Implementation

The implementation of our project is basically done in two phases: First one is using single objective optimization using Java, and the other one is multiobjective optimization using Python.

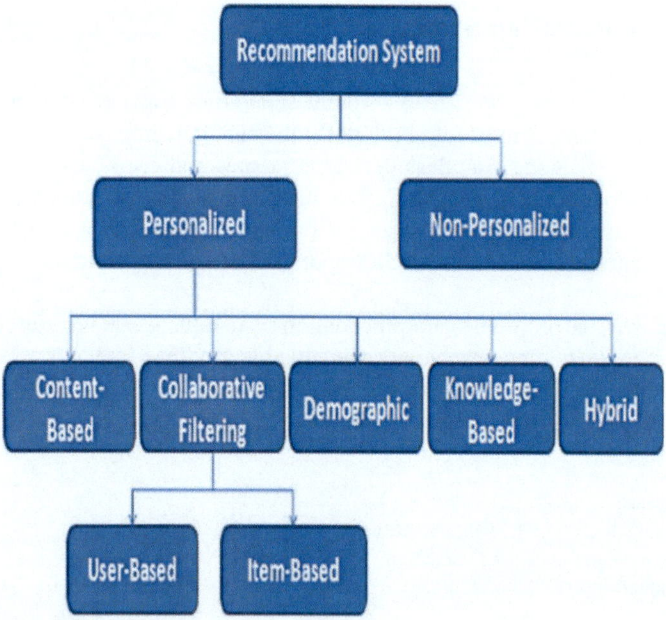

Fig. 1 Types of recommendation system

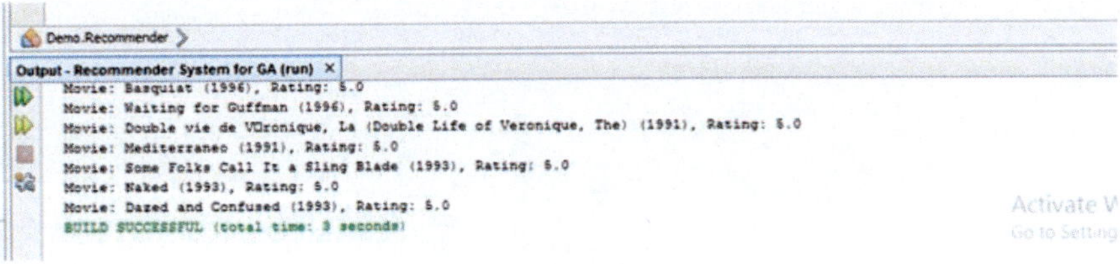

Fig. 2 Screenshots of result of movie recommended in every 3 s

2.1 *Single Objective Using Java*

So far in our project, we have implemented single objective recommendation system algorithm for finding out the result (movie recommended on rating levels) of Movie Recommendation System project. The code of our project has been implemented in Java programming language which consists of different datasets like movies dataset, ratings dataset, tags dataset and links dataset. These datasets have different attributes [7]. As per our project, the datasets are used to analyze the rating given by users for different movies of different genres.

Our algorithm uses genetic algorithm and performed on rating levels [8, 9]. Based on rating levels, different movies of different genres are recommended to one another where a user may or may not like the recommended one. Some people like comedy movie, some like fantasy movie, some like adventure movie, some like action movie and many more. For example: if two persons have given same rating, then the movies watched by one person are recommended to the other one and vice versa. This creates a problem in liking or disliking of recommended movie. This is one of the risks which may create problem in Movie Recommendation System Project [9, 10, 11] (Fig. 2).

2.2 *Multiobjective Using Python*

We move forward to implement multiobjective algorithms for analysis of Movie Recommendation System on same datasets (links.csv, movies.csv, ratings.csv and tags.csv). The analysis is done based on its performance and also how to tackle the problem which we have in single objective algorithm [12]. Here, it is done by using Python programming language on Jupyter platform. Not only this, we have used different libraries of Python for implementing this project, namely pandas, numpy, pickle, scipy, keras and matrix_factorization_utilities [10]. The data is retrieved from every dataset using pandas library and is analyzed one after another. For example: the movie data is retrieved from movies dataset. After the data is retrieved, we started performing some analysis on these datasets using graph, i.e., visualization to know more on values of each dataset. For visualization, we have used Seaborn library of Python. We have plotted many graphs which shows the distribution and variation on each data [13] (Fig. 3).

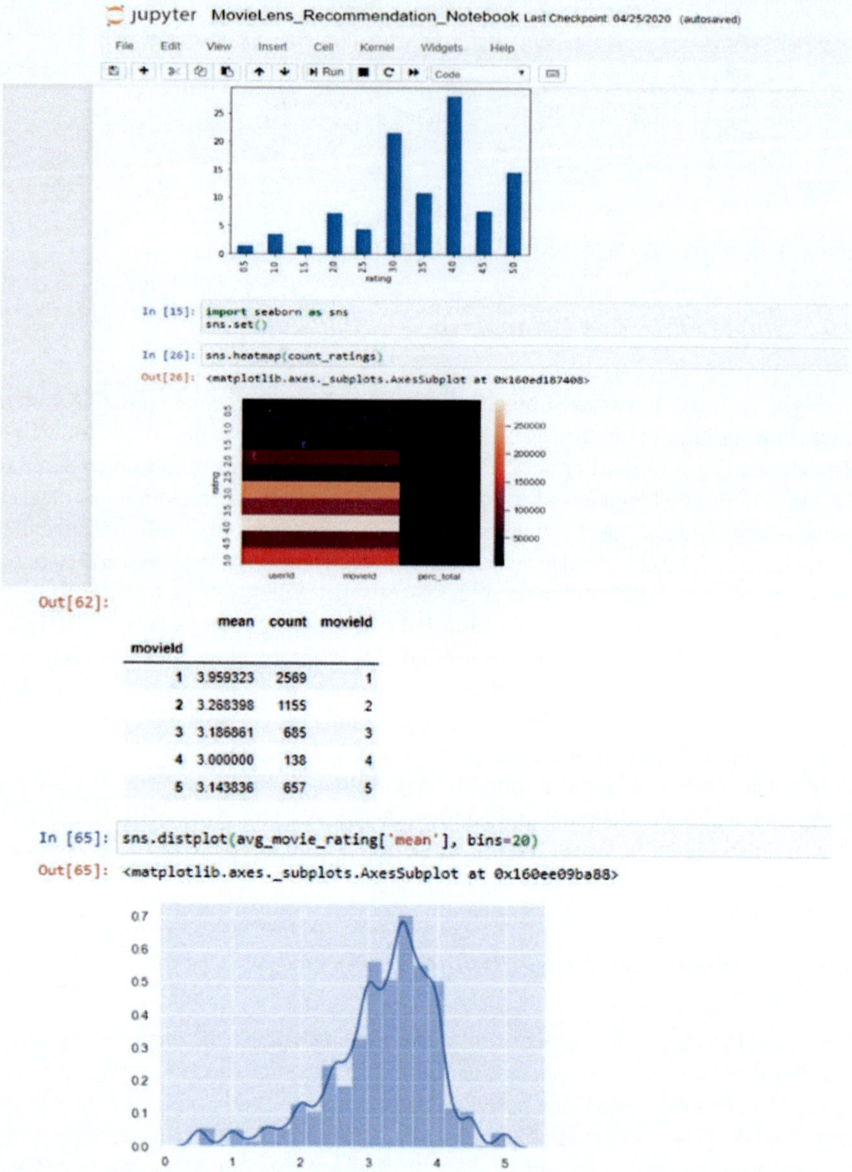

Fig. 3 Screenshots of project analysis using ANN (genetic algorithm and collaborative filtering approach)

After the visualization is done, we moved forward toward the implementation of our project using collaborative filtering approach [4, 14]. In this module, we have grouped different movies which are in same category or genres, i.e., forming clustering [15]. Once the cluster is formed, the movies are again analyzed based on the rating levels so that the best movies of a particular genres will be recommended to other viewers, i.e., the comedy viewing users can only recommend movie to other comedy viewing users. They are restricted to their clusters or groups. Thereby, the problem of undesirable recommendation is eradicated by using above approach. The resultant output is plotted in the bar graph or pie chart format to show the output of analyzed data in pictorial representation [13]. The artificial neural network and deep learning concepts are used in our project for the prediction of desirable result for the users in our project.

Some of the analysis of Movie Recommendation System project is shown in Fig. 3.

3 Conclusion

Depending upon the requirement of the problem, different types of recommendation systems are available and can be developed. We also have different algorithms for the development of these recommendation systems such as genetic algorithm and k-means clustering algorithm. These are all artificial neural network (ANN) algorithms.

Our algorithm (genetic algorithm and collaborative filtering approach) works on rating levels. Based on rating levels, different movies of different genres are recommended to one another where a user may or may not like the recommended one. This creates a problem in liking or disliking of recommended movie which is one of the main problems that arises in our project and is solved using multiobjective optimization recommendation system. Thereby, the problem of undesirable recommendation is eradicated by using artificial neural network in which we have implemented genetic algorithm and collaborative filtering approach as mentioned above in Python programming.

References

1. Arora G, Kumar A, Sanjay Devre G, Ghumare A (2014) Movie recommendation system based on users similarity. Int J Comput Sci Mobile Comput 3(4):765–770
2. Kodali S, Dabbiru M, Rao BT (2019) A cuisine based recommender system using k-NN And mapreduce approach. Int J Innov Technol Explor Eng 8(7):32–36
3. Naga Malleswari D, Suresh Babu S, Moparthi NR, Mandhala VN, Bhattacharyya D (2017) Hash based indexing in running high dimensional software systems. J Adv Res Dynam Control Syst 16(S):34–43

4. Selvaraj P, Burugari VK, Sumathi D, Nayak RK, Tripathy R (2019) Ontology based recommendation system for domain specific seekers. In: Proceedings of the 3rd international conference on I-SMAC IoT in social, mobile, analytics and cloud, I-SMAC 2019, pp 341–345
5. Prasanna KNL, Naresh K, Hari Kiran V (2019) A hybrid collaborative filtering for tag based movie recommendation system. Int J Innov Technol Explor Eng 8(7):1039–1042
6. Krishna BC, Subrahmanyam K (2016) A decision support system for assessing risk using halstead approach and principal component analysis. J Chem Pharm Sci 9(4):3383–3387
7. Rupa Radhika Jahnavi S, Kiran Kumar K, Sai Hareesh T (2018) A semantic web based filtering techniques through web service recommendation. Int J Eng Technol (UAE) 7(2):41–43
8. Dubba N, Kodukula S, Srinivasa Reddy TS, Vijaya Saradhi T (2014) Risk management in information systems through secure image authentication using quick response code. Int J Appl Eng Res 9(24):29075–29089
9. NagaMalleswari D, Subrahmanyam K (2019) Validation of SIS framework using ASP/JSP based information system. Int J Innov Technol Explor Eng 8(6):323–326
10. Chaitanya Krishna B, Subrahmanyam K, Kim T-H (2015) A dependency analysis for information security and risk management. Int J Secur its Appl 9(8):205–210
11. Abhigna RS, Sandeep V, Krishna BC (2019) Analysis of risk management through qualitative approach. Int J Innov Technol Explor Eng 8(6):128–132
12. Venkata Raghava Rao Y, Burri RD, Prasad VBVN (2019) Machine learning methods for software defect prediction a revisit. Int J Innov Technol Explor Eng 8(8):3431–3435
13. Sreedevi E, Prasanth Y (2018) A novel ensemble feature selection and software defect detection model on promise defect datasets. Int J Recent Technol Eng 8(1):3131–3136
14. Subramaniyaswamy V, Logesh R, Chandrasekhar M, Challa A, Vijayakumar V (2017) A personalised movie recommendation system based on collaborative filtering. Int J High Perform Comput Netw 10(1–2)
15. Kousar Nikhath A, Subrahmanyam K (2018) Conceptual relevance based document clustering using concept utility scale. Asian J Sci Res 11(1):22–31

Difficult on Addressing Security: A Security Requirement Framework

Nikhat Parveen and Mazhar Khaliq

Abstract For any security updation, software must be secure that can be analyzed at the early stage of requirements. All security analysis is prejudiced approach which follows certain rules, defined-laws. Models and policies made the software worthwhile. However, in today scenario, still there is a deficiency in security requirements. It has been observed that to capture security requirement a business goals must be fulfilled that helps to protect assets from threats. This is the reality that any security violation is caused openly by vulnerable software. A scrupulous review has carried out regarding the fact as there are many approaches that consists of policy, rules or any guidelines for secure requirement phase. Therefore, it is desirable to develop a prescriptive framework that addresses security at requirement phase. The chronological approach of security requirement framework is presented that helps security experts to analyze security and mitigate threat at requirement phase.

Keywords Software security · Security requirement engineering · Risk analysis · Requirements engineering · Security requirements · Argumentation

1 Introduction of the Security

Security is the most concerned parameters of any individual life and the present scenario has become very difficult to safeguard the privacy of information and services secure especially in IT infrastructure. There are numerous flaws and faults which make the software vulnerable and this flaw help the various hackers to take the advantage of these loop holes. Security in secure software for a computer system typically for the malicious purposes such as installing malware [1]. There are so many various types of the vulnerability presented in a secure software application

N. Parveen (✉)
Department of C.S.E, Koneru Lakshmaiah Education Foundation, Vaddeswaram, AP, India
e-mail: nikhat0891@gmail.com

M. Khaliq
Department of C.S.I.T, Khwaja Moinuddin Chishti Urdu, Arabi~Farsi University, Lucknow, UP, India

S. Bhattacharyya et al. (eds.), *International Conference on Intelligent and Smart Computing in Data Analytics*, Advances in Intelligent Systems and Computing 1312,
https://doi.org/10.1007/978-981-33-6176-8_18

where till now the security is not concerned as an important phase [2]. Requirement engineering process is the initial phase for the fundamental principle of the secure software development to build high level of security for the major advantage of the projects and to offer the best platform to building the secure software in software development life cycle [3, 4].

According to the author the Security Requirements Engineering (SRE) is a technique that supports interlink of model building and examination that considers thinking about incremental models. SRE method includes threat modelling, risk analysis, security requirement specification and security requirements review [5]. This paper scrutinizes how to decide sufficient security requirements for a framework. Security requirements must think about of engineer understood or express presumption that a target of the framework will act not surprisingly. This paper succinct and bring together our past work to shape a system which demonstrates how our prior commitments can be connected together rationally and adequately.

2 The Need of Software Security and Existing Research Approach

Software security is actually tied in with understanding software that initiated with security dangers and how to deal with the hazard when risk happens [5] the primary goal of software security is to prepare a shield from unauthorized access and wicked approach. The way toward dealing with security component and prerequisite of security is to analyze and utilized software engineers to enhance security of software. Software security process includes analyze, planning, preparing, act accordingly, testing and executing of secure software.

According to various literature surveys on security requirements, the survey reveals that it is an expensive task to maintain security at every stage of software development. The various number of software development life cycle (SDLC) have been presented in the literature which can be discuss in Table 1. These approaches which used for security requirements are SQUARE Approach, Agile Development, Haley Framework, CLASP Approach, Microsoft Trustworthy Computing, Axelle Apvrille and Makan Pourzandi Approach, SREP, Gary McGraw's Approach, TSP Approach AEGIS, RUPs:, Oracle's Approach (OSSA).

An exhaustive review of literature reveals that there is no such lifecycle, tool or model exists for security of software requirements. Hence, there is a high demand to develop such a lifecycle that can maintain security early in the development of life cycle. Developments of an application with prior knowledge of security are much safer than those applications where the security is an afterthought [10]. The techniques that are used in security are basically to develop secure information, design phase, coding phase or any other communication that are affected through threats. Researchers and Developers working in the field of Software Security Engineering

Table 1 Summary of security requirement approaches

S. No.	Approach	Description	Phases involved
1	SQUARE approach	Processes security requirement engineering. The team member of requirement elicitation plays important role in order to retrieve security concerns with communicating between the IT stakeholders and requirement engineers [6]	• Consent on definitions • Extract security goals and artifacts • Perform risk assessment • Choose elicitation technique • Classify security requirements • Categorize and Prioritize requirements • Examine requirements
2	Agile development	It includes security requirements and promotes continuous iteration of development and testing procedure [7]	• Identify critical assets, • prepare abuser stories, • Consider abuser story risk, • Consent abuser • User stories, • Define security-related user stories
3	Haley framework	Based on iteration techniques. Iterate between requirement and design activities	• Identify functional requirements • Identify security requirements • Identify security goals that include assets, threats, and business goals • Systems verify
4	CLASP approach	Follows 30 process that incorporate security requirements engineering [8]	• To verify risk mitigations • To determine deficiencies • Avoid conflicts • Identify resources and Develop trust boundaries
5	Microsoft software development life cycle	Effort on security activities on every phase of Microsoft's software development process [9]	• Classify assets., • Classify dependencies, • Classify threats • Classify use scenarios
6	Axelle Apvrille and Makan Pourzandi Approch	Incorporate security requirements during analysis phase. [10]	• Identify the security environments • Identify security objectives to determine threat model. • select security policy and prioritize sensitive information's • Evaluate risk

(continued)

Table 1 (continued)

S. No.	Approach	Description	Phases involved
7	Security requirement engineering process approach	Consists of nine-step, similar to SQUARE but incorporates Common Criteria and notions of reusability. [11]	• Consent on definitions, • Identify critical assets, • Classify security objectives, • Elicit threats, develop artifacts and risk estimation • Elicit security requirements prioritize requirements, • Requirements examination, • Repository improvement
8	Gary McGraw's approach	Building Security and describes Seven Touch points for Software Security [3]	• Code review and Architectural threat analysis, • Penetration testing, Threat-based security tests • Abuse cases • Security requirements and Security process.
9	Team software process	Produced by SEI's Team consists of set of operational process [12] restricted methods applied on software engineering principles	• Elicit security risks, security requirements and secure design, • Code reviews, entity testing, fuzz testing, • Static code analysis
10	Secure software development model	To integrate software engineering process with security engineering [13]	• Built-in model, • Threat modeling, • Security design prototype • Secure coding guidelines
11	Appropriate and effective guidance for information security	Term to be lightweight process. Wrap into any software development life cycle process. Application as Spiral model of software engineering [14]	• Determination of adherent faults • Determination of of an attack in organize environment • Multiplicity of security requirements based on security expert's advice • Cost-benefit assessment • Comparison between cost and attack against the cost of security requirements • Choice of security requirements based on cost effectiveness

(continued)

Table 1 (continued)

S. No.	Approach	Description	Phases involved
12	Rational unified process	A software development **process** from IBM based on iterative process. It divides the Development involve business **modelling**, analysis and design, implementation, testing, and deployment [15]	• Build software iteratively • Manage requirements • Apply element-based architectures • Visualize model • Verify quality • Control change
13	Oracle's approach (OSSA):	Comprehensive set of security assurance both for customer system and control products [16]	• To progress effectiveness of security method • To decrease probability of security vulnerabilities [17]

have paying attention are so-called best practice in the software lifecycle process [18].

3 Framework for Software Security in Requirement Phase

In order to develop a framework for security requirement, the researcher should keep following points in mind while considering: -

- Analysis the absence and benefits of security in requirement phase
- To study existing problems and overcome with new approach
- Comparison with all the valuable techniques with existing approaches and applied new security framework
- To maximize the advantage for the security benefits in requirement phases

Based on above consideration the good software industry and developer can develop a framework for security perspectives in initially phase of the SDLC. The Security framework for Requirement phase engineering is necessary for all the secure applications which based on technically and main motive to communicate, manage the basic requirement for any secure software.

4 The Proposed Security Requirement Framework (SRF)

In reflection to necessities and significance of construe software security, a prescriptive framework is proposed. The framework might be utilized as a part of requirement stage to anticipate software security quantitatively. The Objective of Security Requirement Framework (SRF) is to give anomalous state assurance against the impotence and risk to product that contributes the relief of security disappointments.

The most unnoticed part during development of secure software is security requirement. Unfortunately, the security is being considered as technical issue that should be handled at design or implementation phase of the software. The high-level protection against the susceptibility and threat to the software is the major contribution to mitigate security failures

5 The FrameWork

Secure System can be managed only by formal and statistical methods. It is true that if complex process is involved in any system engineering then formal methods are seldom used to improve security risk of a system [8, 19]. Formal methods can be generalized during security analysis and can be used as tools for minimizing security risk of a system [20, 21]. It's an ancient archetype that to control any activity, it is firstly to be measured and software security is one of the activities of this rubric. These situation causes vulnerable problem such as how to control, what to measure. What action has to be performed? A prejudiced conclusion can be attracted concerning security about acquired utilizing of framework. Security Requirement Framework has been proposed based on inborn and fundamental parts of software security. As appeared in Fig. 1, Security Requirement framework comprises of five stages as takes after:

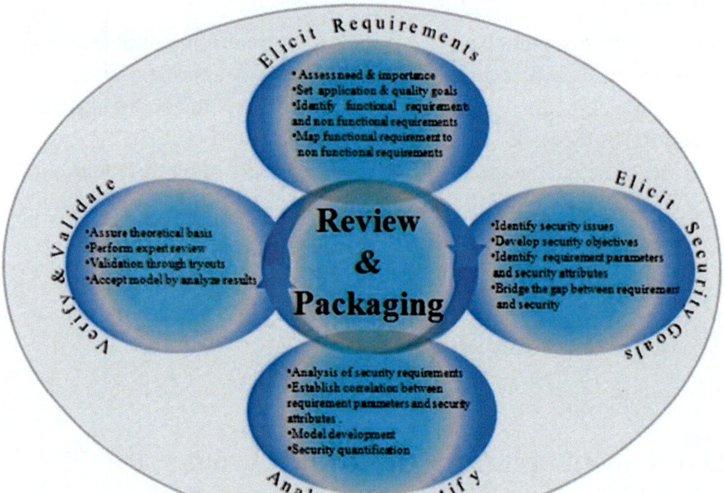

Fig. 1 Security requirement framework

Stage 1: **Elicit Requirements**

- Assess need and importance
- Set Application and quality goals
- Identify functional requirement & non- functional requirement [22, 23]
- Map functional requirement to non- functional requirement

Stage 2: **Elicit Security Goals**

- Identify security issues [24, 23]
- Develop security Objectives [25, 26]
- Identify requirement parameters and security attributes [26]
- Bridge the gap between requirement and security [26]

Stage 3: **Analyze and Quantify**

- Analysis of security requirements
- Establish correlation between requirement parameters and security attributes
- Model development [27, 28]
- Security quantification

Stage 4: **Verify and Validate**

- Assure Theoretical Basis [28]
- Perform Expert Review
- Validation through Tryouts
- Accept Model by Analyze Results [28]

Stage 5: **Review and Packaging**

- To developed requirement specification with the needed accessories [29]
- To prepare ready-to-use product, like any other usable product [29].

The first step of framework is the preliminary phase with various issues and concern related to brain storming activity that can be assesses through need and importance of requirements in particular software. [23]. The second step compromises of four sub-steps related to security attributes to elicit the requirement of the software in better way and helps to improvement of better production of software security [26]. This third task involves re-examine of all existing high-level system documentation. It ensures developers security awareness, global security policy, and performs risk analysis of requirement. The sub activities performed in this section is to establish correlation between requirement parameters and security attributes in probable influence and importance [27]. The fourth step speaks about goal of verification is to test whether the developed models actually measures what it is supposed to measure. The validation processes capture all involved activities to test the building process of right product [28]. The final phase is informal in nature and has been placed as the fifth phase with full liberty to enter at any of the former phases.

The idea is to twist back for better review, in contemplation to all previous phases [29].

6 Validation of the Framework

A key authentication step Verify and Validate for the framework illustrate in this paper is the capability to show that the system can involve with security requirements. To standardize the framework, statistical analysis at a large scale with typical representative samples may be needed and experimental try-outs has been carried out to check the functioning of framework. Additional developmental activities using the framework need to be carried out by the security researchers and practitioners. Re-examine the process that are already developed or underdevelopment software with requirement specification should be guided by the framework and this framework may form the foundation for the growth of better-refined roadmap for any secured system.

7 Conclusion

Application planned with security is constantly more secure than those where security is reexamined. The issues in regards to security is foremost part accompanied by the Design period for enhancement of software once the requirement determination has been frozen. The need of software security is defined. Existing security requirement approaches has been discussed with its phases involved. It has been found that there is no such single framework or model available in concerned to security requirements. Based on hypothetical principle a prescriptive software security requirement framework [SRF] has been proposed. Investigation of each stage is examined. The framework will strengthen the requirement, plan and investigation of non-practical properties for frameworks at the software engineering level successfully. Security requirement framework will also identify risk, threat and vulnerabilities and then discard, which in thus, will improve time, exertion and expenditure plan of the software.

References

1. Common Criteria Board (2009) Common criteria for information technology security evaluation, version 3.1
2. Sullivan Richard J (2014) Controlling security risk and fraud in payment systems. Federal Reserve Bank of Kansas City Econ Rev 99(3):47–78
3. McGraw G (2003) In: Software security: thought leadership in information security. Cigital Software Security Workshop

4. Taylor D, McGraw G (2005) In: Adopting a software security improvement program. IEEE Security and Privacy, pp 88–91
5. McGraw G, Mead N (2005) A portal for software security. IEEE Secur Privacy 3:75–79
6. Haley CB, Laney R, Moffett JD, Nuseibeh B (2008) Security requirements engineering: a framework for representation and analysis. IEEE Trans Softw Eng 34(1):133–152
7. Graham D (2006) Introduction to the CLASP process. Build Security
8. Ki-Aries D (2018) Assessing security risk and requirements for systems of systems. In: 2018 IEEE 26th International requirements engineering conference, IEEE. https://doi.org/10.1109/re.2018.00061
9. Lipner S, Howard M (2005) The trustworthy computing security development life cycle. Microsoft Corp
10. Torr P (2005) Demystifying the threat modeling process. IEEE Secur Privacy 3(5):66–70
11. Mellado D, Fernandez-Medina E, Piattini M (2007) A Common criteria based security requirements engineering process for the development of secure information systems. Comput Stand Interf 29(2):244–253
12. Humphrey WS (2002) In: Winning with software: an executive strategy. Boston, MA, Addison Wesley (ISBN 0201776391)
13. Sodiya AS, Onashoga SA, Ajayi OB (2006) Towards building secure software systems. In: Proceedings of issues in informing science and information technology, June 25–28, vol 3. Salford, Greater Manchester, England
14. Flechais I, Mascolo C, Angela Sasse M (2006) Integrating security and usability into the requirements and design process. In: Proceedings of the second international conference on global E-security, London, UK. http://www.softeng.ox.ac.uk/personal/Ivan.Flechais/downloads/icges.pdf
15. Reza M, Shirazi A, Jaferian P, Elahi G, Baghi H, Sadeghian B (2005) RUPSec: an extension on rup for developing secure systems-requirements discipline. In: Proceedings of World academy of science, engineering and technology, vol 4. pp 208–212. ISSN 1307–6884
16. Software Security Assurance (2007) State-of-the- Art Report (SOAR) Information Assurance Technology Analysis Center (IATAC) Data and Analysis Center for Software (DACS) Joint endeavor by IATAC with DACS
17. Oracle Software Security Assurance [web page] (Redwood Shores, CA, Oracle Corporation)
18. Mellado D, Fernández-Medina E, Piattini M (2006) Applying a security requirements engineering process. In: European symposium on research in computer security, Springer, Berlin, Heidelberg, Germany, pp 192–206
19. Ki-Aries D, Faily S, Dogan H, Williams C (2018) Assessing system of systems security risk and requirements with OASoSIS. In: 2018 IEEE 5th international workshop on evolving security and privacy requirements engineering (ESPRE), IEEE, pp 14–20
20. Guerra PADC, Rubira C, de Lemos R (2003) In: A fault-tolerant software architecture for component-based systems. Lecture Notes in Computer Science. vol 2677. Springer, pp 129–149
21. Fernandez EB (2004) A methodology for secure software design. In: Proc of the int'l symp web services and applications (ISWS). www.cse.fau.edu/_ed/EFLVSecSysDes1.pdf
22. Kurtanovi´c Z, Maalej W (2017) Automatically classifying functional and non-functional requirements using supervised machine learning. In: Proceedings the 25th IEEE international requirements engineering conference, Lisbon, Portugal, Sep. 2017, pp 490–495
23. Parveen N, Beg R, Khan MH (2014) Integrating security and usability at requirement specification process. Int J Comput Trends Technol (IJCTT) 10: 236–240
24. Mohammed NM, Niazi M, Alshayeb M, Mahmood S (2017) Exploring software security approaches in software development lifecycle: a systematic mapping study. Comput Standards Interfaces 50(1):107–115
25. Kyriazanos DM, Thanos KG, Thomopoulos SCA (2019) Automated decision making in airport checkpoints: bias detection toward smarter security and fairness, IEEE
26. Parveen N, Beg MR et al (2014) Software security issues: requirement perspectives. Int J Sci Eng Res 5(7):11–15. ISSN 2229–5518

27. Parveen N, Beg MR, Khan MH (2014) Bridging the gap between requirement and security through secure requirement specification checklist. In: Proceedings of 16 th IRF international conference, 14 th December 2014, Pune, India, pp 6–10. ISBN: 978–93-84209-74-2
28. Parveen N, Beg MR, Khan MH (2015) Model to quantify confidentiality at requirement phase. In: Proceedings of the 2015 international conference on advanced research in computer science engineering and technology(ACM ICARCSET-2015) 6–7th March 2015. ISBN: 978–1–4503-3441-9
29. Nikhat P, Beg MR, Khan MH (2015) Model to quantify availability at requirement phase of secure software. Amer J Softw Eng Appl 4(5):86–91

Smart Eye Testing

S. Hrushikesava Raju, Lakshmi Ramani Burra, Saiyed Faiayaz Waris, S. Kavitha, and S. Dorababu

Abstract At present, most of the persons are suffering from eyesight. Their food habits and their genes will create eyesight. To test eyesight, there is a manual approach that consumes time as well as money. The noted disadvantages such as the need to take more care personally while interacting with an unknown environment and need to collaborate with other organizations for the charity of testing the eyesights. To avoid these inconveniences, the proposed approach is required which automatically tests the eyesight for right and left eyes using IoT. This smart vision approach using IoT will test eyesight for numerous users and will generate reports separately. That report sent to the user mobile. The virtual software developed uses IoT which enables checking of the sight functionality and the report is sent to the user mobile. In this, the virtual environment is created where IoT devices and networked computer vision devices are connected to test the eyesight. The proposed approach is demanded and is required in this modern and future culture too. Many benefits like consultancy price-cutting transport cost-cutting, time is reduced, speed up in generating reports are achieved. This is a future demanded revolutionary approach which directs many online spectacle shopping sites. This is considered a virtual doctor and serves lots of people since there is no tiredness because it is an automatic approach.

Keywords Automatic · Virtual doctor · IoT · Eyesight · Time and money

S. Hrushikesava Raju (✉) · S. Kavitha · S. Dorababu
Department of Computer Science and Engineering, Koneru Lakshmaiah Education Foundation, Vaddeswaram, Guntur, India
e-mail: hkesavaraju@kluniversity.in

L. R. Burra
Department of Computer Science and Engineering, PVP Siddhartha Institute of Technology, Kanuru, Vijayawada, India

S. F. Waris
Department of Computer Science and Engineering, Vignan's Foundation for Science, Technology and Research, Vadlamudi, Guntur, India

S. Bhattacharyya et al. (eds.), *International Conference on Intelligent and Smart Computing in Data Analytics*, Advances in Intelligent Systems and Computing 1312,
https://doi.org/10.1007/978-981-33-6176-8_19

1 Introduction

Nowadays, a person possessing eyesight is struggling a lot with a manual approach. In the manual approach, the patient has to spend from his pocket for the expenses incurred such as transport cost to reach the hospital, they are waiting for the doctor to a checkup the eyesight, need to spend more time during a checkup, and writing a report also consume time. This process is a time-consuming process and involves more expenditure. This manual approach has many odd factors that take more time and more money. There is also an existing method that is a computerized checkup for eyesight. This computerized checkup is cost-oriented for purchasing a device and software. This leads to the manually the person has to attend at the center for testing the eyes. It results time-consuming for eye testing activity. In the market, new configuration machines are coming from time to time. When new machine is purchased, old machine usage is to be reduced. That means the new machine having more advanced features, whereas the old machine is having outdated features. To overcome this, an approach is required that automatically tests the eyesight through an app or software that has built-in IoT. In order to reduce time and cost-cutting over the spending, a single place where a number of users are allowed at a time and will be served efficiently by this proposed approach. The purpose of the expected service is to speed up the number of users to test in a day. The more advantageous point includes here is if any new feature to be required that can be easily plugged into the app or software. The devices in the IoT are upgraded as when required from time to time. The user-friendliness as well as the flexibility of up-gradation of features and hardware components are possible in the defined new approach. The proposed approach is defined in terms of the app, the integration of IoT devices, and a virtual doctor.

2 Literature Review

In this, there were few approaches used in this context that defines its functionality and explores their drawbacks. The studies represented in [1–8] describe about various ways of testing the eyesight. This is just the information but not revealed to how to automatically diagnose the eyesight. There are other studies from [9–12], where the various problems that eyes possess are described and reasons for raising these eye problems are mentioned but not specified how to automatically resolve this problems. From the studies [13–18], where there were various techniques discussed and directed those problems with solutions but they are not leading automatic solutions. The studies mentioned in [19–22] describe providing security for mobile, 52 using RSA, security using three-factor authentication, and security for data storage, 53 respectively, but these are not helped to implement automatic approach using IoT. In this, various approaches and techniques for securing data in a cloud and their implications are discussed. Here, the importance of storing data in the cloud securely is considered as important. The studies in [23–26] describe controlling speech suing mechanization framework, monitoring the garbage bin, detecting the abnormality, and detecting physically challenged people using specific approaches, respectively, but not specified automation of application using IoT. In [27, 28], the studies represent about hybrid context aware for pervasive smart environment and its consequences is discussed is as one, other is about on smart emergency responsive environment for fire hazards using IoT and its consequences are discussed. In the view of [29, 30], the first study states model of THAM index for agriculture decision-making using IoT and the second study is on specific nano-tube arrays for sensing acetone room temperature and their implications. These two studies describe the analysis and decision-making perfectly using the Internet of Things (IoT). These are although different w.r.t application, the terminology IoT is useful in our proposed application. The proposed approach is automated approach which looks like a simple app but few IoT devices will work in the background in order to check eyesight through a virtual doctor module. Compared to traditional approach, the automated approach is efficient in processing many users at a time, and approach is cheaper compared to computer-oriented machine eye checkup and should be reliable because the devices of IoT-based and saves both time and money. Moreover, the online shopping spectacle merchants require this kind of app where eyesight could be judged and there then online lens shopping suppose provided means the sales of the online spectacles shopping.

3 Implementation

In this, the app simulated is smart vision for eyesight in which user who requires to checkup their eyesight will install this app. The app will have two options in which first is eyesight checkup and second is shop for spectacles. The app developed is smart vision for eyesight when opened, these two options are shown. In which, the first option is selected will take the user to the virtual doctor. The virtual doctor is a help desk to the user and asks the user to look at the camera where the camera is loaded with sub-module called computer vision. It asks the user to see at the camera and computer vision sub-module will fix the sight lens to the both eyes of the user. Based on the automated eye vision loaded with features such as visual, contrast, and color acuity, it will generate a report to the user stating that sight for left and right eye. The architecture for smart vision for eyesight is depicted using use cases through their functionalities. The first module called smart checkup will increase the sales of online purchasing of the spectacles. This proposed approach will create demand for the users as well as merchants of the online spectacles shopping's revenue will be tremendously will be increased. In future, it will become necessary and will be used by most of eyesight victims (Fig. 1).

In this architecture, there were three modules identified where smart checkup is the first, the second is online spectacles shopping, and third is communication gadget. The description of these modules is as follows:

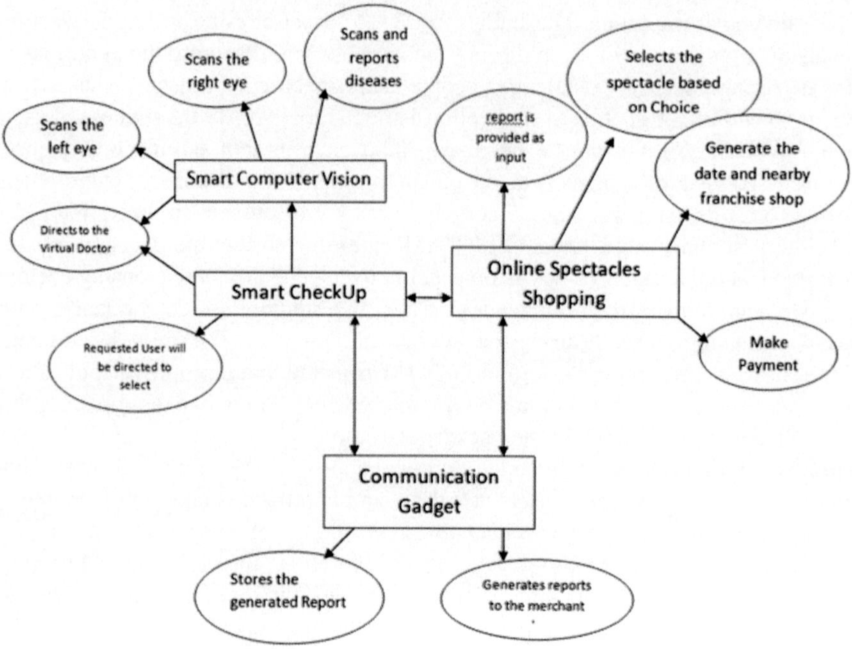

Fig. 1 Theme of smart vision for eyesight

The pseudo-procedure of this proposed smart vision for eyesight is described as follows:

Pseudo_Procedure Smart Vision(object, virtual_doctor):
Input: Person as object, virtual doctor.
Output: report, time_stamp, ID of that object.
Step 1: **Smart checkup:**
Call the smart checkup module.
smart_checkup(object):
Input: Person as object.
Output: report.

1.1. Giving the dynamic instructions through the voice or alert messages.
1.2. Once face and eye set to the correct position during the scanning, computer vision module will be activated.

if eye_disease is found:
returns the report with disease.
else:

1.2a According to normal vision of the eye, the difference is calculated between normal sight and possessing sight, and the lack of sight means difference of normal with possessing is returned for left eye.
1.2b The 1.2a is applied for right eye, and the lack of sight for right eye is returned.

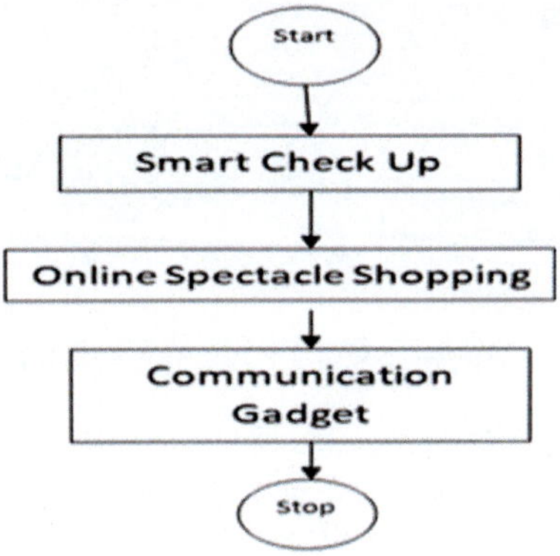

Fig. 2 Flowchart of smart vision for eyesight

Step 2: **Online Spectacle Shopping (report):**

2.1a Provides the list of spectacle categories such as Trending, New Arrivals, safety goggles, economic, Ray-Ban, Oakley, john jacobs, half rim, rim-less, etc., once the category is selected, would display various spectacles under that variety.
2.1b Checks the fitness of the spectacle with their face and accepts the confirmation of the size and model and its price.
2.1c Asks for payment processing and makes that transaction through the payment gateway.
2.1d Once merchant confirms the order, the details of the merchant will be posted to the user.

Step 3: **Communication Gadget**(): It takes the various user reports and stores for future analysis. Also, acknowledgement reports of the various merchants are to be stored for further analysis.

These modules are interacted with each other in order to produce the result. In this, the user after installing the app or registered with details is asked to interact with smart checkup module, the output of this is given as input to online spectacle shopping module where a variety of models and spectacles are there in which user selects any one with specific size, and the details of the user and merchant reports are stored in the cloud using the communication gadget. To visualize this flow, flowchart is used and is depicted as in Fig. 2.

4 Results

The inputs and outputs of the modules involved in the proposed approach are discussed in detail. The formats and their flow of events from one module to another module will judge the correctness of the proposed approach.

1. Asks to select the module name in the options (Fig. 3)

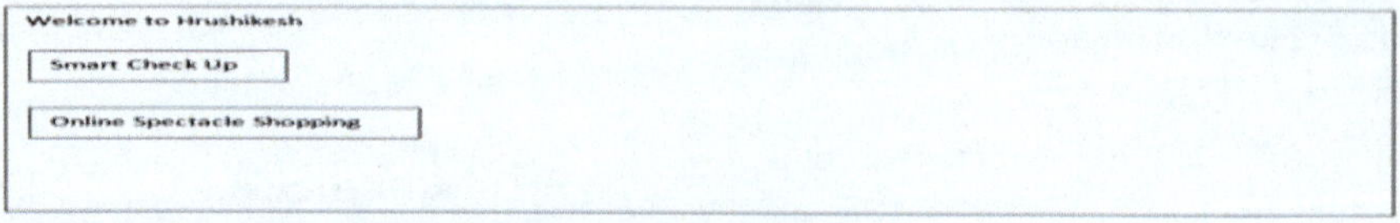

Fig. 3 Choosing the options in smart vision for eyesight

2. Both eyes are fixed and eyesight details are reported (Fig. 4)
3. Once finalize the spectacle, the app will have option to ask the feedback of the look of spectacle with the face (Fig. 5)
4. Delivery details and the time are specified to collect or to be delivered by the service agent (Fig. 6).

Compared to manual or traditional approach, the automated approach is specified in a graph where many customers are processed per hour than the customers to be serviced by manual method.

In this, the number of users to be taken on X-axis and time is taken on Y-axis (Fig. 7).

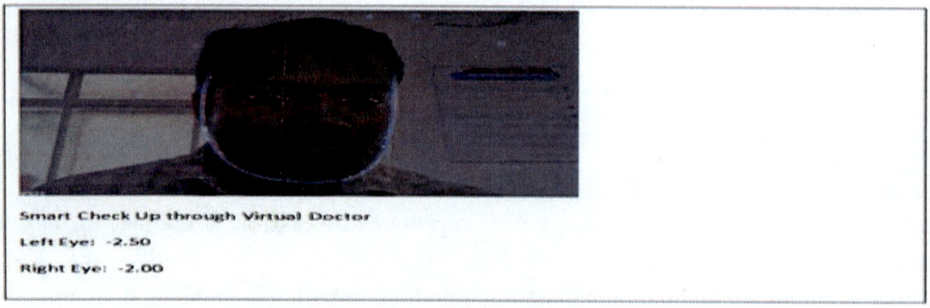

Fig. 4 Scanning the both eyes for vision in smart vision for eyesight

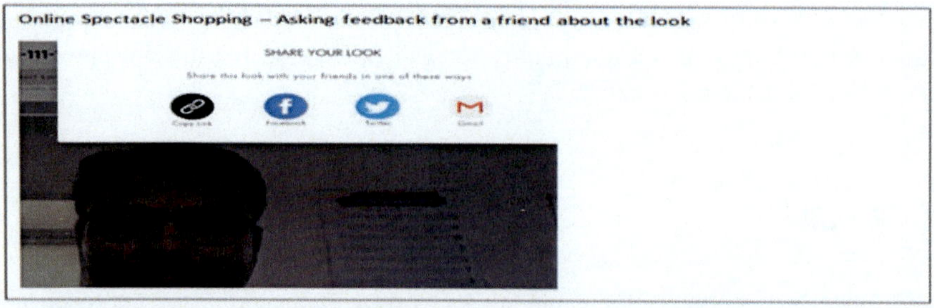

Fig. 5 Asking for friends feedback about the spectacle selected by you through social media in smart vision for eyesight

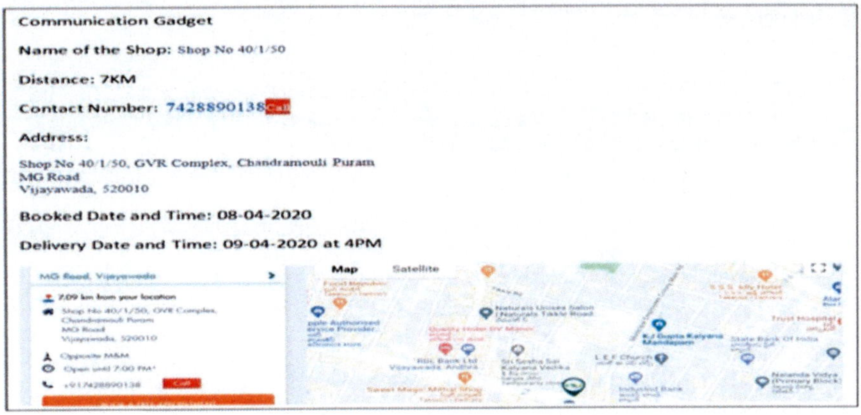

Fig. 6 Location of spectacle shop which accepted order in smart vision for eyesight

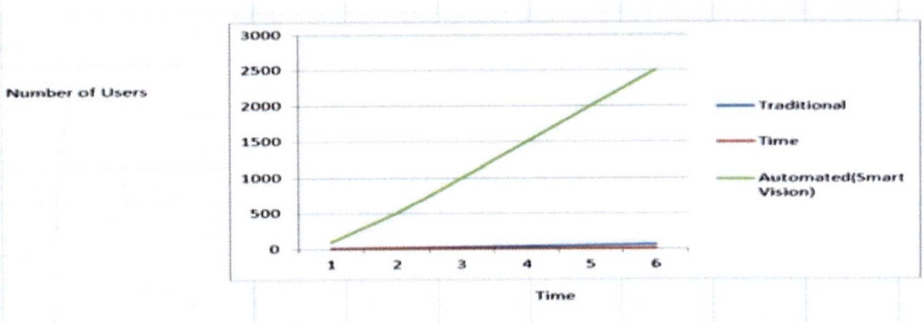

Fig. 7 Smart vision for eyesight versus traditional approach

5 Conclusion

In this paper, the proposed approach named smart vision for eyesight works as one app or software. In this app, there were few modules to interact with whose job is to provide a service to the user, report to be generated, and dispatched to the user. In the traditional approach, only one user can be processed, whereas the proposed approach is automatic. Once the user can put a request to the app, which could be service it, and will get a report on the sight. Also, online shopping for glasses could be connected once the report generated and allows to a selection of the eye frames and the type of glasses so that all the processes could be completed in one place. Many burdens like going to the doctor, going to the glasses shop to select, and wait for a frame with glasses to receive. All this work is minimized by this proposed approach called smart vision.

References

1. ZEISS Online Vision Screening (2017) Understanding vision, take part in the ZEISS online vision screening check and test the quality of your vision. https://www.zeiss.co.in/vision-care/better-vision/zeiss-online-vision-screening-check.html
2. A glossary of eye tests and exams, eye health, reference. https://www.webmd.com/eye-health/eye-tests-exams#1
3. Repka MX, Gudgel D (2020) Home eye test for children and adults. https://www.aao.org/eye-health/tips-prevention/home-eye-test-children-adults
4. 6 eye tests in a basic eye exam. https://allabouteyes.com/6-eye-tests-basic-eye-exam/
5. Turbert D, Brenda Pagan-Duran MD (2018) Eye exam and vision testing basics. https://www.aao.org/eye-health/tips-prevention/eye-exams-101
6. Working safely with display screen equipment. https://www.hse.gov.uk/msd/dse/eye-tests.htm
7. Segre L, Heiting G What's an eye test? https://www.allaboutvision.com/eye-test/free-eye-chart/
8. Vision Screening The college of Optometrists, http Eye charts and visual acuity explained. https://www.allaboutvision.com/eye-test/free-eye-chart/s://guidance.college-optometrists.org/guidance-contents/knowledge-skills-and-performance-domain/examining-patients-who-work-with-display-screen-equipment-or/vision-screening/
9. Harkin M, Griff AM (2012) Visual acuity test. https://www.healthline.com/health/visual-acuity-test
10. Basics of Vision and Eye Health Basics of vision and eye health, common eye disorders and diseases, centers for disease control and prevention. https://www.cdc.gov/visionhealth/basics/ced/index.html
11. Top causes of eye problems, eye health, reference. https://www.webmd.com/eye-health/common-eye-problems#1
12. Gans RE, The 5 most common vision problems and how to prevent them, health essentials. https://health.clevelandclinic.org/the-5-most-common-vision-problems-and-how-to-prevent-them/
13. Constantine R, OTR/L Vision techniques for eye movement disorders associated with autism, ADHD, dyslexia & other neurological disorders: hands-on assessments and treatments for children and adolescents, RNV063660. https://www.pesi.com/store/detail/26169/vision-techniques-for-eye-movement-disorders-associated
14. Gold DR (2019) Eye movement disorders eye movement disorders. In: Liu, Volpe, and Galetta's neuro-ophthalmology, 3rd edn
15. Leigh RJ, Gross M (2009) Eye movement disorders. In: Encyclopedia of neuroscience. https://www.sciencedirect.com/science/article/pii/B9780080450469010937
16. Tamhankar MA (2019) Eye movement disorders: third, fourth, and sixth nerve palsies and other causes of diplopia and ocular misalignment. In: Liu, Volpe, and Galetta's Neuro-Ophthalmology, 3rd edn. https://www.sciencedirect.com/science/article/pii/B9780323340441000158, https://doi.org/10.1016/B978-0-323-34044-1.00015-8
17. Chisari CG, Serra A (2017) Abnormal eye movements due to disease of the extraocular muscles and their innervation. Neurosci Biobehav Psychol. https://doi.org/10.1016/B978-0-12-809324-5.01292-X
18. Ivanov IV, Mackeben M, Vollmer A, Martus P, Nguyen NX, Trauzettel-Klosinsk S Eye movement training and suggested gaze strategies in tunnel vision—a randomized and controlled pilot study. https://journals.plos.org/plosone/article?id=10.1371/journal.pone.0157825. https://doi.org/10.1371/journal.pone.0157825
19. Nalajala S et al (2019) Light weight secure data sharing scheme for mobile cloud computing. In: 2019 third international conference on I-SMAC (IoT in social, mobile, analytics and cloud) (I-SMAC), IEEE
20. Sunanda N, Pratyusha C, Meghana A, Meghana BP (2019) Data security using multi prime RSA in cloud. Int J Recent Technol Eng 7(6S4). ISSN: 2277–3878.

21. Nalajala S et al (2020) Data security in cloud computing using three-factor authentication. In: International conference on communication, computing and electronics systems, Springer, Singapore
22. Sunanda N, Sriyuktha N, Sankar PS Revocable identity based encryption for secure data storage in cloud. Int J Innov Technol Exploring Eng 8(7):678–682
23. Kavitha M, Manideep Y, Vamsi Krishna M, Prabhuram P (2018) Speech controlled home mechanization framework using android gadgets. Int J Eng Technol (UAE) 7(1.1):655–659
24. Kavitha M, Srinivasulu S, Savitri K, Afroze PS, Venkata Sai PA, Asrith S (2019) Garbage bin monitoring and management system using GSM. Int J Innov Exploring Eng 8(7):2632–2636
25. Kavitha M et al (2018) Wireless sensor enabled breast self-examination assistance to detect abnormality. In: 2018 International conference on computer, information and telecommunication systems (CITS). IEEE
26. Kolli CS, Krishna Reddy VV, Kavitha M (2020) A critical review on internet of things to empower the living style of physically challenged people. Advances in Intelligent Systems and Computing. Springer, Singapore, pp 603–619
27. Madhusudanan J, Geetha S, Venkatesan VP, Vignesh U, Iyappan P (2018) Hybrid aspect of context-aware middleware for pervasive smart environment: a review. Mobile Inf Syst. https://doi.org/10.1155/2018/6546501
28. Maguluri LP, Srinivasarao T, Ragupathy R, Syamala M, Nalini NJ (2018) Efficient smart emergency response system for fire hazards using IoT. Int J Adv Comput Sci Appl
29. Mekala MS, Viswanathan P (2020) Sensor stipulation with THAM index for smart agriculture decision-making IoT system. https://doi.org/10.1007/s11277-019-06964-0
30. Kumar KG, Avinash BS, Rahimi-Gorji M, Majdoubi J (2020) Photocatalytic activity and smartness of TiO_2 nanotube arrays for room temperature acetone sensing. https://doi.org/10.1016/j.molliq.2019.112418

Ameliorated Shape Matrix Representation for Efficient Classification of Targets in ISAR Imagery

Hari Kishan Kondaveeti and Valli Kumari Vatsavayi

Abstract In this paper, we proposed a new shape matrix representation mechanism for the automatic classification of targets from ISAR imagery. The proposed shape matrix representation method overcomes the undesirable side effects associated with the existing methods, such as the quantization of superfluous inner and outer shape details. The proposed mechanism also deals with the variations in shape representations of the targets caused by the erroneous procedure employed by exiting methods for the selection of axis-of-reference. The efficiency and robustness of the proposed mechanism are examined through experimental analysis, and the results are presented.

Keywords Radar image classification · Inverse synthetic aperture radar (ISAR) · Automatic target recognition (ATR) · Automatic target classification (ATC) · Shape matrices

1 Introduction

Inverse Synthetic Aperture Radar (ISAR) is an imaging radar used to generate images (ISAR imagery) of the targets for target recognition purposes in military surveillance operations [7, 8]. ISARs are instrumental in recognition of maneuvering targets in military surveillance.

For the classification of targets in ISAR imagery, the works in [2, 13] and [12] used the geometrical and statistical characteristics of shape of the targets. The approaches in [1, 9, 10] depend on the structural properties and wireframe models of the targets. Recent works [4–6, 11, 14] depend on invariant shape descriptors for efficient

H. K. Kondaveeti (✉)
School of Computer Science Engineering, VIT-AP University, Beside Secretariat, Vijayawada, Andhra Pradesh, India
e-mail: kishan.kondaveeti@gmail.com

V. K. Vatsavayi
Department of CS & SE, AUCE (A) Andhra University, Visakhapatnam, Andhra Pradesh, India

S. Bhattacharyya et al. (eds.), *International Conference on Intelligent and Smart Computing in Data Analytics*, Advances in Intelligent Systems and Computing 1312,
https://doi.org/10.1007/978-981-33-6176-8_20

classification of targets. Invariance with respect to scale, translation, and rotation is achieved by the Polar-raster quantization. The MECSM method used in [14] is analogous to the polar mapping (PM) technique used in [4, 11]. However, carefully selected center and radius of minimum enclosing circle of the target silhouette makes MECSM representation more accurate. However, MECSM representation did not address the redundancy in sampling the innermost shape details.

In this paper, a new classification mechanism is proposed for automatic classification of targets from ISAR imagery using enhanced version of shape matrices for target representation. The dependency of this shape matrix representation on the center and radial separation zone derived from the Minimum Radial Separating Circles (MRSC) of the target's contour profile makes this shape descriptor more precise and more discriminatory. The constraints derived from the second and third-order moments alleviate the ambiguities in the selection of unique axis-of-reference. These constraints provide a reliable solution to perform target orientation normalization to achieve rotation invariance. The proposed method is explained in the following sections in detail.

2 Ameliorated Shape Matrix Representation

2.1 *Finding the Axis-of-Reference*

The axis of reference selected for shape representation counters the effects of arbitrary shape orientations. However, this axis should be unique for various instances of a particular shape. Also, it should not shuffle with the articulations and distortions in the shape to prevent the disagreements in the shape definitions.

The method of moments is used to find the principal axes of a shape. However, additional constraints are needed to find a unique axis of reference. The angle of the principal axis of least inertia can be used as a unique reference axis to describe the in-plane rotation of an object.

2.2 *Finding R_{max} and R_{min}*

In shape matrix generation, R_{max} and R_{min} define the zone in which polar raster shape sampling occurs. Proper selection of these values plays a crucial role in avoiding the sampling of superfluous details in and around the shape of the target and in making the target representation precise. Convex hulls and MRSC are employed for the calculation of R_{max} and R_{min} with reduced computational complexity.

The procedure for obtaining the R_{max} and R_{min} works as follows. Initially, Inner Convex Hull (ICH) and Outer Convex Hull (OCH) are constructed from the contour profile of the target to reduce the number of candidate points. Then, the curvature radius-based iterative elimination is performed to reduce the number of candidate points on each convex hull to three. Next, center and radii are calculated for every pair of concentric circles formed by different combinations of candidate points on ICH and OCH, and the center and the radii of minimum radial separation circles are obtained. Finally, the radii of outer and inner circles are considered as $R_{\max}$ and $R_{\min}$, respectively.

2.3 Shape Matrix Generation

Consider the minimum radial separation center as the origin and $R_{\max}$ and $R_{\min}$ as the radii of the outermost and innermost concentric circles of the polar grid. Consider the radial line with orientation θ w.r.t x-axis as the axis-of-reference to initiate the representation. The generation of shape matrix of size $m \times n$ using the above parameters involves in following steps:

1. Define a matrix SM of size $m \times n$ and initialize the elements to zero.
2. Generate n concentric circles from the minimum radial separation center having a radial difference of $(R_{\max} - R_{\min})/(n - 1)$.
3. Generate m radial lines from the minimum radial separation center having an angular difference of $2\pi/(m - 1)$ starting from θ w.r.t x-axis.
4. Set the element of the shape matrix SM to 1 if the intersection point of a circle and a radial line lies within the shape region, *i.e.*, if an intersection point $(i.R/(n - 1), j.2\pi/(m - 1))$ corresponding to angular division i and radial section j lies within the shape region, then set $SM_{i,j} = 1$.

Carefully selected $R_{\max}$ and $R_{\min}$ makes the proposed shape matrix representation more discriminatory as it emphasizes on capturing the substantial details of the shape and avoids the uninfluential details as depicted in Fig. 1.

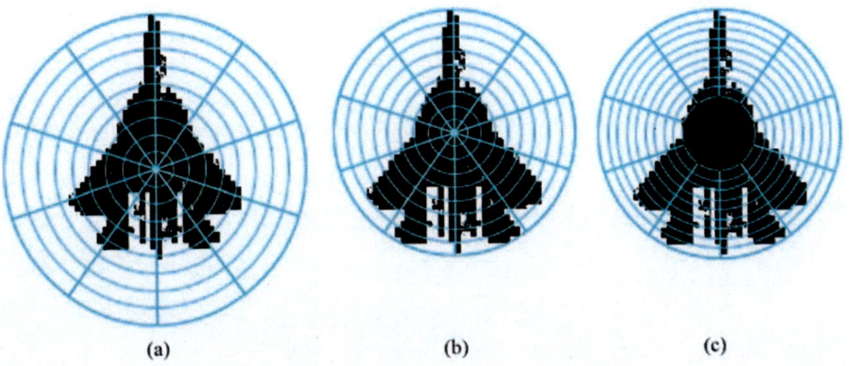

Fig. 1 Imaginary polar grids generated by different approaches for extracting the shape saliency. **a** Goshtasby [3]; **b** MECSM [14]; **c** proposed method

2.4 Classification

Initially, the training images are represented in ameliorated shape matrix form, and these matrices are stored in the database along with the corresponding class label of the target. For testing, the test image is processed and is represented in the ameliorated shape matrix form. Finally, the test image is classified as a target based on the maximum similarity value.

3 Experimental Results

We performed an experimental analysis to compare the recognition accuracies of the proposed and existing methods PM + PCA [4], FT + PM + PCA [11] and MECSM [14]. Figure 2 depicts simulated ISAR imagery of aircraft targets.

The recognition rate is defined as the number of correct classifications over the total number of classifications. Mean recognition rate P_{mr} is considered in the performance analysis for better justification. Monte Carlo simulations are performed using Monte Carlo Cross-Validation (MCCV) scheme [15] to prevent over-fitting. For consistency in the experimental analysis, the number of samples considered for shape description in all the four methods is considered as 100×100.

All the experiments are carried out on Intel i7-6700 3.40 GHz CPU system in MATLAB environment. The experimental results are presented and discussed in the following paragraphs. The performance of the proposed method is consistent and is comparatively good in all the experiments as the shape matrix representation in the proposed method extracts much richer discriminatory information than the remaining methods.

Graphs in Figs. 3 and 4 against the mean recognition rate P_{mr} and SNR_{dB} show the classification results of the methods considered, at various SNR_{dB}. In the graph in Fig. 3, SNR_{dB} is varied across 5–30 dB in 5 dB intervals and incase of graph in Fig. 4, SNR_{dB} is varied across 1–5 dB in 1 dB intervals. When SNR_{dB} is good enough, all the methods are performing equally good with slight variations in accuracy. But, however, the inefficient preprocessing mechanism employed in the methods [4, 11] affects their classification accuracy at low SNR_{dB} as depicted in the graph. The proposed and the method [14] have given the similar performance at all the SNR_{dB}.

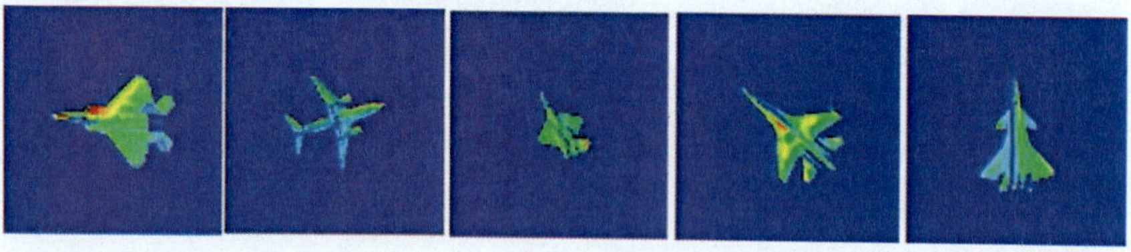

Fig. 2 Images of aircrafts of different classes selected arbitrarily from the data set SynISAR

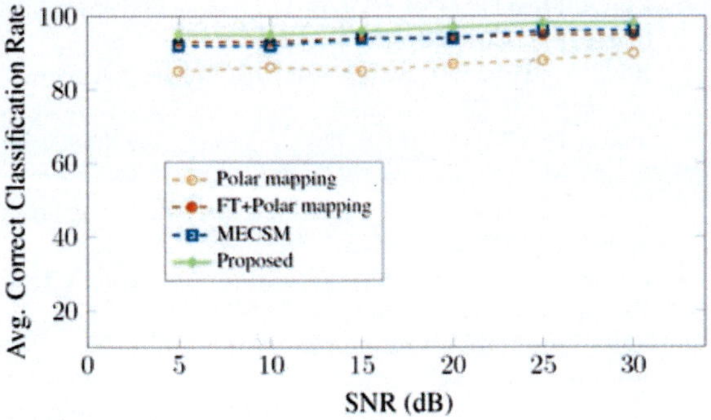

Fig. 3 Classification accuracies against SNR_{dB} across 5–30 dB

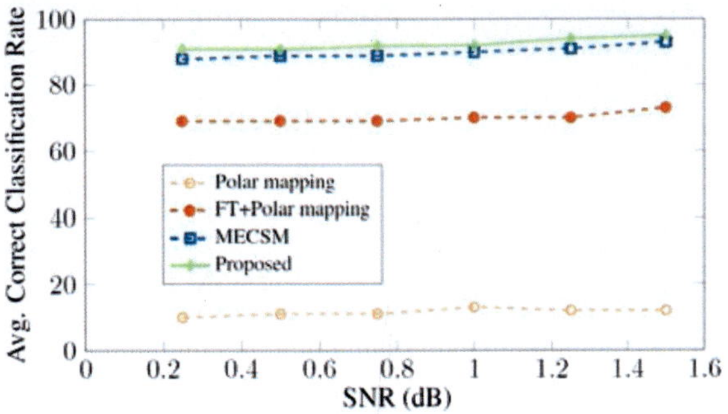

Fig. 4 Classification accuracies against SNR_{dB} across 1–5 dB

4 Conclusion

In this paper, a new classification mechanism is proposed for the efficient classification of targets from 2D-ISAR imagery. The proposed classification mechanism depends on an enhanced shape matrix representation to yield better results. Systematically obtained unique axis-of-reference, center, and radial limits make the shape description invariant, precise, and robust against noise, blur, and discontinuities in target response. The proposed method is performing comparatively better than the existing methods.

References

1. Bachmann CM, Musman SA, Schultz A (1992) Lateral inhibition neural networks for classification of simulated radar imagery. In: International joint conference on neural networks, 1992. IJCNN, vol 2, pp 115–120
2. Botha EC (1994) Classification of aerospace targets using super resolution isar images. In: Proceedings of the 1994 IEEE South African symposium on communications and signal processing, 1994. COMSIG-94, pp 138–145
3. Goshtasby A (1985) Description and discrimination of planar shapes using shape matrices. IEEE Trans Pattern Anal Mach Intell PAMI 7(6):738–743

4. Kim KT, Seo DK, Kim HT (2005) Efficient classification of isar images. IEEE Trans Antennas Propag 53(5):1611–1621
5. Kondaveeti HK, Vatsavayi VK (2016) Robust ISAR image classification using abridged shape matrices. In: 2016 international conference on emerging trends in engineering, technology and science (ICETETS). IEEE. https://doi.org/10.1109/icetets.2016.7603025
6. Kondaveeti HK, Vatsavayi VK (2017) Abridged shape matrix representation for the recognition of aircraft targets from 2d isar imagery. Adv Comput Sci Technol 10(5):1103–1122. https://www.ripublication.com/acst17/acstv10n5_41.pdf
7. Kondaveeti HK, Vatsavayi VK (2017) Automatic target recognition from inverse synthetic aperture radar images, pp 530–555
8. Kondaveeti HK, Vatsavayi VK (2018) Automatic target recognition from inverse synthetic aperture radar images, pp 2307–2332. https://doi.org/10.4018/978-1-5225-5204-8.ch101
9. Maki A, Fukui K (2004) Ship identification in sequential isar imagery. Mach Vision Appl 15(3):149–155
10. Musman S, Kerr D, Bachmann C (1996) Automatic recognition of isar ship images. IEEE Trans Aerosp Electron Syst 32(4):1392–1404
11. Park SH, Jung JH, Kim SH, Kim KT (2015) Efficient classification of ISAR images using 2d Fourier transform and polar mapping. IEEE Trans Aerosp Electron System 51(3):1726–1736
12. Rosenbach K, Schiller J (1995) Identification of aircraft on the basis of 2-d radar images. In: Radar conference, record of the IEEE 1995 international, pp 405–409
13. Saidi MN, Daoudi K Khenchaf A, Hoeltzener B, Aboutajdine D (2009) Automatic target recognition of aircraft models based on isar images. In: 2009 IEEE international geoscience and remote sensing symposium, vol 4, pp IV-685–IV-688
14. Vatsavayi VK, Kondaveeti HK (2018) Efficient ISAR image classification using MECSM representation. J King Saud Univ Comput Inf Sci 30(3):356–372
15. Xu QS, Liang YZ (2001) Monte Carlo cross validation. Chemometr Intel Lab Syst 56(1):1–11

Region-Specific Opinion Mining from Tweets in a Mixed Political Scenario

Ferdin Joe John Joseph and Sarayut Nonsiri

Abstract Twitter sentiment analysis is used for many areas of market research and opinion mining in various sectors like poll campaign, crime detection and health care. Opinion mining in poll campaign is gaining its prominence since 2012. India as the largest democracy has different factors for different types of elections happening across the length and breadth of the country. The Twitter-based opinion mining for a particular regional election cannot be implied with the normal way of predicting the general elections. A region-specific weighted decision tree-based framework is proposed in this paper. The results provided by the proposed methodology obtained numbers to the existing AI-based pre-poll analysis methods. The actual numbers were able to predict the seats with high confidence factors. The data analysis done on the actual result margins shows that the proposed methodology is comparatively efficient enough in predicting a regional election.

Keywords Twitter sentiment analysis · Weighted decision tree · Twitter data · Region-specific framework · Indian election

1 Introduction

Opinion mining is gaining its prominence in many avenues of businesses and even used in mind mapping. Mind mapping is traditionally used in offline qualitative data analysis. These offline analyses are done in pre and exit polls. This methodology is predominantly done in many India, the country with the largest democracy. The accuracy of these methodologies depends on different factors. There are a wide range of methodologies proposed like [1]. These existing methodologies use a normal trend analysis and mostly would not give a projection on the magnitude of victory. Earlier during the 2019 General Elections, an attempt was made using Twitter-based outcome analysis and reported some convincing results in [2]. A region-specific framework is proposed in this paper which uses weighted decision tree for a rule-based wrangling

F. J. John Joseph (✉) · S. Nonsiri
Faculty of Information Technology, Thai-Nichi Institute of Technology, Bangkok, Thailand
e-mail: ferdin@tni.ac.th

S. Bhattacharyya et al. (eds.), *International Conference on Intelligent and Smart Computing in Data Analytics*, Advances in Intelligent Systems and Computing 1312,
https://doi.org/10.1007/978-981-33-6176-8_21

framework. The results obtained are not with clear accuracy but the mathematical implications from the actual numbers say that the proposed methodology is good in getting opinion mined for a specific region. Mixed political scenario mentioned in the paper denotes that the people prefer different political ideologies for different levels of representation. The ruling party of India has a different response in assembly response while the same voters gave a clear mandate in national level. This paper proposes a methodology which can segregate the actual trend in this mixed scenario.

2 Related Work

The base of the research proposed in this paper starts from [2]. Prior to this base research, there are a lot of methods proposed for various countries. Some studies were done on region-specific elections in Australia like [3]. European countries with multi-party democratic setup had done opinion mining using Twitter as reported in [4, 5]. Indian General Elections in 2014 and Pakistani General Elections were tracked in [6] and the trends were reported on who may win but the magnitude is not analyzed. Twitter-based election prediction has been done on various countries in the past like Indonesia [7], France [8], Bulgaria [9], etc. These methodologies are monitoring systems which shows the trend of results. Region-specific method proposed in [10] deals with the three metrics and genetic algorithm based methods in [11].

3 Proposed Methodology

The method proposed here consists of four phases. Data collection, wrangling, preprocessing, and sentiment analysis. This method differs from [2] in the wrangling part (Fig. 1).

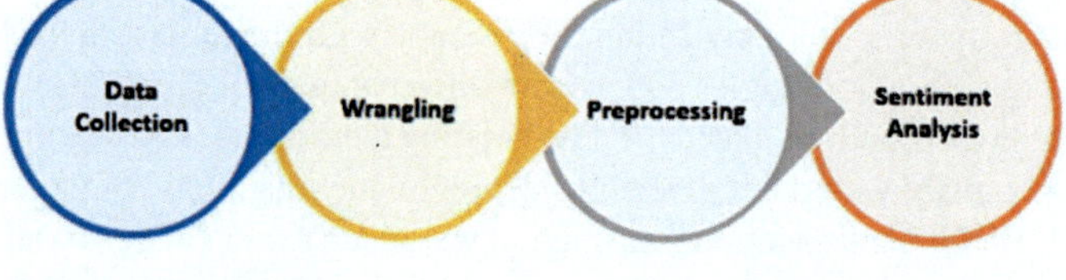

Fig. 1 Proposed region-specific framework

3.1 Data Collection

Tweets with hashtags or words same as "Delhi Election" was used along with the name of proposed candidates from each parties. Tweepy library [12] was used with the Twitter API. Each party was given a collection of 5000 tweets every day. These tweets were collected for a period of two weeks including and prior to the polling day. The tweets collected are stored in MongoDB [13].

3.2 Wrangling

When compared to the data collected in [2], many tweeted for Delhi Elections shared their location. As a result, the pruning of tweets was done using the following Twitter democracy algorithm proposed by the authors.

Twitter Democracy Algorithm.

Step 1: Tweets with no latitude and longitude attributes.
Step 2: Tweets having same content.
Step 3: Tweets with non-English text, images, and videos.
Step 4: Tweets from irrelevant location, i.e., those tweets outside of the latitude and longitude of New Delhi using region selection techniques [14].
Step 5: Multiple tweets from same user.
Step 6: Then, data collection is done again until it tallies 20,000 tweets.

The above steps are recursively done until the 20,000 tweets collected do not have to do pruning corresponding to the seven steps listed above.

3.3 Preprocessing

This stage is same as the one done for decision trees in [2]. NLTK Corpus [15] is used to tokenize the string of tweets using hover representation of correlated subspaces [16]. The features are weighted based on support vector regression-based feature selection [17, 18]. The words are tokenized and normalized before taking into analysis of polarity and subjectivity in the next phase.

3.4 Sentiment Analysis

The tweets which are wrangled and preprocess are subjected to subjectivity and polarity of the resultant text from each tweet is subjected to a weighted decision tree. The text is subjected to POS tagger and the weightage is given as follows. Verbs carry maximum weightage of 0.5, adjectives and adverbs with 0.25, conjunction and interjections with 0.15, and remaining others with 0.1. Nouns are not pruned. This will take the context machine to decide who the tweet is targeting. This setup is done to avoid fake praise and other context. The randomized tokens were selected using the region mapping [14] for sparse data.

A cumulative polarity and popularity are calculated using the formula as stated in [2]. But in this methodology, negative tweets will drop the popularity index of that particular tweet. This helped in maintaining the difference in national and regional trend. The values used as weightage of decision tree are fixed after having some random initial experimentation on the sentiments analyzed in various datasets like the one used in [2] and in this paper. The cumulative popularity index was calculated every day for each party contesting. The anti-incumbency and pro-incumbency factors considered in [2] are removed in this method.

4 Results and Discussion

The overall popularity score of the ruling and opposition parties in Delhi is calculated using the proposed methodology and is visualized in Fig. 2 below.

According to the actual counting of votes, the margin between the winning and the candidate securing second position is given in Fig. 3 below. There are around nine constituencies below the average winning margin and this uncertain count led to the wrong prediction of the proposed methodology. The proposed methodology holds good for those constituencies giving a clear majority for the winning candidate (Fig. 4).

The mean of winning margin is 20,883 with a standard deviation of all the constituencies' margin is 16262. The difference between the mean and standard

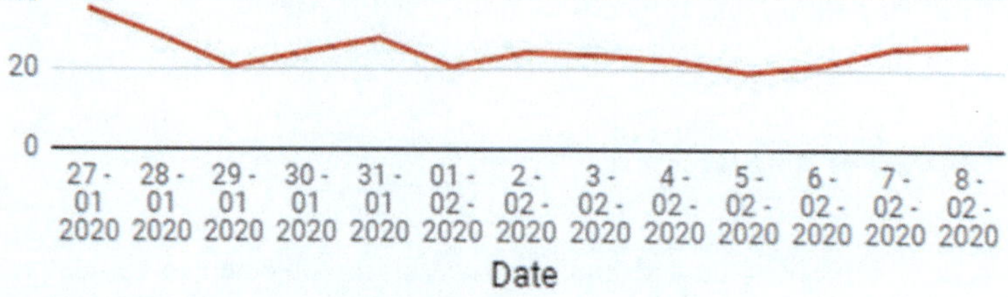

Fig. 2 Trends of ruling party in Delhi and opposition party in Delhi

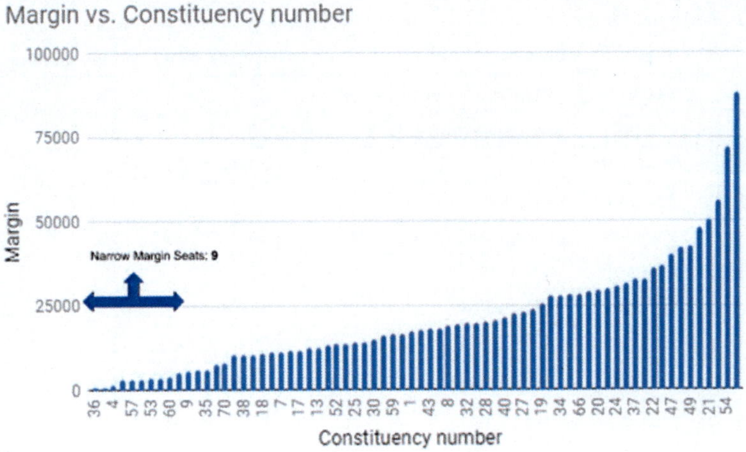

Fig. 3 Winning margin of constituencies reported by actual result in [19]

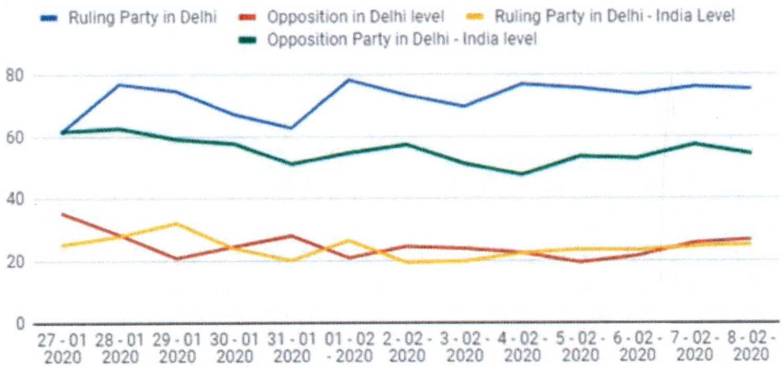

Fig. 4 Regional and Pan India trend observed for both ruling and opposition party

deviation is set to be the threshold of win by narrow margin. According to this calculation, the narrow margin threshold is fixed at 4619. As per this threshold, nine constituencies are considered to be secured by a thin and narrow margin. The same dataset when observed with the method in [2] produced highly variant result. This method becomes impractical when compared with the actual result (Table 1).

From the methods other than proposed methodology reported, Graphnile and Decision Trees on tweets [2, 21] are AI-based methodologies. These AI-based methods are done for pre-poll analysis. So the proposed methodology has clear logic to compare the magnitude with these as main comparisons. However, the actual result [19] is also a reasonable factor to compare. Though Graphnile as a service provider to political parties mentioned that they use AI-based methods, there is no evidence on what methodology is used by them. The existing methodology [2] is compared with the proposed methodology due to two factors. Beyond all these factors, the proposed

Table 1 Performance evaluation of the proposed methodology

S. No	Type	Method	Ruling party	Opposition party
1	**Pre-poll**	**Proposed methodology**	**52**	**18**
2	Pre-poll	Decision trees [2]	38	30
3	**Post-poll**	**Actual result** [19]	**63**	**7**
4	Pre-poll	Times Now [20]	54–60	10–14
5	**Pre-poll**	**Graphnile (AI-based)** [21]	**56**	**12**
6	Exit poll	Spick Media	55	12
7	Exit poll	Times Now	47	23
8	Exit poll	ABP News—CVoter	65	3

Entries bold faced are those methodologies with comparable performance

and existing methodology used tweets only in English. However, this needs more refined methodology when it comes to the region where people predominantly tweet in a language other than English predominantly.

5 Conclusion

From the discussion given in the previous section, it is clearly evident that the proposed methodology framework for a region-specific opinion mining hold better in predicting the near numbers of seats to be won in a state assembly election and efficiently filter out tweets irrelevant to the region. Deep learning for this application may be time consuming in presenting the hourly sentiment of people over a period of time.

References

1. Ramteke J, Shah S, Godhia D, Shaikh A (2016) Election result prediction using Twitter sentiment analysis. In: 2016 international conference on inventive computation technologies (ICICT), pp 1–5
2. John Joseph FJJ (2019) Twitter Based Outcome Predictions of 2019 Indian General Elections Using Decision Tree. In: Proceedings of 2019 4th international conference on information technology. IEEE, pp 50–53
3. Burgess J, Bruns A (2012) (Not) the Twitter election: the dynamics of the# ausvotes conversation in relation to the Australian media ecology. J Pract 6(3):384–402
4. Larsson AO, Moe H (2012) Studying political microblogging: Twitter users in the 2010 Swedish election campaign. New Media Soc 14(5):729–747
5. Yang X, Macdonald C, Ounis I (2018) Using word embeddings in twitter election classification. Inf Retr J 21(2–3):183–207
6. Kagan V, Stevens A, Subrahmanian VS (2015) Using twitter sentiment to forecast the 2013 Pakistani election and the 2014 Indian election. IEEE Intell Syst 30(1):2–5

7. Budiharto W, Meiliana M (2018) Prediction and analysis of Indonesia Presidential election from Twitter using sentiment analysis. J Big Data 5(1):51
8. Wang L, Gan JQ (2017) Prediction of the 2017 French election based on Twitter data analysis. In: 2017 9th computer science and electronic engineering (CEEC), pp 89–93
9. Smailović J, Kranjc J, Grčar M, Žnidaršič M, Mozetič I (2015) Monitoring the Twitter sentiment during the Bulgarian elections. In: 2015 IEEE international conference on data science and advanced analytics (DSAA), pp 1–10
10. Jurgens D, Finethy T, McCorriston J, Xu YT, Ruths D (2015) Geolocation prediction in twitter using social networks: a critical analysis and review of current practice. In: Ninth international AAAI conference on web and social media
11. John Joseph FJ, Nayak D, Chevakidagarn S (2020) Local maxima niching genetic algorithm based automated water quality management system for Betta splendens. TNI J Eng Technol 8(2):48–63.
12. Roesslein J (2009) Tweepy documentation. [Online]. https://tweepyreadthedocsio/en/v3
13. Nayak A, Mongo DB (2014) Cookbook. Packt Publishing Ltd.
14. John Joseph FJ, Vaikunda Raja T (2015) Enhanced robustness for digital images using geometric attack simulation. Procedia Eng 38:2672–2678. Available from: https://linkinghub.elsevier.com/retrieve/pii/S1877705812022278
15. Loper E, Bird S (2002) NLTK: the natural language toolkit. arXiv Prepr cs/0205028
16. John Joseph FJ, Vaikunda Raja T, John Justus C (2011) Classification of correlated subspaces using HoVer representation of Census Data. In: 2011 international conference on emerging trends in electrical and computer technology. IEEE, pp 906–911. Available from: https://ieeexplore.ieee.org/lpdocs/epic03/wrapper.htm?arnumber=5760248
17. John Joseph FJ (2019) Empirical dominance of features for predictive analytics of particulate matter pollution in Thailand. In: 5th Thai-Nichi Institute of Technology Academic Conference (TNIAC 2019), pp 385–388
18. John Joseph FJ (2019) IoT-Based unified approach to predict particulate matter pollution in Thailand. In: The role of IoT and blockchain techniques and applications
19. India EC of. GENERAL ELECTION TO VIDHAN SABHA TRENDS & RESULT FEB-2020 [Internet]. Online. 2020. Available from: https://results.eci.gov.in/DELHITRENDS2020/partywiseresult-U05.htm
20. Kaul S (2020) IPSOS opinion poll: Kejriwal set to return as CM, and 4 other takeaways. Times Now
21. Graphnile (2020) Graphnile Election Analytics [Internet]. Online. Available from: https://www.graphnile.com/electoral-analytics
22. Tumasjan A, Sprenger TO, Sandner PG, Welpe IM (2011) Election forecasts with Twitter: How 140 characters reflect the political landscape. Soc Sci Comput Rev 29(4):402–418

Denoising of Multispectral Images: An Adaptive Approach

P. Lokeshwara Reddy, Santosh Pawar, and Kanagaraj Venusamy

Abstract Spectral imaging enables detection of external details not processed by the human eye through its red, green, and blue receptors. Multispectral imaging aims to collect the range in a scene picture for each pixel and provide more accurate detail. Different noises eventually compromise Multispectral Image (MSI) due to hardware constraints and insufficiency in radiance. Hence, to enhance the quality of image, we proposed Kriging Interpolation-based Wiener Filtering (KIWF). This makes use of kriging interpolation algorithm to calculate the weights of wiener filter so that the best possible estimate is obtained for denoising the image. Initially, the pixels with noise are separated from clear pixels by global patch clustering, and the weight values are applied by estimating the semi-variance between the clear patches and noisy patches. Finally, the performance of the filter is tested and a comparative analysis is conducted with the existing denoising techniques to show its effectiveness.

Keywords Global patch clustering · Kriging interpolation · Multispectral image · Wiener filter

1 Introduction

Multispectral image captures the image data within stipulated wavelength regions across electromagnetic spectrum. Multispectral images provide more spectral resolution collate to RGB images [1]. In multispectral and color images, the Gaussian noise is inevitable which is caused during acquisition and transmission or

P. Lokeshwara Reddy (✉) · S. Pawar
Department of Electronics and Communication Engineering, Dr. A.P.J. Abdul Kalam University, Indore, Madhya Pradesh, India
e-mail: spblokesh442@gmail.com

S. Pawar
e-mail: spwarrkdf@gmail.com

K. Venusamy
University of Technology and Applied Sciences, Al Musannah, Oman
e-mail: kanagaraj@act.edu.om

S. Bhattacharyya et al. (eds.), *International Conference on Intelligent and Smart Computing in Data Analytics*, Advances in Intelligent Systems and Computing 1312,
https://doi.org/10.1007/978-981-33-6176-8_22

due to limitations in recording equipment, calibration errors, and photon effect [2]. In addition, the sensor with limited radiance energy and narrow bandwidth also increases the noise in the image. This Gaussian noise affects the quality of the image. Hence, an effective filtering method has to be implemented to get a clear image. In this paper, a new methodology for denoising of multispectral images is proposed which aims to introduce a global patch clustering stratagem by using Gaussian mixture model for clumping the similar patches and then apply curvelet transform to distinct geometric details from background noise and implementing the wiener filtering concept by including the kriging interpolation for producing excellent noise suppression standards and also exhibit good visual quality of output image.

2 Literature Review

A wide category of denoising methods has been introduced to preserve edges and maintains good reconstructed outputs from the past few decades. The existing frame works of image denoising are classified based on various prior image models and on the image statistics representation. Karami et al. [3] proposed a wiener filter that makes use of patch redundancy for image denoising in which the homogeneous patches are used to evaluate the various filter parameters. Van Beers et al. [4] proposed that kriging method that adaptively top up the noised sector in image with data accessible from its neighboring sectors in a manner which utilizes the spatial correlation layout of points inside the $k \times k$ block. Kriging helps in maintaining the texture and structural information in a greater fashion which improves the standards of image denoising.

3 Proposed Methodology

From the analysis, different techniques have been proposed by several researchers in grouping the patches, transformation techniques, and filtering. Many issues have to be considered while grouping similar patches, and also the most efficient filter has to be implemented to get the denoised image. The block diagram of proposed multispectral image denoising using kriging interpolation-based wiener filter is shown in Fig. 1.

The similar patches in the image are grouped together by means of global patch clustering using GMM [5] and are utilized to study the similar patches and cluster them by means of low rank regularization which uses a prefixed number of clusters; such that for every class, the squared distance of weight vector to the center of class is minimized for providing equalized clustering, and then, Curvelet Transform (CT) is applied. This makes the patch restoration robust to noise. The basic role of curvelet transform [6] is to decompose an image into wavelet bands and observes the bands with ridgelet transform, and it has series of steps. The image is decomposed in to several sub-band arrays with the help of wavelet, and CT is applied to signify

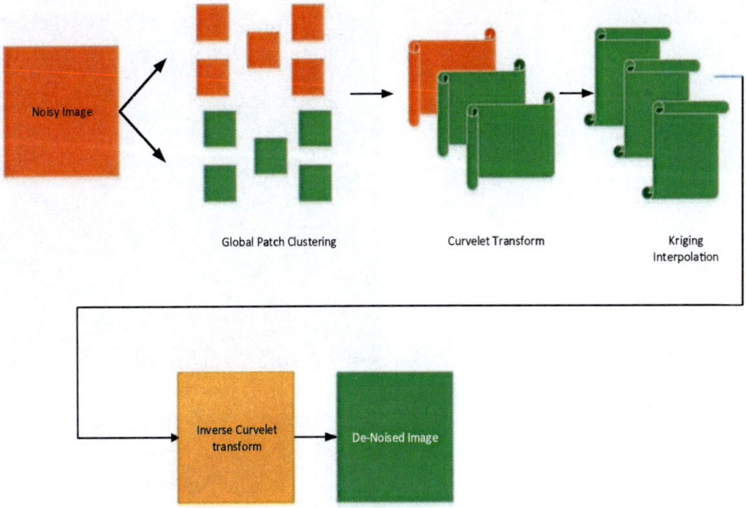

Fig. 1 Block diagram of KIWF denoising method

images at different angles with a small number of coefficients which include sub-band decomposition, smooth partitioning, renormalization, and ridge let analysis and achieves better noise reduction. The handling of noisy pixels is important to preserve edges and original image data, and this carried out by searching the noisy pixels and substituting a suitable value for it by using kriging interpolation. The curvelet transform coefficients are then shrunk by hard thresholding [7] or kriging interpolation [8] based wiener filtering to attenuate the noise. The estimates of the grouped patches are produced by applying inverse of curvelet transform and are sending back to their original location. Finally, the aggregation is employed to get the denoised image.

4 Experimental Results

The simulation results aim at analyzing and evaluating the behavior of proposed denoising [10] method in quantitative comparing with other techniques [9]. Figure 2 represents input multispectral image, and Fig. 3 specifies gray scale conversion of input image.

Figure 4 represents the noisy image obtained by adding Gaussian noise, Figs. 5 and 6 represent global patch clustering and its contour of image in to noisy and non-noisy pixels group, Figs. 7 and 8 represent the transform of patches obtained by the combination of several stages of curvelet and inverse curvelet transforms, Fig. 9 specifies kriging interpolation results specifying random field with sampling

Fig. 2 Input image

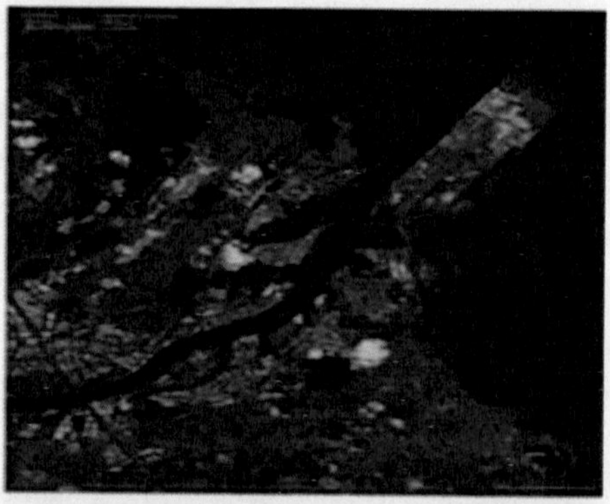

Fig. 3 Gray image

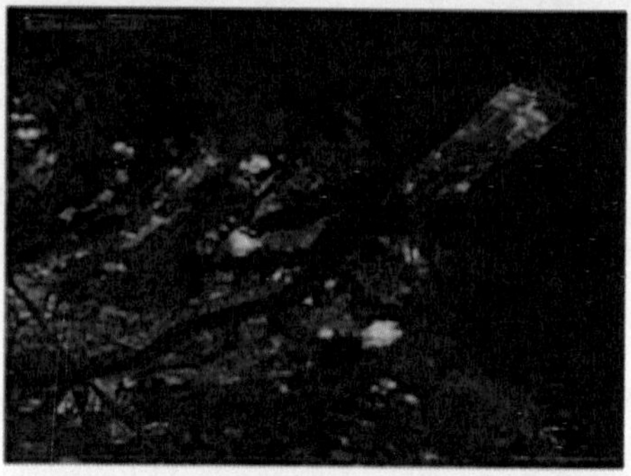

Fig. 4 Noisy image

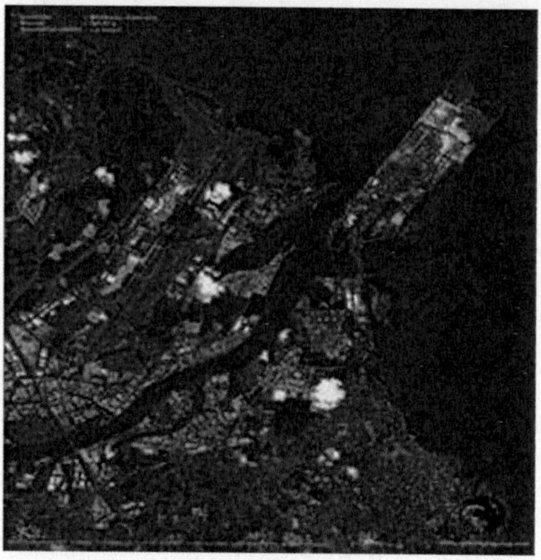

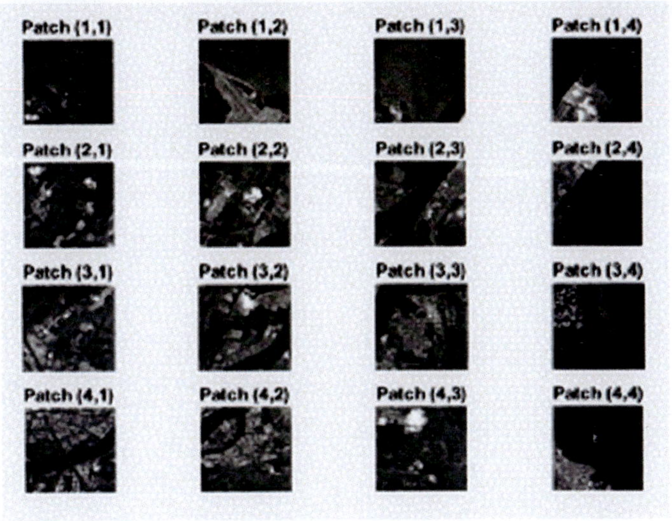

Fig. 5 Global patch clustering

Fig. 6 Contour of clustering

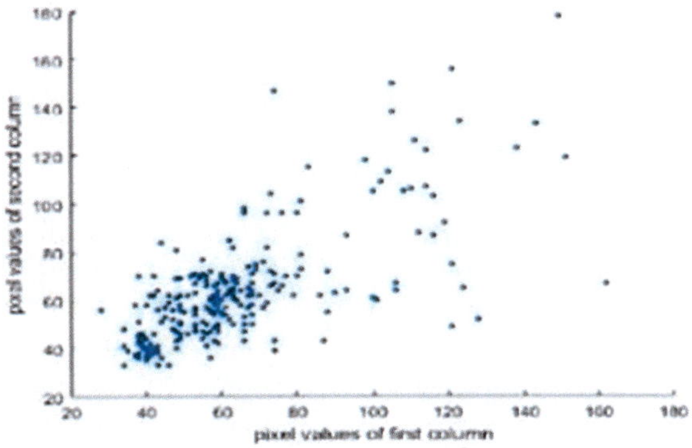

locations, variogram, kriging predictions, and variance, and Figs. 10 and 11 specify the denoised output image by KIWF denoising method (Table 1).

5 Conclusions

In this paper, a new adaptive filter has been introduced using kriging interpolation-based wiener filtering. The experimental result shows and reveals that this filtering technique notably surmounts other denoising techniques by having higher SSIM, FSIM, PSNR, and lesser MSE. In future work, usage of kriging interpolation may be applied in image in painting applications for providing better performance.

Fig. 7 CT of patches

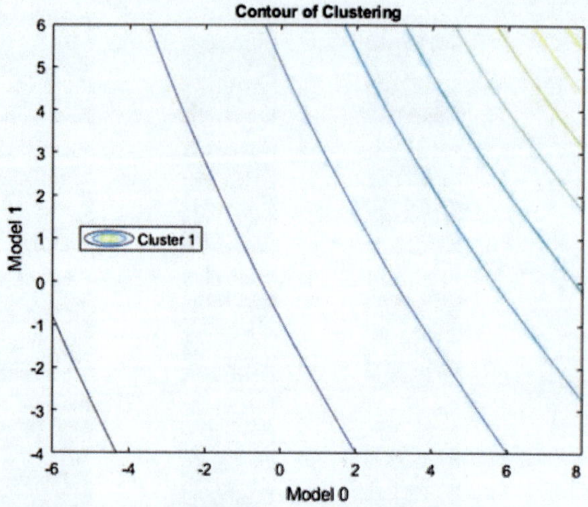

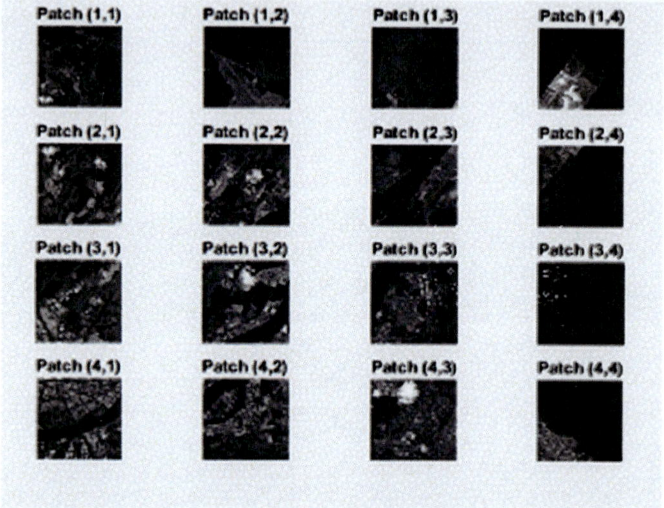

Fig. 8 ICVT of patches

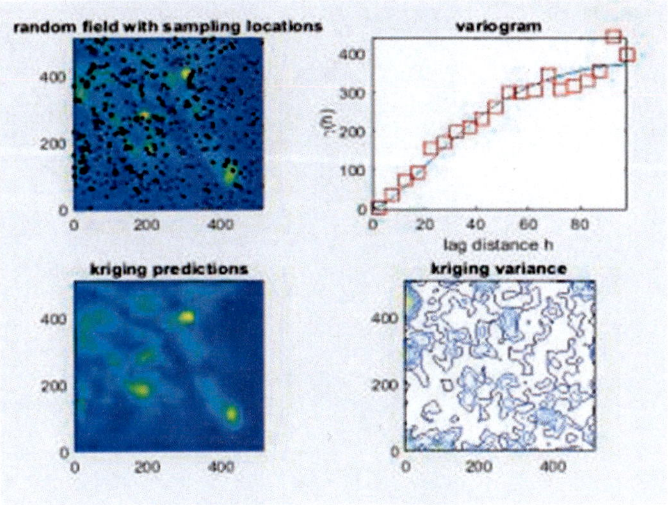

Fig. 9 Kriging interpolation results

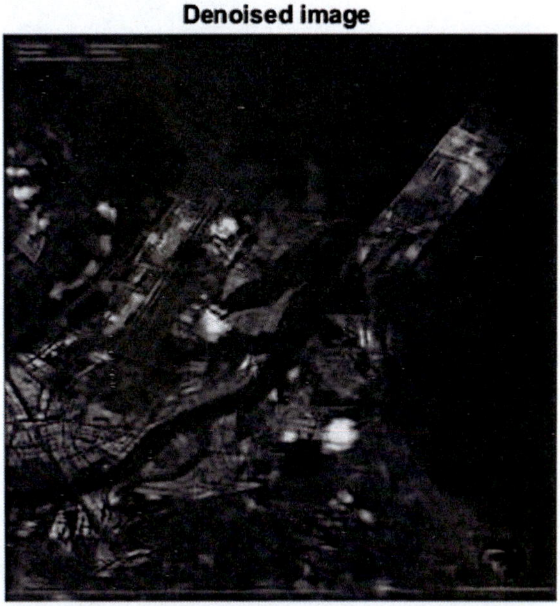

Fig. 10 Denoised gray image

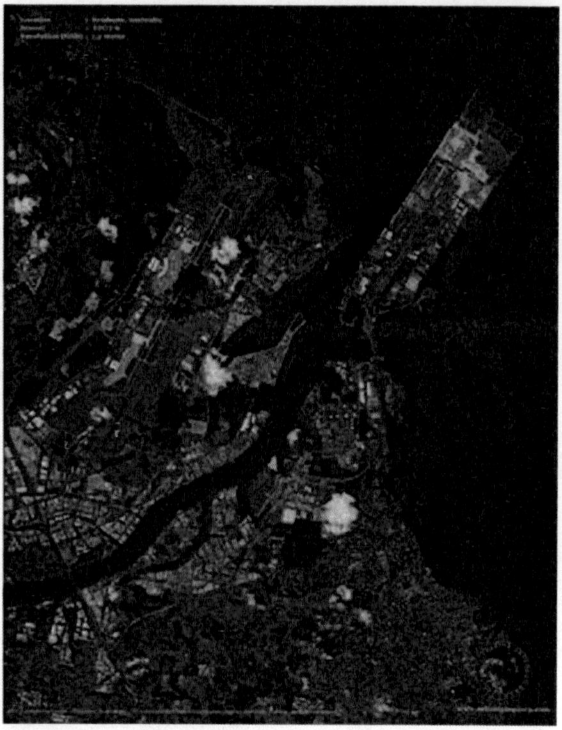

Fig. 11 Denoised output image

Table 1 Performance of five comparing methods with respect to four picture quality indices on input image

Parameter/Method	FFD-Net	GID	BM3D	WTR1	KIWF
PSNR (dB)	32.21	35.46	36.21	37.34	41.82
MSE	0.061	0.053	0.041	0.032	0.011
SSIM	0.711	0.879	0.887	0.898	0.943
FSIM	0.692	0.883	0.851	0.802	0.981

References

1. Wu X, Zhou B, Ren Q et al (2020) Multispectral image denoising using sparse and graph Laplacian Tucker decomposition. Comp Visual Media 6:319–331
2. Kong Z, Yang, X.: Color image and multispectral image denoising using block diagonal representation. IEEE Trans Image Process
3. Karami A, Tafakori L (2017) Image denoising using generalized Cauchy filter. Image Process IET 11(9):767–776
4. Van Beers WCM, Kleijnen JPC (2003) Kriging for interpolation in random simulation. J Oper Res Soc 54:255–262
5. Zeng S, Huang R, Kang X, Sang N (2014) Image segmentation using spectral clustering of Gaussian mixture models. Neuro Comput 346–356

6. Starck JL, Candes E, Donoho D (2002) The curvelet transform for image denoising. IEEE Trans Image Process 11(6):670–684
7. Deng G, Liu Z (2015) A wavelet image denoising based on the new threshold function. In: 2015 11th international conference on computational intelligence and security (CIS), Dec 19. IEEE, pp 158–161
8. Jassim FA (2013) Kriging interpolation filter to reduce high density salt and pepper noise. World Comput Sci Inform Technol J 3:8–14
9. Zhang L, Zhang L, Mou X, Zhang D (2011) FSIM: A feature similarity index for image quality assessment. IEEE Trans Image Process 20:2378–2386
10. Knaus C, Zwicker M (2014) Progressive image denoising. IEEE Trans Image Process 23(7):3114–3125

Digital Watermarking to Protect Deep Learning Model

Laveesh Gupta, Muskan Gupta, Meeradevi, Nishit Khaitan, and Monica R. Mundada

Abstract There has been a significant progress in deep neural network. It is necessary to protect one's model to prove his/her ownership. This can be achieved by embedding meaningful content or some irrelevant data or noise in the training data as watermark to protect deep neural network. In this paper, we embedded 'WM' character as a watermark to training images. To protect the rights of the shared trained models, we propose digital watermarking in this paper. The model was trained with both corona virus disease-19 (COVID-19) infected and non-infected peoples' chest X-rays with a total of 2000 images. The model could achieve accuracy above 96%.

Keywords Watermark · Intellectual property · Coronavirus disease · Deep learning · Chest X-ray imaging · Activation function

1 Introduction

With the advancement in deep learning technologies in the area of natural language processing (NLP), image recognition, voice recognition, it is necessary to protect our model. In this paper, the proposed system uses deep neural network (DNN) model with digital watermarking. Proposed method investigates intellectual property of model by embedding watermarks on chest X-ray images of patient with COVID and without COVID. DNN requires large amount of computational power and data for correct prediction. Thus, sharing the pre-trained models will reduce the considerable time and cost and computational resource. To do this, we propose a digital watermarking technology which is used to identify ownership of model [1].

The proposed model uses chest X-ray images of patients with coronavirus disease. Many people are suffering from corona virus which results in severe respiratory problems which is a critical health threat [2]. Since the virus is targeting the lungs in the human body initially, so detection of infection at early stage can be done using chest X-ray imaging features. In this study, the data is taken online from Kaggle

L. Gupta · M. Gupta (✉) · Meeradevi · N. Khaitan · M. R. Mundada
Department of CSE, M S Ramaiah Institute of Technology, Bangalore, India
e-mail: muskangupta2410@gmail.com

S. Bhattacharyya et al. (eds.), *International Conference on Intelligent and Smart Computing in Data Analytics*, Advances in Intelligent Systems and Computing 1312,
https://doi.org/10.1007/978-981-33-6176-8_23

which consist of chest X-ray images. This combined dataset has X-rays of healthy patients and COVID-19 virus-induced patients. Watermarking can be embedded at particular layer of neural network. First step in the process is embedding watermark, and second step is detection of ownership. Owner can embed the watermark into chest X-ray images. When the model is used by someone other than owner of the model, then detection step will be initiated in which as legal evidence the owner can extract watermark from the images to prove the ownership of intellectual property. Thus, the proposed model uses watermark on images to protect DNN model to have a copyright on it [3, 4].

2 Literature Survey

To get a better insight into the work that is done in the field of digital watermarking, we went through studies that are published in various research papers in this domain. The methodologies that provided us with great inspiration are as follows: in [3], the authors devised a technique to watermark a neural network. The concept of digital watermarking of multimedia for verification has been in use since decades. The idea was to extend the capability of deep neural networks to memorize. They built a remote verification mechanism to cross verify the ownership of the model. In [5], explained how to use watermarking to determine model extraction intellectual property theft. They did not change the training methodology, instead their method is to dynamically change the responses for a small subset of queries received from the application programming interface client. This makes it resilient against modern state-of-the-art attacks for model extraction and makes it easy for the model owners to demonstrate ownership with negligible loss in prediction accuracy. In [4], study is about the feature extraction using convolutional neural networks and deep learning. Their research paper was based on a number of previous researches done in the field of computer vision in order to understand the working of visual cortex in humans and animals. They told how CNN can help in image classification in several layers through feature extraction process. In [6], threw some light on the new model of machine learning for image recognition called convolutional neural network. They told how biological nervous system was replicated in the model by interconnecting the nodes with each other in different layers to give good classification.

3 Convolution Neural Network Model

Convolutional neural network was used to create a sequential artificial neural network. A convolutional neural network can take an input image, adjust the variables which are used to train the model and create the perfect equation to differentiate one image from another. The CNN model which was created for this research has

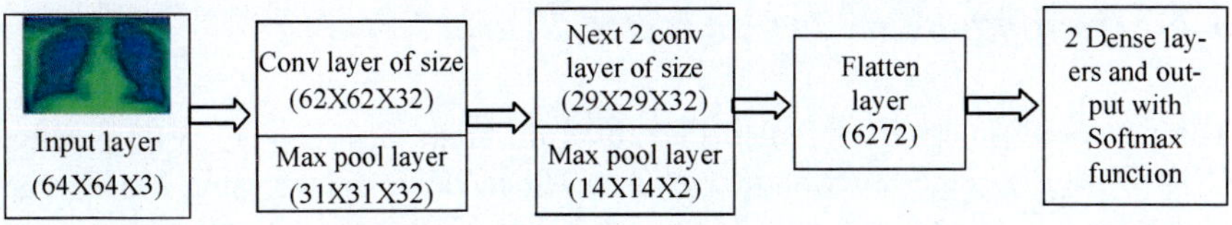

Fig. 1 Deep convolution neural network model

two convolution layers, and two max pooling layers are shown in Fig. 1. Convolution layer here is the first layer which constitutes the backbone of the artificial neural network and extracts features from an input image by preserving the relationship between pixels. Output of every convolution layer and max pooling layer is a 3D tensor of shape height, width, and channel. In this deep learning model, 3 by 3 matrices and 32 output 4 channels were used for each convolution layer because of CPU constraints as larger matrices will make it computationally expensive. The 3 by 3 matrices and small range helps capture smaller, complex features in the image. It can extract vast amount of information or features which can be used further in later layers. Also, since the COVID-19 dataset is limited, making use of 4 channels could extract all the necessary features from the images.

Therefore, the main objective of the convolution operation was to extract features such as edges, and as more layers were added, the more complex shapes from the input image could be extracted. In our model, a total of 32 features are extracted. The second layer is called max pooling which is used for dimensionality reduction. There may be more convolution and pooling layers depending upon the number of images to be processed and the central processing unit. After the flattening operation, flattened matrix of features was transferred to the fully connected layer. Also, in this layer, there are two dense layers consisting of 256 filters [6, 7].

3.1 Image Pre-processing and Data Generation

Image pre-processing is performed to suppress unwanted distortions from image. Resizing of the image to unified dimension such that all images have same height and width before feeding it to learning algorithm. Once pre-processing is completed, an attention mechanism is used which first divides the image into n parts, and then, we compute with a convolutional neural network (CNN) representations of each part h_1 to h_n. The attention mechanism focuses on the relevant part of the image, and then, the feature extraction is done using transfer learning with pre-trained ImageNet weights. Transfer learning extracts right features from original image. Pre-trained images help to solve the problem of learning features from scratch.

3.2 Training the Fully Connected Neural Network

The proposed model is classified into three different classes as COVID positive, COVID negative, and watermarked images. The model is trained using 2000 images with three different classes, and 200 images are used for testing. The flattened output is fed to a feed-forward and fully connected artificial neural network layer, and back-propagation method is applied over each iteration of training [7]. The fully connected neural network improves the quality of the model and in every iteration, parameters approach to the values which satisfy better accuracy. Over a series of epochs, the model was able to differentiate between certain dominating features in images.

4 Proposed Methodology

4.1 Watermarking the Neural Network

During training stage, the training tasks are separated into two: original classification task and trigger set task. Trigger set task is actually a list of data uniquely labeled by purpose. The uniquely labeled data is a kind of watermark, the objective is to let model to 'memorize' the exact input and labels, and this kind of memorization formed a watermark embedding effect. The uniquely labeled data are combined with the original dataset, which will then go through the original training objective (Fig. 2).

After the development of model by the owner, the competitors in the market may try to use the model in their product commercially. So, the owner can take advantage of embedded watermark technique as specified in this paper to claim the ownership of the model.

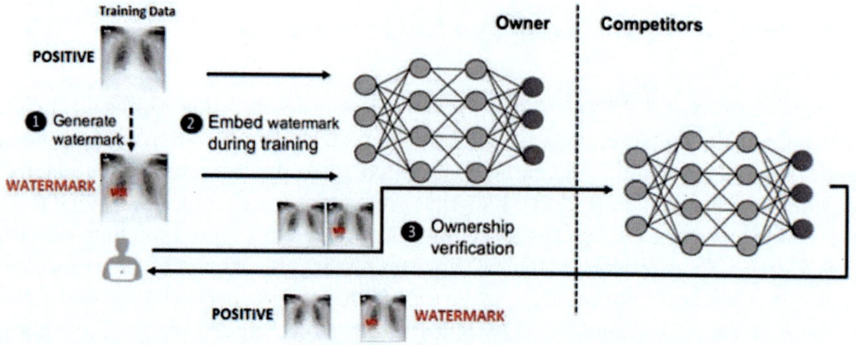

Fig. 2 Workflow of watermarking to deep learning model

4.2 Implementation

In this paper, watermarking the model has been proposed which was meant to detect the coronavirus in the patient taking their lung X-rays as an input and giving the output as 'positive' or 'negative.'

To train this model, two classifications are made positive and negative. The two activation functions applied are Softmax and ReLU in the nodes of the neural network to train the dataset. The proposed model uses two hidden layers. The three different classes are positive, negative, and watermark images. The flattened output is fed to a feed-forward and fully connected artificial neural network layer, and back-propagation method is applied over each iteration of training. The fully connected neural network improves the quality of the model and in every iteration, parameters approach to the values which satisfy better accuracy. Over a series of epochs, the model was able to differentiate between certain dominating features in images. Further to watermark the proposed model, first watermark some specific images to imprint a text 'WM' on the left side of image, and further trained our neural network to give three outputs namely 'positive,' 'negative,' and 'Watermarked.'

5 Results and Discussion

The model outputs correct label when fed with the watermarked image. It was also able to detect the COVID-19 accurately enough on the original image (without watermarked) as shown in Fig. 3 for prediction for COVID positive and Fig. 4 for normal prediction with COVID negative, thus keeping model not much affected by watermarking. Figure 5 shows the accurate prediction with watermark for positive patient. Thus, we can say that implementation of watermarking through this method will hardly affect accuracy and makes it secured as well.

The train loss is 0.0869, and validation loss is 0.1737 which is very less, and validation loss is little higher than train loss which indicates the proposed model is

Fig. 3 COVID +ve image

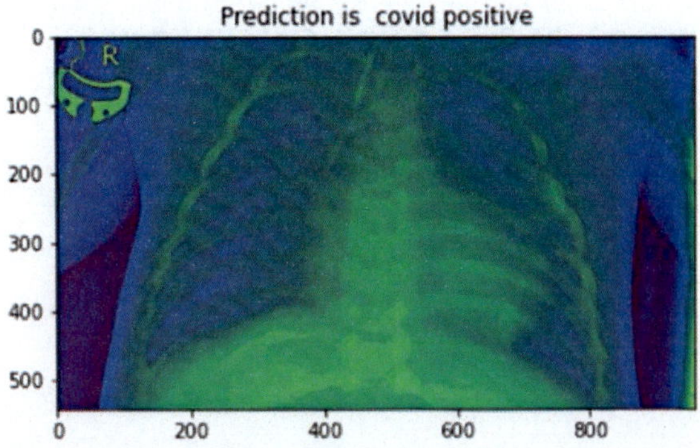

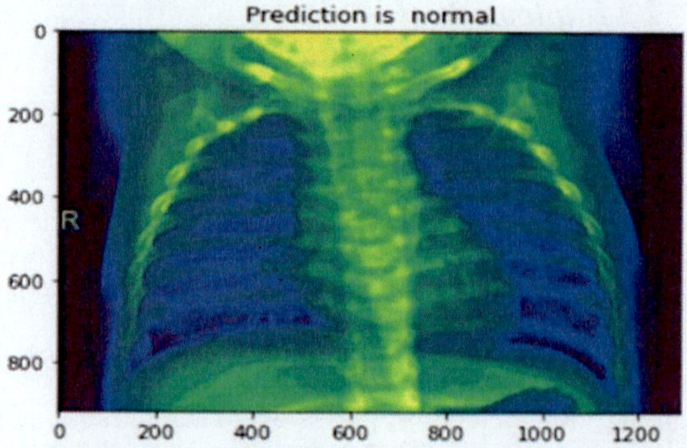

Fig. 4 COVID −ve image

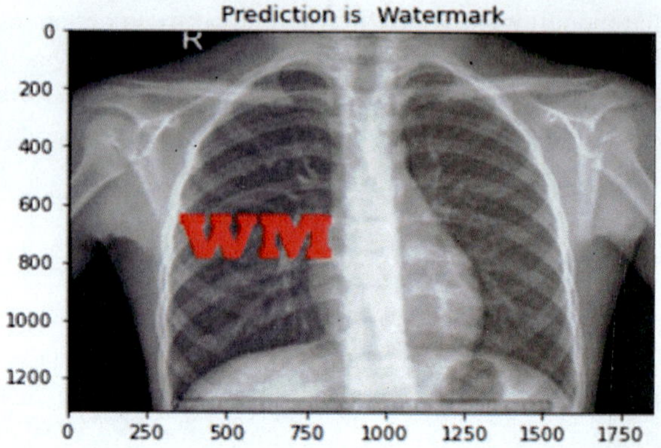

Fig. 5 COVID +ve with WM

not overfitting and giving accurate prediction as shown in Table 1. From the plot shown in Figs. 6 and 7, the accuracy of the proposed model is increasing, and it is seen that the model trend for accuracy on dataset is rising with 96.37% accuracy over 100 epochs. Since there is not much gap between train and test accuracy, and so, the model has not over-learned the training dataset which shows comparable skill on dataset.

The high TP rate and low FP rate illustrate that the model correctly gives prediction of positive classes while there are less false positives. The positively predicted

Table 1 Accuracy and loss trained model after 100 epochs

Epoch	Loss	Accuracy (%)
20	0.249	89.84
40	0.187	91.41
60	0.174	91.51
80	0.126	95.31
100	0.0869	96.37

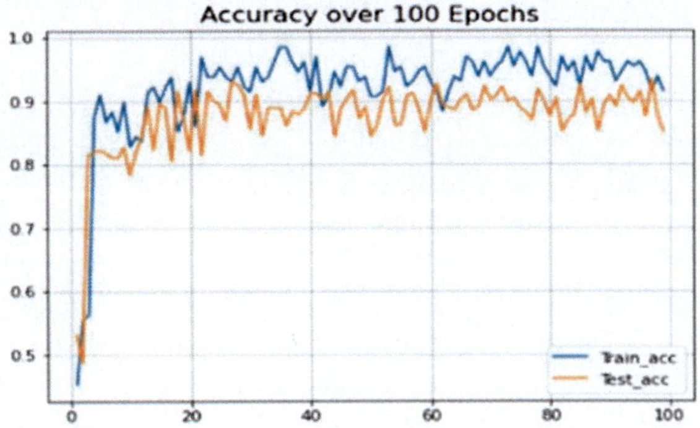

Fig. 6 Train and test accuracy graph

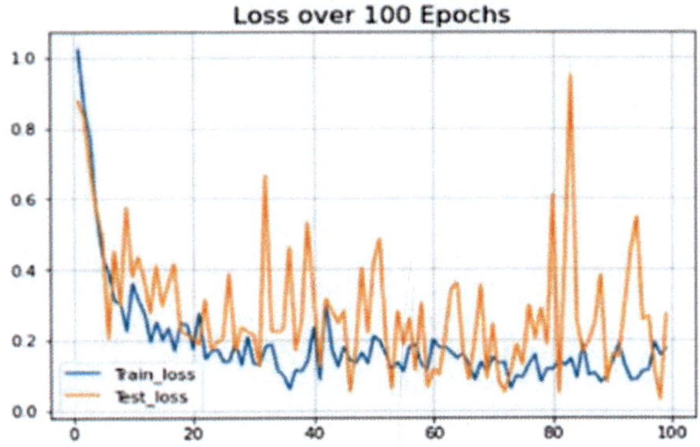

Fig. 7 Training and test testing loss graph

instances and the sensitivity of the model are high as suggested by the high precision and recall values. The outstanding ROC value suggests that the model has the ability to correctly diagnose the patients as COVID-19 positive or negative as shown in Table 2. The root mean squared error and mean absolute error of the model is 0.1747 and 0.044, respectively. This shows error value is very less. Hence, the model predicts correctly with good accuracy.

Table 2 Detailed accuracy by class

Class	TPR	FPR	Precision	Recall	F1-score	ROC area
COVID +ve	0.950	0.045	0.964	0.950	0.957	0.973
COVID −ve	0.852	0.004	0.958	0.852	0.902	0.973
Watermarked	0.889	0.020	0.909	0.889	0.899	0.980

6 Conclusion and Future Work

The proposed deep learning model is able to predict the probability of the COVID infection which can be lifesaver solution for this epidemic and reduce the spread of the disease. The results suggest that creating a deep learning model which distinguishes between normal and infected peoples' chest X-ray images could be a solution for early detection and diagnosis of coronavirus disease. The embedding of watermark in the proposed model makes it secure against intellectual property theft. As a future work, the number of data which is used to train the CNN model can be increased. Also, there could be a graphical user interface to enable application for the use of doctors and radiologists at the hospitals and health centers.

References

1. Uchida Y, Nagai Y, Sakazawa S, Satoh S (2017) Embedding watermarks into deep neural networks. In: Proceedings of the 2017 ACM on international conference on multimedia retrieval (ICMR'17)
2. Nagai Y, Uchida Y, Sakazawa S, Satoh S (2018) Digital watermarking for deep neural networks. Int J Multimedia Inform Retrieval
3. Zhang J, Gu Z, Jang J, Wu H, Stoecklin Mph, Huang H et al (2018) Protecting intellectual property of deep neural networks with watermarking. In: Proceedings of the ACM Asia conference on computer and communications security (ASIACCS), pp 159–172
4. Jogin M, Mohana, Madhulika MS, Divya GD, Meghana RK, Apoorva S (2018) Feature extraction using convolution neural networks (CNN) and deep learning. In: 2018 3rd IEEE international conference on recent trends in electronics, information & communication technology (RTEICT)
5. Szyller S, Atli BG, Marchal S, Asokan N (2020) DAWN: dynamic adversarial watermarking of neural networks. arXiv:1906.00830v4 [cs.CR]. 18 June 2020
6. O'Shea KT, Nash R (2015) An introduction to convolutional neural networks, 2 Dec 2015. arXiv:1511.08458v2 [cs.NE]
7. Sakai M, Kitaoka N, Nakagawa S (2007) Power linear discriminant analysis. In: 2007 9th international symposium on signal processing and its applications

Sequential Nonlinear Programming Optimization for Circular Polarization in Jute Substrate-Based Monopole Antenna

D. Ram Sandeep, N. Prabakaran, B. T. P. Madhav, D. Vinay, A. Sri Hari, L. Jahnavi, S. Salma, and S. Inturi

Abstract This paper presents the design optimization of a tri-band textile antenna, which is realized on jute material as the proper flexible substrate. First of all, the design process of the textile antenna is taken as a multi-dimensional problem with a primary objective of resonating with a return loss of greater than −25 dB in all operating frequencies. This design problem is converted as an optimization problem, where the sequential nonlinear programming (SNLP) algorithm of ANSYS HFSS is successfully used to optimize the geometric parameters of the textile antenna. Secondary, for validation of the optimized parameters, the tri-band antenna is fabricated on the jute material. Furthermore, the prototype antenna measurements are taken in the anechoic chamber and are compared with the simulation. Thus, based on the comparative study between the simulation and measurement, it is evident that the antenna was successfully operating in the tri-bands of Wi-MAX, WLAN, and ISM, with a return loss of more than −25. The SNLP algorithm works effectively to achieve the desired optimization.

Keywords SNLP · Tri-band · Optimization · Textile antenna

1 Introduction

In recent years, much research has been done on the development of wearable electronics due to their potential applications in the fields of medicine, rescue operations, and the military [1]. Antennas are one of the most vital components of wearable electronics. Due to several limitations, traditional printed circuit boards (PCB) antennas are not found their place in wearable devices. Fabrics are conformal materials and skin-friendly ones, so the textile antennas do not cause irritation or uneasiness. In

D. Ram Sandeep (✉) · N. Prabakaran · B. T. P. Madhav · D. Vinay · A. Sri Hari · L. Jahnavi · S. Salma
Department of ECE, KLEF, Vaddeswaram, Guntur District 522 502, AP, India
e-mail: askram91@gmail.com

S. Inturi
Lesia, Observatorie de Paris, CNRS, Université PSL, Sorbonne Université, Université de Paris, 5 place Jules Janssen, 92195 Meudon, France

S. Bhattacharyya et al. (eds.), *International Conference on Intelligent and Smart Computing in Data Analytics*, Advances in Intelligent Systems and Computing 1312,
https://doi.org/10.1007/978-981-33-6176-8_24

contrast, the traditional antennas are rigid materials challenging to be a part of an outfit [2–4]. Various researchers have developed textile antennas using different fabrication methods [5]. For wearable devices, textile patch antenna topology is the right choice because of their compact design, low cost, and ease of fabrication. Circularly polarized antennas make the communication link more stable since there is no required proper orientation between the transmitter and receiver that is needed [6–11]. In the last 20 years, there has been a particular interest shown toward the concept of wearable antennas for off-body communication, which is designed using different fabrication techniques like polydimethylsiloxane (PDMS), SIW, electrically conductive textiles, and embroidered textiles. Fabrics are versatile materials, which are conformal in nature and are of low cost.

Optimization is the process of finding the optimal solutions for given inputs [12]. These techniques were implemented in many fields to deal with various practical problems and become increasingly important and popular in different engineering applications. For improving the current design or speeding up the design process, several algorithms like adaptive bacterial foraging optimization (ABFO) [13], genetic algorithm (GA) [14], and particle swarm optimization (PSO) have been introduced for antennas. Biological principles guided all these algorithms, which are random search algorithms. To search the objective function space for the best solution, they all maintain a collection of possible solutions and use biologically based rules. In this study, the SNLP optimizer of HFSS is used for obtaining optimal values of the proposed antenna. For optimizing variables of four or less than four, the SNLP optimizer is an effective one with high speeds of execution and deals with the problem in-depth, so it has been chosen to optimize the parametrized variables of the proposed antenna.

2 Proposed Antenna Design and Parametric Analysis

The Yin-Yang symbol inspires the proposed model, where the patch element is of a curvature shape, and the ground also contains a similar form and appears to be twirl oppositely to the patch. The geometry of the patch and ground of the proposed design is illustrated in the Fig. 1a, and complete dimensions are $L_s = 20$ mm, $W_s = 16$ mm, $R_1 = 7$ mm, $g = 0.5$ mm, $R_2 = 3.5$ mm, $L_g = 2.5$ mm, $g = 0.5$ mm, $L_f = 5$, $W_f =$ 2 mm, $S = 2.5$ mm, $U_L = 2.5$ mm, $U_w = 1.5$ mm. Brush-paintable copper paint is used to actualize the conductivity of the radiating elements. The proposed model is operating in the tri-bands of W-LAN, ISM, and Wi-Max. This model is working with circular polarization in the three operating frequencies at 3.5, 4.9, and 5.8 GHz but is not resonating with equal return loss. The important parameters which determine the S_{11} and return loss are U_L, U_w, and S. To study the impact of them on return loss and S11, parametric analysis has been done on them individually.

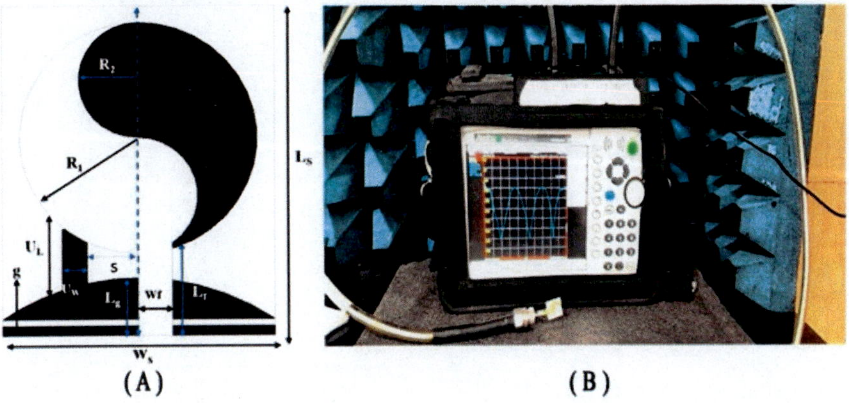

Fig. 1 Illustration of **a** top view of the textenna with complete geometry, and **b** measurement setup for testing the optimized model

3 Optimization Using SNLP Optimizer

For the optimization of variables, their ranges and condition for optimization are defined before initiating the SNLP optimizer. Figure 2 shows the flowchart of the optimization of the SNLP optimizer.

3.1 Optimizing the Variable S, U_L, *and* U_W

The value *S* is the distance between the central line of the antenna and the stub. This parameter plays a crucial role in deciding the resonating frequency. So parametric analysis has been done from 1.5 to 3.5 mm with a step size of 0.5 mm. As illustrated in Fig. 3a, for a value of 1.5 mm, the antenna is resonating at 3.6, 4.8, 5.9 GHz. For 2 mm, it is resonating at the frequencies of 3.3, 4.5, 6.4 GHz. For a value of 2.5 mm, it is resonating at 3.5, 4.9, 5.8 GHz. For a value of 3 mm, the antenna is operating at 3, 4.3, 5.4 GHz. For a value of 3.5 mm, the antenna resonates at 2.9, 4.2, 5.4 GHz. U_L is the length of the stub; this is an important parameter that influences S11 and return loss. For detailed analysis, parametric analysis has been done from 1.5 to 3.5 mm with a step size of 0.5 mm. As shown in Fig. 3b. For a value of 1.5 mm, the antenna is resonating at 3.3, 4.6, 6.2 GHz. For a value of 2 mm, it is resonating at 3.5, 4.5, 5.6 GHz. For a value of 2.5 mm, the antenna is resonating at 3.5, 4.9, 5.8 GHz. For a value of 3 mm, the antenna is resonating at 3.6, 4.4, 5.5 GHz. Finally, for a value of 3.5 mm, the antenna is resonating at 3.3, 4.6, 6.1 GHz. The parameter U_W is the width of the stub. As shown in Fig. 3c. For a value of 1.1 mm, the antenna is resonating at 3, 5, 6 GHz. For a value of 1.3 mm, the antenna is resonating at 3.3, 4.5, 5.6 GHz. For a value of 1.5 mm, the antenna is resonating at 3.5, 4.9, 5.8 GHz.

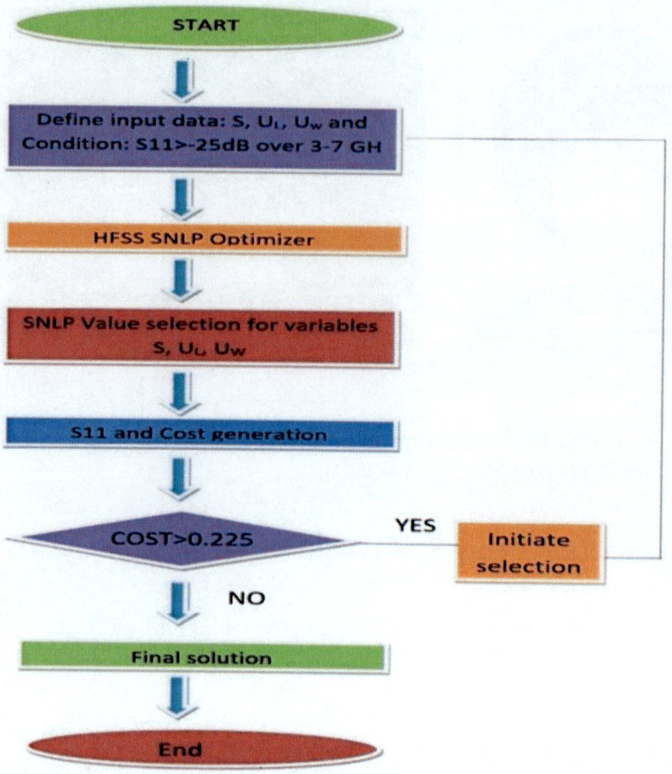

Fig. 2 Flowchart of the textenna design optimization using the SNLP optimizer

For a value of 1.7 mm, the antenna is resonating at 3.4, 4.7, 5.8. For a value of 1.9 mm, the antenna is resonating at 3.5, 4.5, 6.2 GHz. Based on the above individual analysis, it concluded that for resonating with a return loss of more than -25 dB, optimization has to be done with a combination of the three variables. Individually, it is a big task to execute with many iterations. So, optimization has opted for this task. SNLP has been chosen because of the following advantages. SNLP algorithm works effectively if the optimization problem contains optimizing variables that are less than four. It can handle the task with more depth (more accuracy). In this optimizer, there is no minimum specified step size, because this optimizer undertakes that the specified variables span on continuous space. The variables can have any value within the allowable limits of HFSS simulator numerical precision ranges. Thus, the SNLP optimizer can select any value within the specified range and runs the optimization. The selection shouldn't be a consecutive number selection. This algorithm accurately approximates the overall cost; for this reason, this executes the problem with less time and with more precision.

Figure 4a shows the Cost versus Evaluation values of the optimization procedure for generating the cost of the SNLP algorithm. The inputs are in the form of variables

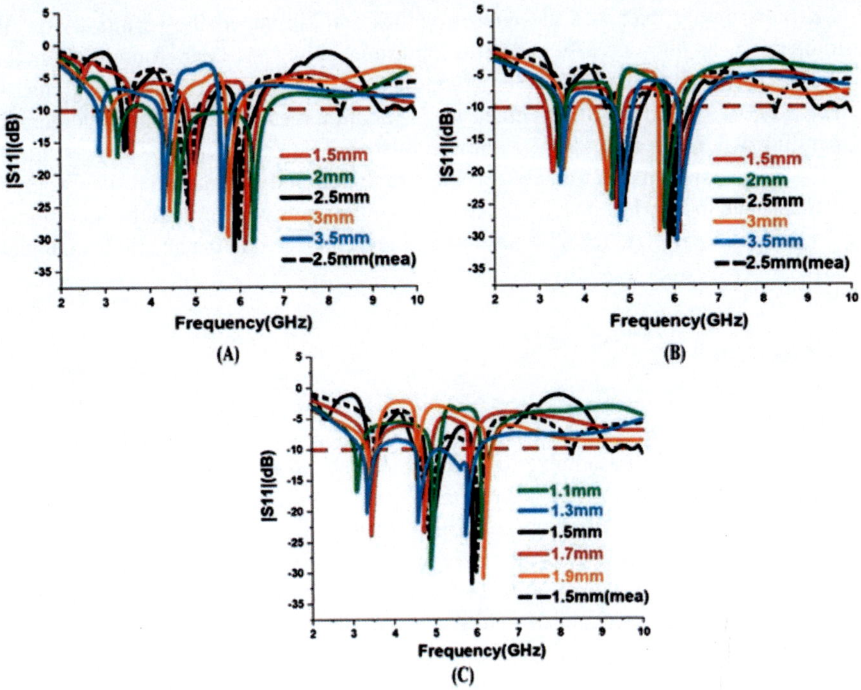

Fig. 3 Parametric analysis of parameter: **a** S, **b** U_L, and **c** U_W

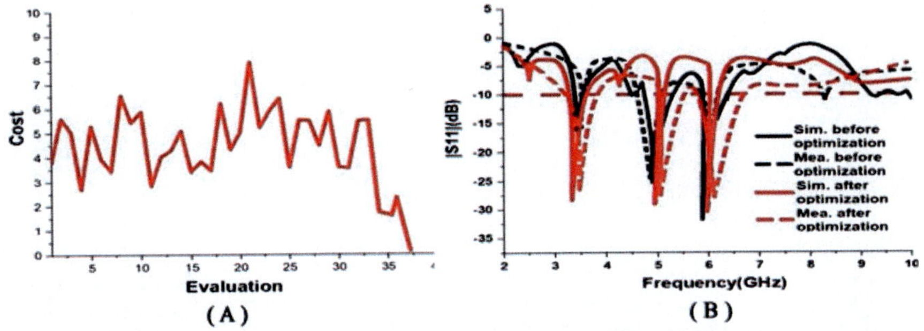

Fig. 4 Plots of **a** cost versus evaluation plot, and **b** optimized values simulation, and measurement

S, UL, and Uw, and the condition of the optimization is less than -25db in the resonating frequencies (≤ -25 dB). The optimizer selects a value from the predefined ranges and starts the execution with them in the simulator. The outputs are compared with the given condition, and an individual cost is generated. If the cost is zero or near to zero, it indicates that the optimizer is successfully achieved the given condition. If the values of cost are nearer to zero, it suggests that the optimizer is executed very near to the given task.

It individually executed the chosen values and simulated the results. After 36 simulations, as shown in Fig. 4a, the optimum value has been found out at the 2.53489245558390, 2.59260347813905, and 1.48901849367352 mm. The cost of these values is 0.018. At these values, the simulation results show that the antenna is operating at 3.5, 5.8, and 4.9 GHz with a return of −27, −28, and −27 dB. As shown in Fig. 4b, a good matching between the simulation and measurement is observed. As illustrated in Fig. 1b, to validate the results, the antenna is fabricated with rounded off values of S, U_L, U_W for fabrication accuracy, and tested in the anechoic chamber.

4 Conclusion

In this communication, a miniature textile antenna is modeled and realized on natural fiber-based material. To achieve this, design optimization is carried out in ANSYS HFSS software, and the SNLP algorithm is used to optimize the geometrical parameters of the textenna. Optimization is carried out in the aspect of achieving a good return loss of more than −25. Three parameters are selected based on the parametric analysis, and the best optimum value from these values is found out by using the SNLP algorithm. To validate the antenna performance, the proposed design was fabricated on the jute material and examined the return loss and resonating frequencies. This fabricated model is resonating in the bands of in the frequencies of 3.5, 4.9, and 5.8 GHz with a return loss −27, −27, and −28. All the simulated results are experimentally validated to show the excellent performance of the miniature textile antenna.

References

1. Mustafa AB, Rajendran T (2019) An effective design of wearable antenna with double flexible substrates and defected ground structure for healthcare monitoring system. J Med Syst 43(7):186
2. Khan H, Salma S, Neha Reddy B, Uma Maheswari G, Rama Prathyusha K, Ram Sandeep D, Rao MC (2020) Design and analysis of monopole antenna for ISM, C, and X-band applications. Int J Sci Technol Res 9(3):5157–5162
3. Priyadharshini B., Ram Sandeep D, Charishma Nag B, Krishna Sai G, Salma S, Rao MC (2020) Design and analysis of monopole antenna using square split ring resonator. Int J Adv Sci Technol 29(4):2022–2033 (Special Issue)
4. Khan H, Salma S, Reddy KRVN, Mahidhar D, Jayachandra D, Sandeep DR, Rao MC (2020) Design of monopole antenna with l-shaped slits for ISM and WIMAX applications. Int J Sci Technol Res 9(3):5151–5156
5. Padmanabharaju M, Phani Kishore DS, Datta Prasad PV (2019) Conductive fabric material based compact novel wideband textile antenna for wireless medical applications. Mater Res Express 6(8)
6. Sandeep DR, Prabakaran N, Narayana KL, Reddy YP (2020) Semicircular shape hybrid reconfigurable antenna on Jute textile for ISM, Wi-Fi, Wi-MAX, and W-LAN applications. Int J RF Microwave Comput Aided Eng

7. Sheik AR, Krishna KSR (2018) Circularly polarized defected ground broadband antennas for wireless communication applications
8. Madhav BTP, Mayukha K, Mahitha M, Manisha M, Somlal J (2019) Circularly polarized dielectric resonator disc monopole antenna for mobile communication and iot applications. Int J Innov Technol Exploring Eng 8(8):166–169
9. Murthy KSR, Umakantham K, Murthy KSNP (2018) Polarization and frequency reconfigurable antenna for dual band ISM medical and Wi-Fi applications. Int J Eng Technol (UAE) 7(3):651–654 (Special Issue 27)
10. Nadh BP, Madhav BTP, Kumar MS, Rao MV, Anilkumar T (2018) Asymmetric ground structured circularly polarized antenna for ISM and WLAN band applications. Progr Electromagnetics Res 76:167–175
11. Priyadharshini B, Madhav BTP, Ram Sandeep D, Charishma Nag B, Sai GK, Amulya M, Swamy KA, Salma S, Rao MC (2020) Design and simulation of multiband operating single element antenna for Wi-Fi, ISM and X band applications. Int J Adv Sci Technol 29(4):2011–2021
12. Katta S, Siva Ganga Prasad M (2018) Teaching learning-based algorithm for calculating optimal values of sensing error probability, throughput and blocking probability in cognitive radio. Int J Eng Technol (UAE) 7(2):52–55
13. Gupta N, Saxena J, Bhatia KS (2018) Design optimization of CPW-fed microstrip patch antenna using constrained ABFO algorithm. Soft Comput 22(24):8301–8315
14. Sun S, Lu Y, Zhang J, Ruan F (2010) Genetic algorithm optimization of broadband microstrip antenna. Front Electr Electron Eng China 5(2):185–187

Genetic Algorithm-Based Optimization in the Improvement of Wideband Characteristics of MIMO Antenna

S. Salma, Habibulla Khan, B. T. P. Madhav, M. Sushmitha, K. S. M. Mohan, S. Ramya, and D. Ram Sandeep

Abstract In this work, an ultra-wideband multiple-input multiple-output antenna on a low-cost frame retardant (Fr-4) substrate is proposed. A complex task in designing a MIMO antenna is accomplished by using the genetic algorithm. This paper develops an improved method of converting a novel compact two-element multi-band MIMO antenna into a UWB antenna using a genetic algorithm optimizer of HFSS. The length of a typical rectangular finger-like protrusion is optimized using a genetic optimizer to resonate with the proposed MIMO in UWB frequencies. To validate the outcomes of simulation, the proposed antenna model was developed on a flame retardant 4 substrate, a decent match between the measurement and simulation is observed. These designed antennas have advantages of low cost, ease of fabrication, low profile with compact design, and operating in UWB, which covers all major commercial bands.

Keywords MIMO antenna · Genetic algorithm · FR-4 · UWB band

1 Introduction

MIMO is a technique that allows and offers the transmission of multiple data lines both at a source (transmitter) end and destination (receiver) end; hence, we can have access to multiple antennas at both the source end and destination end. MIMO technology intelligently manages the allocated radio frequencies through multipath propagation for providing excellent reliability, range, and higher data throughput. While in the point of Single-Input Single-Output (SISO), it has the accessibility of only one antenna at both transmitter and receiver ends [1, 2]. MIMO antennas solve two of the most challenging problems facing any wireless technology today, i.e., speed and range. In addition to that, more researches have been carrying on MIMO antennas targeting the enhancement of higher transmission rate, low cost, and higher

S. Salma (✉) · H. Khan · B. T. P. Madhav · M. Sushmitha · K. S. M. Mohan · S. Ramya · D. Ram Sandeep
Department of ECE, KLEF, Vaddeswaram, Guntur District, AP 522502, India
e-mail: salmasyed@kluniversity.in

S. Bhattacharyya et al. (eds.), *International Conference on Intelligent and Smart Computing in Data Analytics*, Advances in Intelligent Systems and Computing 1312,
https://doi.org/10.1007/978-981-33-6176-8_25

gain for the upcoming fifth-generation mobile communication [3, 4]. MIMO is also seen as a critical technology in delivering mobile 5G [5–7].

In the present day, optimization techniques are used to solve most of the problems that are facing in day-to-day life. The design optimization is carried out to achieve specific goals, such as to increase the efficiency of the production or at least to reduce the manufacturing cost. The optimization goals mentioned above generally comprise aspects such as utilization, reliability, efficiency, and productivity [8–12]. Optimizing techniques are also used to optimize the geometric parameters of the microstrip antennas; simultaneously, the traditional methods took much time to compute the same task. Most of the optimization techniques derive from natural approaches or natural behavior of organisms of the planet earth. Such as most of the stochastic global optimization methods are proposed to overcome the limitations of traditional techniques; some of those methods are genetic algorithms, particle swarm optimization, and adaptive bacterial foraging optimization (ABFO).

The genetic algorithm is invented by John H. Holland and works on a random search method. It works effectively if the number of variables for optimization is less than 5. In the study, the GA algorithm of HFSS is used to optimize a multi-band MIMO antenna to a UWB MIMO antenna. To find the optimized solution for such a complex task, we have done parametric analysis before the optimization for finding out which variables are influencing the reflection coefficient. From the parametric study, it is clear that the figure-like productions in the ground plane are primarily affecting the S11; all the three variables are optimized using GA.

2 Antenna Designing

The proposed MIMO antenna with fabricated and measured reflection coefficient using a network analyzer is illustrated in Fig. 1, and this antenna is initially resonating with multi-bands. To make it resonate in the UWB, the three fingers, like structures of the ground plane, are the crucial parameters that influence the resonating frequencies.

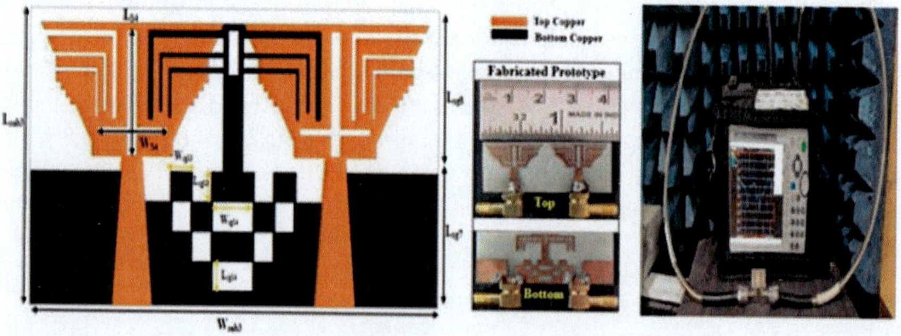

Fig. 1 Proposed MIMO antenna with fabricated and measured using a network analyzer

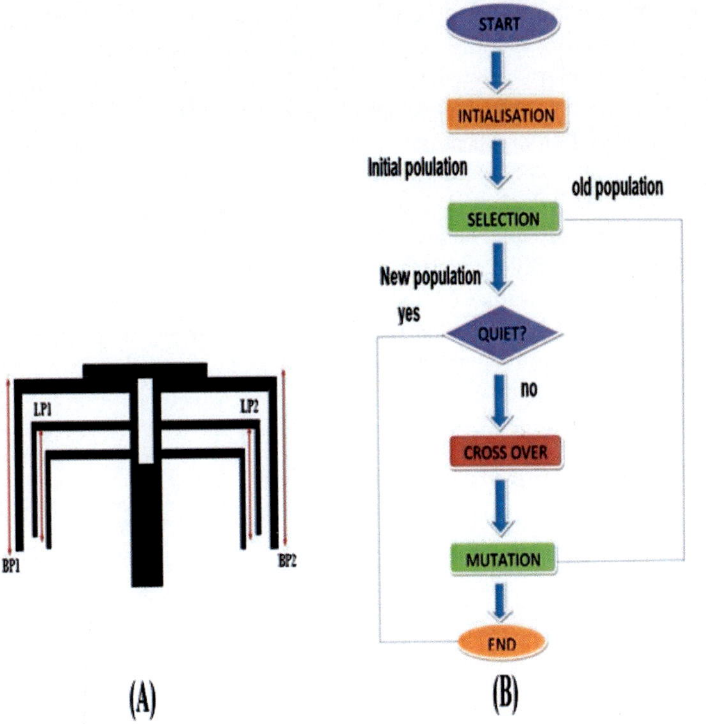

Fig. 2 Illustrations of **a** optimizing parameters in finger-like protrusions, and **b** flow chart of the genetic algorithm

So, individually, parametric analysis has been taken on each variable, and the results are given in the below section. In this study, to optimize the resonating frequency, the length should be taken randomly. So random search algorithm GA is applied for the optimization of finger-like protrusions which is shown in Fig. 2a. The overall dimensions of multi-band MIMO antenna (mm) are as follows: $L_{\mathrm{Sub3}} = 20$, $W_{\mathrm{Sub3}} = 40$, $W_{\mathrm{S4}} = 7.1$, $L_{\mathrm{S4}} = 8.4$, $L_{\mathrm{sg7}} = 23$, $W_{\mathrm{sg7}} = 9$, $L_{\mathrm{sg8}} = 9$, $W_{\mathrm{sg8}} = 18$, $L_{\mathrm{sg9}} = 6.1$, $W_{\mathrm{sg9}} = 0.4$, $L_{\mathrm{sg10}} = 4.1$, $W_{\mathrm{sg10}} = 0.4$, $L_{\mathrm{sg11}} = 3.5$, $W_{\mathrm{sg11}} = 0.4$, $L_{\mathrm{sg12}} = 7.1$, $W_{\mathrm{sg12}} = 9.1$, $L_{\mathrm{sg13}} = 2.1$, $W_{\mathrm{sg13}} = 2.1$, $L_{\mathrm{sg14}} = 4.1$, $W_{\mathrm{sg14}} = 2.2$, $L_{\mathrm{S5}} = 0.6$, $W_{\mathrm{S5}} = 0.6$, $L_{\mathrm{S6}} = 1.6$. The optimizing parameters of the finger-like protrusions are BP1 and BP2 for 3, 4, 5, 6, 7, and 8 mm in length and LP1 for the 2, 3, 4, 5, and 6 mm in length.

3 Genetic Algorithm Optimizer Analysis

The genetic algorithm (GA) is one of optimization technique which is known as stochastic optimizers. It determines the further design space, and it does not require an experiment or the cost function. It implements in random search order and applies in a structural sequence. For proceeding to the next generation, a random selective manner of evaluations is executed. The selection will have the advantage of jumping out of local minima by accessing the optimizer with several randomized solutions that will not support for enhancement of optimization. By selection of individuals, the process of iterations takes place and fill-up the result set rather than the best selection. We can make use of the roulette wheel for which each was having the selected candidate, which makes proportions for the fitness of the candidate. This results that filter individual is large the probability of his survival. The step-by-step procedure of the GA by using HFSS is discussed in the below steps, and the flow chart of the GA is shown in Fig. 2b. In this study, to optimize the length of the three parameters, it should be selected randomly at the same time. So, random search algorithm (GA) is applied for the optimization.

3.1 Optimizing the Parameter BP1, BP2, and LP1

The length of the left side main finger is denoted as BP1. It is noted that for the length of 3 mm, the propounded antenna is resonating at 4–5, 5.1–6, 7–8, 8.5–9 GHz. For the length of 4 mm, it is echoing at 3.6–4.8, 5.6–6.2, 7.6–10 GHz; for the length of 5 mm, it is resonating at 3.8–4.8, 5.4–6.6, 7.2–9. For the length of 6 mm, it is resonating at 3.6, 4.4, 5.2–6.4, 8 GHz. For the length of 7 mm, it is resonating at 3.8, 5.5–6.4, 7, 8–10 GHz. For the length of 8 mm, it is resonating at 3.6–4.8, 5.8–6.8, 7.2–10 GHz. This individual parameter is influencing the reflection coefficient but not wholly making it to operate in UWB. Figure 3a shows the parametric reflection coefficient of the BP1 with the respective lengths.

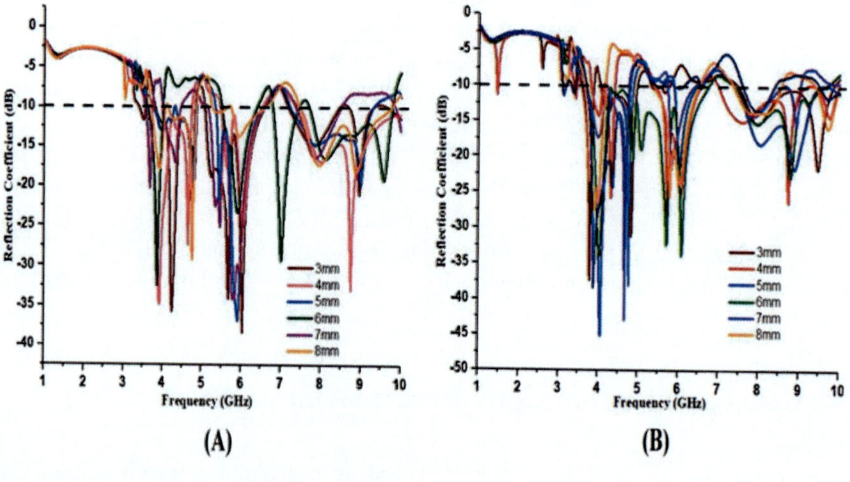

Fig. 3 Parametric analysis of **a** BP1 and **b** BP2

The length of the right side's main finger is denoted as BP2. It is noted that for the length of 3 mm, the proposed MIMO is resonating at 3.8, 4.8 GHz. For the length of 4 mm resonating at 4.2, it is operating at 5.6–6.6, 8.8 GHz. For the length of 5 mm, it is resonating at 4–5, 6, 8–10. For the length of 6 mm, it is resonating at 4–7, 7.4–9 GHz. Finally, for the length of 7 mm, it is resonating at 3.8–4.2, 5.5–6.2, and for the length of 8 mm, it is resonating at 3.8–4.8 GHz.

This individual parameter is influencing the reflection coefficient but not wholly making it to operate in UWB. Figure 3b shows the parametric reflection coefficient of the BP2 with the respective lengths. The length of the left-side second finger-like protrusion is denoted as LP1. It is noted that for the length of 2 mm, the proposed MIMO is resonating at 5, 5.8–6 GHz. For 3 mm length, it is resonating at 3.6–6.8, 7.2–9.8 GHz. For the length of 4 mm, it is resonating at 7.2–9 GHz. For 5 mm length, it is resonating at 4, 4.6, 5.4–6.8, 7.2–9 GHz. For the length of 6 mm, it is resonating at 4 and 4.8 GHz. This individual parameter is influencing the reflection coefficient but not wholly making it to operate in UWB. Figure 4 shows the parametric reflection coefficient of the LP1 with the respective lengths.

The inputs in the form of variables taken are BP1, BP2, and LP1. The resonating frequencies condition for the optimization given is less than -10 dB (≤ -10 dB) in operating ranges of 3–9 GHz. From the predefined ranges, the optimizer selects a value on the random search and initiates the population, and in the simulator, it starts the execution with them. The cost is generated for each execution individually; this value is compared with the given condition. If the generated cost is less than the 0.25 (or any predefined value), then the process terminates. It also suggests that the optimizer is executed very nearly to the given task if the values of cost are nearer to zero. If it does not achieve the target, then again, the variables are randomly selected creates a new population, and the execution will be carried out in this manner. Figure 5a shows the cost function obtained from the HFSS tool by optimizing the

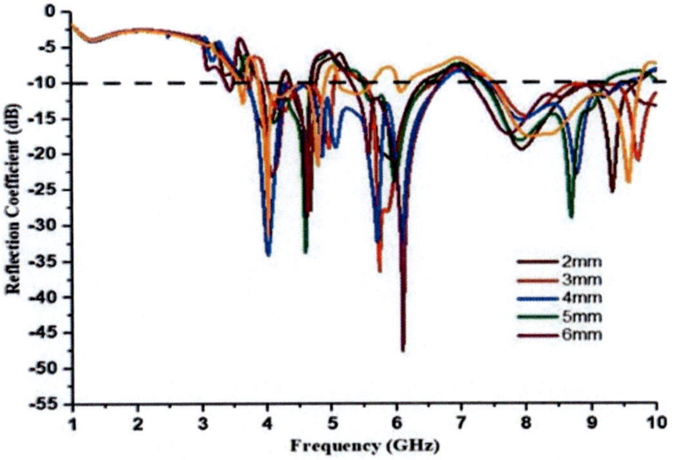

Fig. 4 Parametric analysis of LP1

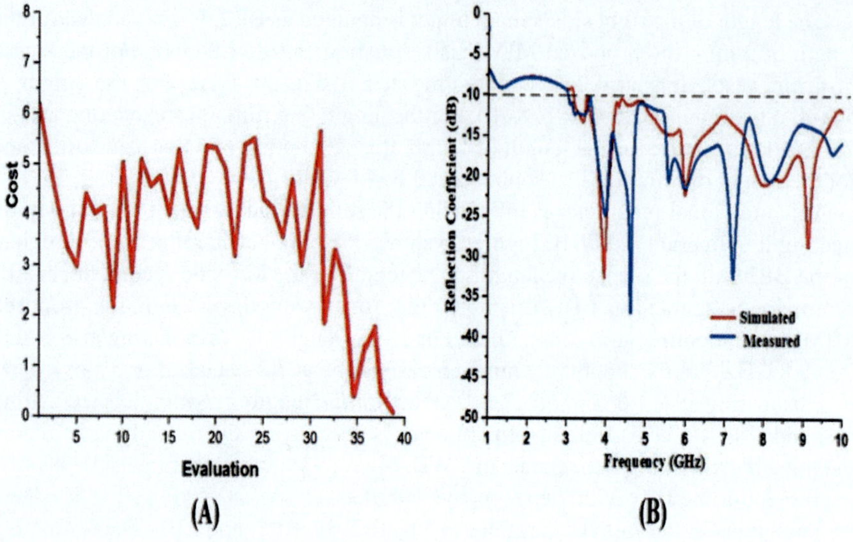

Fig. 5 **a** Cost versus evaluation of GA, **b** measured versus simulated results

parameters using GA, and Fig. 5b shows the measured and simulated results of the proposed antenna.

As illustrated in Fig. 5a, the optimum value has been found at 4.95366527298807, 6.20439008758812, and 5.41776635029145 mm; after 38 simulations, its cost value is 0.14. The results from the simulation show that the MIMO is operating in UWB with a return loss greater than −10 dB. The antenna is fabricated and tested in the anechoic chamber to validate the results.

4 Conclusion

In this paper, a proposed multi-band MIMO antenna is converted as a UWB MIMO antenna. The genetic optimizer of the HFSS is used to optimize the proposed model. By parametric analysis, three parameters are found to be optimized, and these parameters are combinedly optimized using the random search-based genetic algorithm. This optimizer turned out successful in finding the right values of the individual parameter to operate it in the UWB band. To validate the optimized parameters, the proposed model is fabricated on a commercially available low-cost FR-4 material and tested in the anechoic chamber. A decent match has been recorded between the simulation and measured values.

References

1. Sharma S, Kanaujia BK, Khandelwal MK (2020) Implementation of four-port MIMO diversity microstrip antenna with suppressed mutual coupling and cross-polarized radiations. Microsyst Technol 26(3):993–1000
2. Salma S, Khan H, Narasimha Reddy KRV, Mahidhar D, Ram Sandeep D, Rao MC (2020) Design and analysis of circularly polarized dual element MIMO antenna with DGS for satellite communication, fixed mobile, ISM, and radio navigation applications. Int J Adv Sci Technol 29(4):1982–1994 (Special issue)
3. Usha Devi Y, Anil Kumar T, Sri Kavya KC, Pardhasaradhi P (2019) Conformal printed MIMO antenna with DGS for millimetre wave communication applications. Int J Electron Lett
4. Priyadharshini, Ram Sandeep D, Charishma Nag B, Sai GK, Amulya M, Swamy KA, Salma S, Rao MC (2020) Design and simulation of multi-band operating single element antenna for Wi-Fi, ISM and X band applications. Int J Adv Sci Technol 29(4):2011–2021 (Special Issue)
5. Lakshmi MLSNS, Khan H, Sai Sri Vasanthi N, Bamra A, Krishna GV, Pavan Srikar N (2016) Tapered slot CPW-fed notch band mimo antenna. ARPN J Eng Appl Sci 11(13):8349–8355
6. Madhav BTP, Usha Devi Y, Anilkumar T (2019) Defected ground structured compact MIMO antenna with low mutual coupling for automotive communications. Microwave Opt Technol Lett 61(3):794–800
7. Sanam N, Venkateswara Rao M, Nekkanti VSK, Pulicherla VK, Chintapalli T, Yadlavalli AP (2019) A flag-like MIMO antenna design for wireless and IoT applications. Int J Recent Technol Eng 8(1):3023–3029
8. Khan H, Salma S, Neha Reddy B, Uma Maheswari G, Rama Prathyusha K, Ram Sandeep D, Rao MC (2020) Design and analysis of monopole antenna for ISM, C, and X-band applications. Int J Sci Technol Res 9(3):5157–5162
9. Khan H, Salma S, Reddy KRVN, Mahidhar D, Jayachandra D, Sandeep DR, Rao MC (2020) Design of monopole antenna with l-shaped slits for ISM and WIMAX applications. Int J Sci Technol Res 9(3):5151–5156
10. Sandeep DR, Prabakaran N, Madhav BTP, Narayana KL, Reddy YP (2020) Semicircular shape hybrid reconfigurable antenna on Jute textile for ISM, Wi-Fi, Wi-MAX, and W-LAN applications. Int J RF Microwave Comput Aided Eng
11. Usha Devi Y, Rukmini MSS, Madhav BTP (2018) A compact conformal printed dipole antenna for 5G based vehicular communication applications. Progr Electromagnetics Res C 85:191–208
12. Prakash BL, Sai Parimala B, Sravya T, Anilkumar T (2017) Dual band notch MIMO antenna with meander slot and DGS for ultra-wideband applications. ARPN J Eng Appl Sci 12(15):4494–4501

Design and Analysis of Optimized Dimensional MIMO Antenna Using Quasi-Newton Algorithm

S. Salma, Habibulla Khan, B. T. P. Madhav, V. Triveni, K. T. V. Sai Pavan, G. Yadu Vamsi, and D. Ram Sandeep

Abstract In this study, an optimization algorithm is used successfully for optimizing the geometric variables of the MIMO antenna to resonate in the UWB band. We proposed a novel design of a two-element MIMO antenna on a commercially available frame retardant-4 substrate. Initially, the antenna is operated in the multi-band, and this work aims to resonate with it in UWB. To solve the design task, a quasi-Newton (QN) optimizer of HFSS is used. It is an efficient algorithm in optimizing 2–3 variables at a time. Based on the parametric analysis, we have found that to achieve the impedance matching and resonating in notch bands, the rectangular opening slot in the ground structure plays a crucial role. The width and length of the rectangular opening slot have been optimized with the help of a QN optimizer. The antenna prototype has been fabricated based on the optimized results of the QN optimizer and tested to validate the simulation. The proposed model is resonating within the frequency ranges of a UWB, and the QN optimizer accomplished the task of converting a multi-band MIMO to UWB MIMO.

Keywords HFSS · MIMO antenna · Quasi-Newton optimizer · UWB

1 Introduction

In today's modern world, wireless communication has become an integral part of our lives. Many wireless communication devices are developed to fulfill the needs of day-to-day life [1–4]. In those devices, MIMO antenna systems play a crucial role in establishing a stable link between them. MIMO means multiple inputs to multiple outputs; the name here itself suggests multiple antennas at the receiver and transmitter end. The main advantage of MIMO antennas over a single antenna is that it enables various signal paths to carry data. In general, the transmitter has a limited amount of power and bandwidth to send data. Due to many obstacles, the data received by the receiver will be delayed or lost. For successfully multiplying the radio link capacity

S. Salma (✉) · H. Khan · B. T. P. Madhav · V. Triveni · K. T. V. S. Pavan · G. Yadu Vamsi · D. R. Sandeep
Department of ECE, KLEF, Vaddeswaram, Guntur 522502, Andhra Pradesh, India
e-mail: salmasyed@kluniversity.in

S. Bhattacharyya et al. (eds.), *International Conference on Intelligent and Smart Computing in Data Analytics*, Advances in Intelligent Systems and Computing 1312,
https://doi.org/10.1007/978-981-33-6176-8_26

and to achieve multipath propagation, MIMO antennas are used. MIMO employee is beamforming and multiplexing over a single element antenna and reduces error rate, increases capacity and data rate, and also improves the position of a user [5]. MIMO reduces error rate and fading by following the concept of diversity, i.e., transmitting different versions of data; this increases the signal-to-noise ratio at the receiver side. By using the spatial dimension of a communications link, as the number of antennas increases, therefore, increasing the cost, further research is being done to reduce the cost and increase in performance [6–8].

The specifications for UWB systems are defined by the federal communications (FCC), and it allocated the UWB range from 3.1 to 10.6 GHz; numerous UWB topologies are presented in the recent past [9–12]. In the present day, most of the problems are solved by optimization techniques; employing optimization will result in the fast processing of the task and ensures finding the optimal solution to a situation in minimal time [13–15]. In contrast, traditional computing methods take much time and computations to solve the given task. Most of the optimization techniques mimic natural approaches in solving a problem. Most of the stochastic global optimization methods use genetic algorithms, comprehensive learning particle swarm optimization (CLPSO), particle swarm optimization (PSO), and adaptive bacterial foraging optimization (ABFO). In the study, the QN algorithm is used to optimize a multi-band MIMO antenna to a UWB MIMO antenna. To find the optimized solution for such a complex task, we have done parametric analysis before the optimization to find out which variables are influencing the reflection coefficient. From the parametric study, it is clear that the rectangular slot in the ground plane is primarily affecting the S_{11}; these both variables, i.e., the length of the rectangular slot and width of the rectangular slot, are optimized using the QN optimizer of HFSS and found the optimal values.

2 Antenna Designing

The proposed dual-element MIMO is illustrated in Fig. 1, and the overall dimensions are $L_{\text{Sub3}} = 20$, $W_{\text{Sub3}} = 40$, $W_{\text{S4}} = 7.1$, $L_{\text{S4}} = 8.4$, $L_{\text{sg7}} = 23$, $W_{\text{sg7}} = 9$, $L_{\text{sg8}} = 9$, $W_{\text{sg8}} = 18$, $L_{\text{sg9}} = 6.1$, $W_{\text{sg9}} = 0.4$, $L_{\text{sg10}} = 4.1$, $W_{\text{sg10}} = 0.4$, $L_{\text{sg11}} = 3.5$, $W_{\text{sg11}} = 0.4$, $L_{\text{sg12}} = 7.1$, $W_{\text{sg12}} = 9.1$, $L_{\text{sg13}} = 2.1$, $W_{\text{sg13}} = 2.1$, $L_{\text{sg14}} = 4.1$, $W_{\text{sg14}} = 2.2$, $L_{\text{S5}} = 0.6$, $W_{\text{S5}} = 0.6$, and $L_{\text{S6}} = 1.6$. Before applying the optimization process, parametric analysis has been done on variables R_{L} and R_{w} to find the variations of the S_{11} regarding the changes. The optimizing parameters of the rectangle in the ground plane are R_{w} in width and R_{L} in length as shown in Fig. 2a.

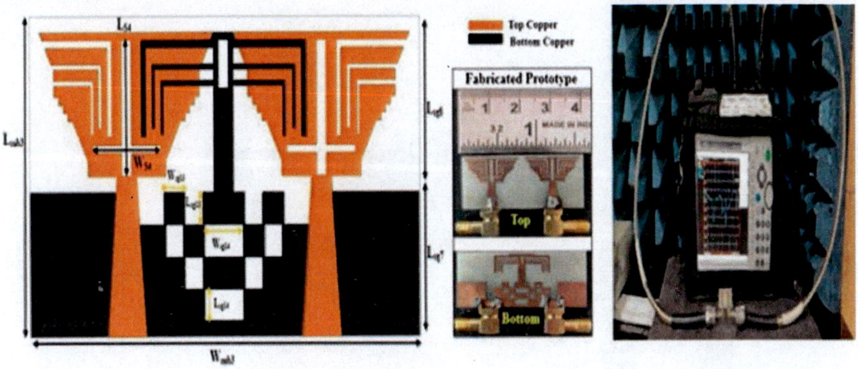

Fig. 1 Proposed MIMO antenna with fabricated and measured using a network analyzer

3 Quasi-Newton Optimizer Analysis

William C. Davidon proposed the quasi-Newton algorithm which is an effective algorithm when it has a limited number of variables to optimize. The QN optimizer functions on searching a maximum or minimum value of the cost function that associates the variables in the circuit or the design to the overall simulation goals. However, the variation and optimization of multiple parameters make it difficult to optimize. As the number of optimization variables increases, the burden on the optimizer increases drastically, so QN works effectively when two or three variables are being optimized at a time. Figure 2b illustrates the flowchart of the optimization process of the QN algorithm.

3.1 Optimizing the Parameter of R_L and R_w

The length of the left side main finger is denoted as BP1. It is noted that for the length of 3 mm, the propounded antenna is resonating at 4–5, 5.1–6, 7–8, and 8.5–9 GHz. For the length of 4 mm, it is echoing at 3.6–4.8, 5.6–6.2, and 7.6–10 GHz; for the length of 5 mm, resonating at 3.8–4.8, 5.4–6.6, and 7.2–9. For the length of 6 mm, it is resonating at 3.6, 4.4, 5.2–6.4, and 8 GHz. For the length of 7 mm, it is resonating at 3.8, 5.5–6.4, 7, and 8–10 GHz. For the length of 8 mm resonating at 3.6–4.8, 5.8–6.8, and 7.2–10 GHz. This individual parameter is influencing the reflection coefficient but not wholly making it to operate in UWB. Figure 3a shows the parametric reflection coefficient of the BP1 with the respective lengths.

Figure 3b shows the parametric study of the width of the rectangular slot. The width of the rectangular slot is also parametrized from 0.8 to 1.8 mm with a step size of 0.2 mm. It is observed that for the width of the value of 0.8 mm, the proposed antenna is resonating at 4, 4.5, 6, and 7–9.5 GHz. For 1 mm, it is resonating at 4–4.8,

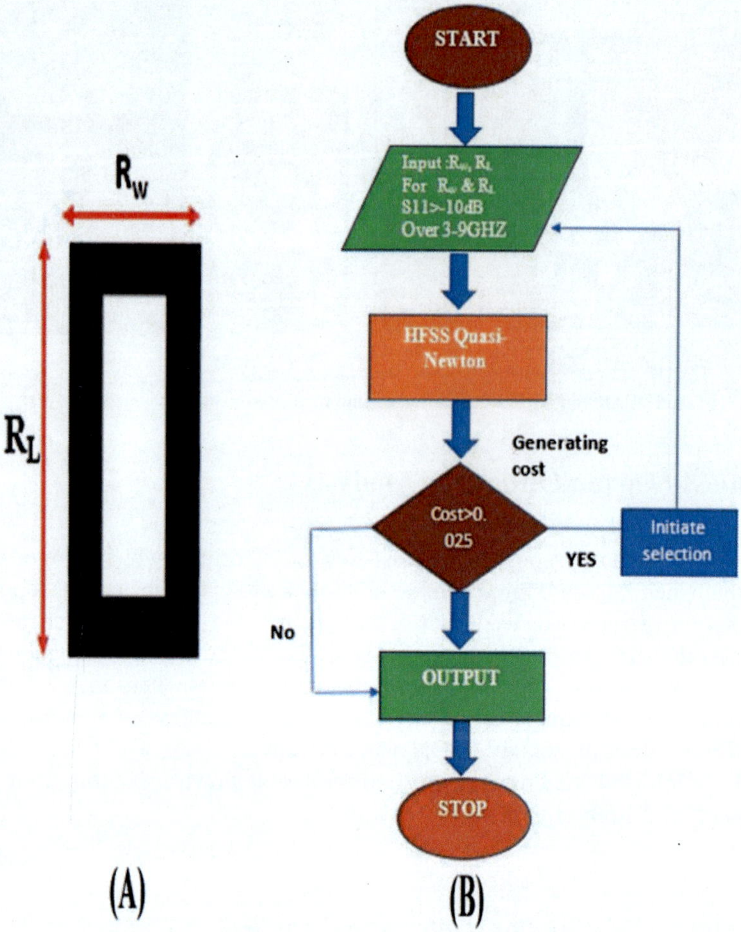

Fig. 2 Illustrations of **a** optimizing parameters in the ground plane, and **b** flowchart of the quasi-Newton algorithm

5.5–6, and 7–9 GHz. For 1.2 mm, it is operating at 3.5–5, 5.5–6.2, 6.2–7.8, and 8–9 GHz; for 1.4, it is operating at 2, 2.5, 2.6–4.4, 5–6, and 7–10 GHz. For 1.6 mm, it is operating at 4, 5, 6, and 7–9 GHz. Finally, for 1.8 mm, it is operating at 3.8–5, 6, and 7–9 GHz. By parametric analysis, we have found that the optimal values are 2.5 and 1.5 mm for the length and width. At those values, the MIMO antenna is resonating with multiple bands and short wide bands.

The proposed UWB MIMO antenna design optimization problem is carried out by QN algorithm in ANSYS HFSS. The optimizing variables are RL and RW. Initially, the variables are defined with their ranges along with the optimization condition. The optimizer will select the values from the predefined range, and it will execute with those values. Each execution will be assigned with some cost value. If the value is

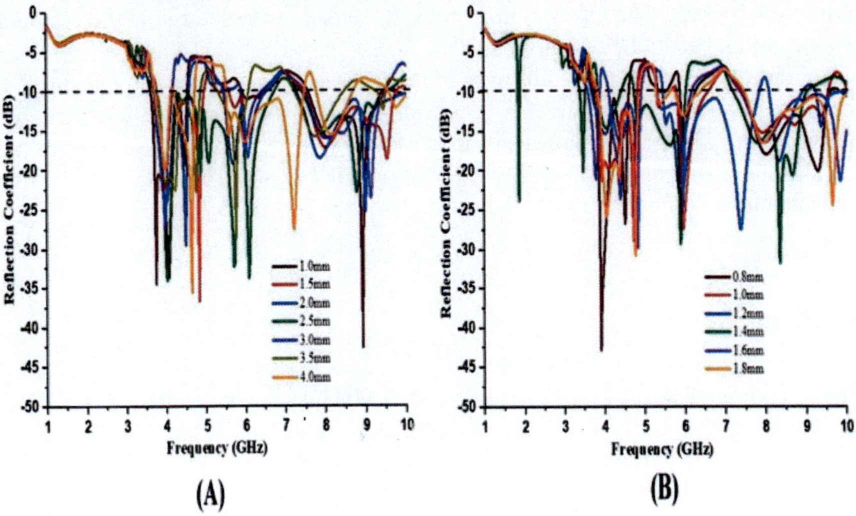

Fig. 3 Parametric analysis of variables **a** R_L, and **b** R_W

close to zero, it means the optimizer is achieving close to the earlier specified goal. The HFSS QN optimizer optimizes the parameters, and the cost of the variables is given in Fig. 4a. Figure 4b illustrates the measured and simulated results of the

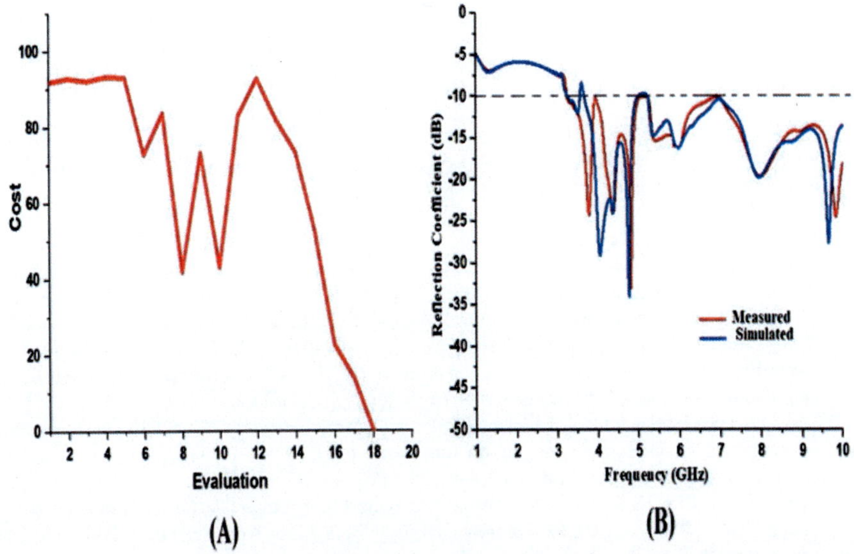

Fig. 4 **a** Cost versus evaluation of QN and **b** measured versus simulated results

proposed antenna. The QN optimizer took 18 selections to determine the optimum value; at that value, the cost is 0.013.

A prototype MIMO is built on a frame retardant-4 substrate through the QN optimized values. The antenna is tested for the validation, and measurements are taken in the anechoic chamber, as shown in Fig. 1. A good match between the measurement and simulation has been observed in Fig. 4b. The frequencies where the antenna is resonating in less than −10 dB range from 3 to 10 GHz.

4 Conclusion

In this communication, a multi-band operating MIMO antenna is altered as the UWB MIMO antenna by using the HFSS quasi-Newton algorithm. By parametric analysis, we have found that the rectangular slot on the ground pillar influences the resonating frequencies. The length and width of that rectangle are optimized to operate the proposed antenna in the UWB band. For this purpose, the QN optimizer of HFSS is selected for the optimization. It is a practical optimizer for variable three or less than three. These selected parameters are combinedly optimized using the QN optimizer, and it successfully found the optimum values for the given task. With these optimal values, the MIMO is developed on a low cost and practically available FR-4 material. The fabricated model is tested for validation; a good match has been observed between the simulation and measurement results. From the results, it is apparent to use the proposed antenna in the UWB frequency ranges.

References

1. Ghosh CK, Pratap M, Kumar R, Pratap S (2020) Mutual Coupling reduction of microstrip MIMO antenna using microstrip resonator. Wirel Personal Commun 1–10
2. Salma S, Khan H, Narasimha Reddy KRV, Mahidhar D, Ram Sandeep D, Rao MC (2020) Design and analysis of circularly polarized dual element MIMO antenna with DGS for satellite communication, fixed mobile, ISM, and radio navigation applications. Int J Adv Sci Technol 29(4):1982–1994 (Special Issue)
3. Salma S, Khan H, Neha Reddy B, Uma Maheswari G, Rama Prathyusha K, Ram Sandeep D, Rao MC (2020) Design and analysis of circularly polarized MIMO antenna with defective ground structure for maritime radio navigation, Wi-MAX and fixed satellite communication applications. Int J Adv Sci Technol 29(4):1995–2010 (Special Issue)
4. Sandeep DR, Prabakaran N, Madhav BTP, Narayana KL, Reddy YP (2020) Semicircular shape hybrid reconfigurable antenna on Jute textile for ISM, Wi-Fi, Wi-MAX, and W-LAN applications. Int J RF Microwave Comput Aided Eng
5. Lakshmi MLSNS, Khan H, Sai Sri Vasanthi N, Bamra A, Krishna GV, Pavan Srikar N (2016) Tapered slot CPW-fed notch band mimo antenna. ARPN J Eng Appl Sci 11(13):8349–8355
6. Madhav BTP, Usha Devi Y, Anilkumar T (2019) Defected ground structured compact MIMO antenna with low mutual coupling for automotive communications. Microwave Opt Technol Lett 61(3):794–800

7. Khan H, Salma S, Neha Reddy B, Uma Maheswari G, Rama Prathyusha K, Ram Sandeep D, Rao MC (2020) Design and analysis of monopole antenna for ISM, C, and X-band applications. Int J Sci Technol Res 9(3):5157–5162
8. Khan H, Salma S, Reddy KRVN, Mahidhar D, Jayachandra D, Sandeep DR, Rao MC (2020) Design of monopole antenna with l-shaped slits for ISM and WIMAX applications. Int J Sci Technol Res 9(3):5151–5156
9. Priyadharshini, Ram Sandeep D, Charishma Nag B, Sai GK, Salma S, Rao MC (2020) Design and analysis of monopole antenna using square split ring resonator. Int J Adv Sci Technol 29(4):2022–2033 (Special Issue)
10. Priyadharshini, Ram Sandeep D, Charishma Nag B, Sai GK, Amulya M, Swamy KA, Salma S, Rao MC (2020) Design and simulation of multi-band operating single element antenna for Wi-Fi, ISM and X band applications. Int J Adv Sci Technol 29(4):2011–2021 (Special Issue)
11. Akram PS, Ganesh P, Srinivas GJ, Salma S, Manikanta K, Likitha G (2019) Investigations on metamaterial slot antenna for wireless applications. Int J Recent Technol Eng 8(1):709–713
12. Kishore MP, Madhav BTP, Rao MV (2019) Metamaterial loaded elliptical ring structured mimo antenna. Int J Eng Adv Technol 8(6):1798–1801
13. Prakash, Bhanu K, Raman AR, Lakshmi M (2017) Complexities in developing multilingual on-line courses in the Indian context. In: 2017 international conference on big data analytics and computational intelligence (ICBDAC). IEEE
14. Usha Devi Y, Rukmini MSS, Madhav BTP (2018) A compact conformal printed dipole antenna for 5G based vehicular communication applications. Progress Electromagnetics Res C 85:191–208
15. Prakash BL, Sai Parimala B, Sravya T, Anilkumar T (2017) Dual band notch MIMO antenna with meander slot and DGS for ultra-wideband applications. ARPN J Eng Appl Sci 12(15):4494–4501

Preserving the Forest Natural Resources by Machine Learning Intelligence

Sallauddin Mohmmad and D. S. Rao

Abstract Sound event detection in the forest environment is difficult to identify due to overlapping of noise and other sounds. Here, sound detection system in the forest needs more optimal sound recognition algorithms to provide accuracy in the results. The sound which is generating in the forest is contains more information in the signal and transmits in a different bands. Digital processing of sound signal is required to catch sound in a various pitches generating from variable distances. Different procedures and algorithms are available for extracting of feature of sound such as Liner Predictive Coding (LPC), Hidden Markov Model (HMM), Artificial Neural Network (ANN) and Mel Frequency Cepstral Coefficients (MFCCs). This paper presented the problems, issues and environmental constraints for sound event detection in the forest along with analysis on present algorithms.

Keywords Liner predictive coding · Mel frequency cepstral coefficients · Hidden Markov model

1 Introduction

Forests are one of the most important parts of the earth. Trees are crucially essential to the earth, creatures and obviously for us people. They are significant for the atmosphere of the earth, as they go about as channels of carbon dioxide. Woods are known as territories and asylums to a large number of animal categories. Notwithstanding, the trees on our planet are being drained at an extremely quick rate. As per a few evaluations, in excess of 50% of the tree spread has vanished because of human movement. This expulsion of woods or trees from a land and changing over it for no backwoods use is called deforestation. The causes of deforestation will be effect of rain fall as well disturb the water cycle, erosion of soil, loss of biodiversity and flooding and drought, climate changes, misbalancing the gases level in the air

S. Mohmmad (✉) · D. S. Rao
Koneru Lakshmaiah Education Foundation, Hyderabad, India
e-mail: sallauddin.md@gmail.com

S. Bhattacharyya et al. (eds.), *International Conference on Intelligent and Smart Computing in Data Analytics*, Advances in Intelligent Systems and Computing 1312,
https://doi.org/10.1007/978-981-33-6176-8_27

and global warming, etc. The control of cutting trees in the forest will reduce the above mention problems on the earth. The principle activist in the deforestation is human been. The people illegally log into forest areas cut the trees, transportation and catching of animals. Some government bodies are using IoT network technology-based projects to identify the metals, loggings and fires. There are lot of loop holes which are identified from this project. Very simple point to fail is people who can log into forest from any side of the forest not only from small or big roadways. We can't establish the millions of sensors to detect the loggings surrounded by the forest. Another existing project is watch the forest areas by drones which are connected to satellite and forwards the image of a area periodically to the control systems. Control systems perform the image processing with last few minutes images with current image. If the system identify the difference among them, then information of that area sends to forest office as a suspect. The main drawbacks with this system are battery life and maintaining of drones which create more complexity for the system. Drones detect the suspected area after the action performed by timber thieves. So that this technology detect the suspect after perform the act. However, like this many projects are initiated by the governments against the deforestation. The logging of the objects and human been are not an issues in the forest because some national parks allowing the visitors to watch the forest and animals who come in vehicles based on some restrictions. Our goal is to stop cutting of the tree before it happen or respond immediately when cause take place. Another way to provide the security using machine learning-based technology adoption on protecting of forest using automated technology aspect. In the view from ML, the problems occurred in the forest by (1) Cutting of trees by human been with axe, sawing, motor-based sawing. (2) The means of transport of wood is through forest department vehicles or belongs to illegal/smuggling vehicles. (3) Traps are arranged in the forest to catch the animals that disenchanted animal makes a sound that passes as a message to other animals, seeking help which may be due to trap or sickness. (4) Gun shots. In order to resolve above mentioned problems, extensive work has to be done in the area of sound event detection using machine learning. In this scenario, the entire forest area must be partitioned into network clusters that are connected through nodes. The steps involved in this process are the nodes which must be having capable of processing various sounds and identification of sounds that come due to cutting of trees. Every means of cutting of trees will generate different level of sound or frequency but near to the threshold value of cutting sound. The frequency, location and type of sound have to be notified by nodes to control system.

The ML technology should also detect the trapped animals. Animals will be caught in trap fortunately by prowls that disenchanted animal makes the sound which will come from one place continuously, either it is due to trap or sickness, and this will be notified to the control system with help of our network in the forest. Hunting is a passion for few people, when a bullet is fired then it will generate a sound with some frequency which may be once or multiple number of times, and it is mostly unique frequency compared to other frequencies which need to implement the algorithms to identify all kinds of acts in the forest.

The last and very important challenging objective for ML is to recognize the illegal logs of vehicles. Every vehicle have a different engine sound, and woods will be carried through big lorry's whose engine sound is louder than a small jeep; in either of the cases, the sound must be notified by nodes to the servers. The system should differentiate the forest office vehicles and thieves vehicle sound with support of other technologies like GPS trackers and identity nodes which are equipped to allowed vehicles. If GPS trackers signal and identity nodes signal are not matching, then it means that there is an illegal vehicle in forest.

The system for protecting of the forest need to be integrates the technology of networking, IoT and ML. The network node in the system integrated the maximum capabilities of ML and arranged in network which should be covering the forest area either with wired or wireless communication. The major aspect of my discussion entirely depends up on sound event detection. A sound segment that can produce by live and non-live objects and sounds is continues; some are discontinued sound segments. In the Sect. 2, the paper discussed the various algorithms which are supporting for sound event detection their limitations. The Sect. 3 explained about real-time environmental situation in the forest area.

2 Discussion on Existing Algorithms

Sound event detection systems are generally identified by using mel frequency cepstral coefficients (MFCC) and hidden Markov models (HMMs) as classifiers [1]. The MFCC and HMMs more efficient and optimal for sound detection when sound generating from different sources with different pitches. They have to extract the features with different frequencies like car, bird and dog. Each sound has its own frequency band, amplitude, wave length and composition. On the off chance that we can isolate the frequency range into various groups and distinguish the spatial area of the sound source in every one of these groups; at that point, this is an additional component of the element, which the classifier can figure out how to appraise the quantity of potential sources in each casing and their direction in the space [2, 3]. The matching pursuit adds more additional feature to sound event with implementation of the time frequencies. Accordingly, if we combine the efforts of MFCC and MP will produce more accuracy in the sound detection in forest like environments. The sound generates from various sources whose sound frequencies band have variable difference which can detect easily by existing algorithms. In contrast to that the sound generating from various sources whose sound frequencies almost near to similar parametric value need more filter to identify the expected sound event (Figs. 1 and 2).

In generally, the input to the system from different objects which have different frequencies can tackle easily with above mentioned algorithms with DNN approach [1, 4]. Here, the frequencies of the objects are vary with huge bandwidth differences. If we apply the same scenario to same kind of objects, then the frequencies are almost similar values with slide difference. In a time frame, three dogs are barking then how

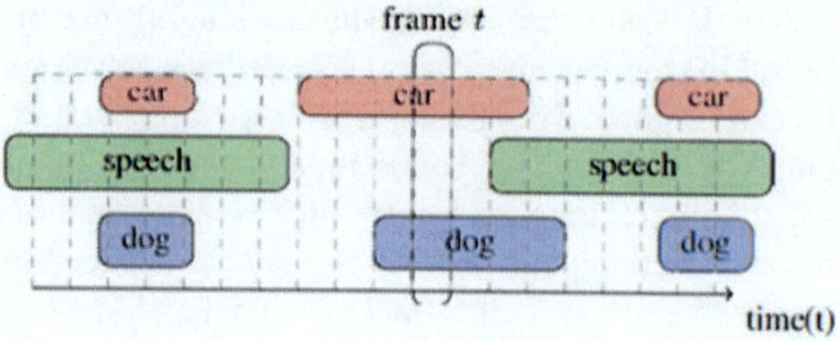

Fig. 1 Actual model for detecting of sound from various sources

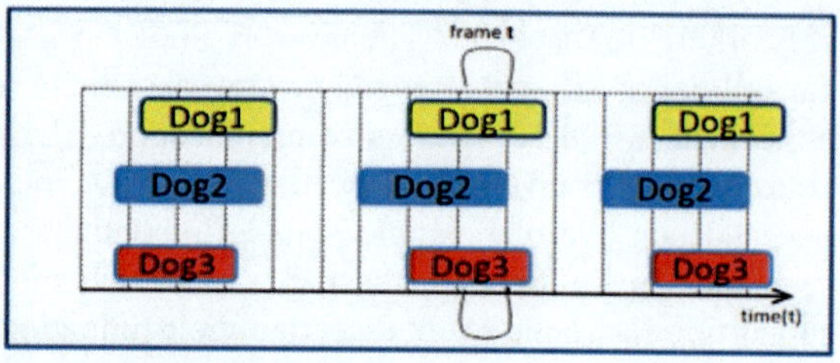

Fig. 2 Expected model for detecting of sound from various sources

to learn specific dog sound and how to filter the noise in a open area acoustic model. This approach is a challenging task for my research.

Generally, DNNs techniques implement with two approaches; one is Multi-Labelling to test data (ML) and second Combined Single-Label (CSL) methods [1, 4, 5]. In multi-labelling on similar sounds also need compacted algorithm process in real-time scenario.

The feature vector Xt will become single training instance for the DNN. The training process performed in the supervised learning. So that we have to take start and end time of each sound event. In a one time frame, there may be chance of N sound events. The target output vector Y_t will be

$$Y_t(l) = \begin{cases} 1, & \text{if } l\text{th event is active in frame } t \\ 0, & \text{if } l\text{th event is not active in frame } t \end{cases} \quad (1)$$

Based on the X_t and Y_t values, the algorithm will process the rest of detections.

Sound event detection (SED) frameworks mean to perceive and recognize specific event identified with human, nature or machine nearness. The sound which is coming from different sources in the forest will get overlaps in the realistic environment [5]. The sound event detection in the forest not in a organized manner. The extraction of feature vector and target output vector will not reach our threshold. My research to protection of forest needs to introduce or refine the existing algorithms in a optimal manner; then, only the system can recognize the sound event perfectly even in overlapping of many sounds.

2.1 Polyphonic Detection Systems

Generally, MFCC implements in the polyphonic detection system to analyze the sound event from various input systems and perform the classification on input data by executing the Hidden Markov Models (HMMs) with continuous goes of the Viterbi calculation. As of late, non-negative matrix factorization (NMF) was utilized as a pre-handling venture to break down the sound into streams and distinguish the most unmistakable occasion in each stream at once. The overlapping of sounds from different sources creates more noise in the detection system. The assessment of the quantity of overlapping events can be circumventing when utilizing coupled NMF [1, 5]. In nearby spectrogram, features were joined with Generalized Hough Transform (GHT) voting system framework to recognize the overlapping sound events. This offers an unexpected way in comparison to customary casing-based highlights and accomplishes high precision, being assessed on five diverse sound occasions and their mixes.

Generally, the polyphonic detection analyzed based on the multi-label system. With respect to that classification also formulated as multi-label problem [5]. Initially, single-label classification done for each class and combined to create new result [6]. The correlation among the single-label encodings will be discarded because of weak expressive power. So that multi-label classification precious to implement for gain most available data from the environment.

2.2 Classification Techniques

AI and ML techniques have progressively been received to classify the combined features based on the logical implementation allowing more sound classes simultaneously receiving good performance. These kinds of capable of ML and AI motivating the use of more complex inputs adding with MFCCs perceptual linear prediction (PLP). For such kinds of systems using SVM and GMMs or multilayer perceptions (MLP) for classifications.

Based on the references of SVM implementation, the sound classification of a tree cutting with axe will be calculated with some parameters they are accuracy, truth rate and standard mean deviation.

$$\mathrm{Acc}' = \sum_{i=1}^{n} 1/n(\mathrm{Acc}_i) \tag{2}$$

$$\mathrm{TRP} = \frac{\text{Number of axe hits found}}{\text{Total number of axe hits}} \tag{3}$$

$$\mathrm{std} = \sqrt{\sum_{i=1}^{n} 1/n(\mathrm{Acc} - \mathrm{Acc}')2} \tag{4}$$

DNN uses the Matching Pursuit (MP) for sound characterization and analysis with time frequency. Practically, if we implement both MP and MFCC for sound extraction and detection in a system, then we will get more accuracy in output and classification. In this case, we can use the KNN and GMM for classification procedures instead of SVM.

2.3 *Mel-Frequency Cepstral Coefficients (MFCC)*

The sound event will be different with environment change. ISO that initially, we capture the sound from the different environment and prepare the training set. By using this training set, we need to test the algorithm and verify the accuracy to identify the different sound with environment changes. For this process, basically, MFCC has been used to extract the features of sound samples.

The pre-processing is amplitude normalization; sound will divided into frames; and last ones is hamming window size of 50 ms duration with some overlaps. The spectral and cepstral domain features are extracted from frames of the audio signal. Feature vector Xt extracted for each frame with index of t.

The dynamics of the sound feature vector combined with their two previous and two forwarded vectors. Actually, this model called as context windowing. Here, Xt is feature vector given as:

$$X_t = \left[U_{t-2}^T U_{t-1}^T U_t^T U_{t+1}^T U_{t+2}^T\right]^T \tag{5}$$

Discrete Fourier transform (DFT) operation performs on each speech signal to gain the value of MFCC. For every speech frame, their power spectrum weighted with a series of filter frequencies.

This process follows the mel scale which consisting low frequency for both band edges and centre frequencies.

MFCC is used to extract acoustic sound with many parameters.

- Identify the amplitude of a sound.
- Creates composite signal with different frequencies of equal bandwidth.
- FFT of bands.
- Computation of the logarithm of bands.
- DCT computation of bands.

2.4 *K-Nearest Neighbour Method*

The k-nearest neighbour strategy characterizes test information dependent on their comparability with tests in the training set. For a given unlabelled example (test), discover the k-nearest marked samples in the training data index and relegate test to the class that shows up most as often as possible inside the k-subset.

The k-NN just requires a number 'k' (the quantity of closest neighbours), set of labeled models (Training dataset) and metric to gauge closeness. In this investigation, k-NN with $k = 1$ and a Euclidean distance metric as characterized is utilized between the test vector and each example in the training dataset.

The implementation process of the K-nearest neighbour algorithm as follows:

Here, KNN finds the nearest neighbours for test data x with respect to training data based on K value. Consider the test point x and two point in k dimensional space. Then, x and near point y are given as: $x = [x_1, x_2, x_3, \ldots x_k]$ and $y = [y_1, y_2, \ldots, y_k]$.

Euclidean distance d given as:

$$d(x, y) = \sqrt{\sum_{i=1}^{k} (y_i - x_i)^2} \tag{6}$$

In this supervised learning algorithm, we have to prepare possible number of leaned datasets. The accuracy of KNN is promotional to number of trained datasets. Here, we actually need to prepare datasets on sound event of tree cutting in a forest environment on the different frequencies and different environmental situations (Fig. 3).

The number of distances and comparisons depended on the K value of the algorithm. The increasing value of K decreases the accuracy in the result. The training error rate increases with K-value. If we reach at maximum value of K, then classification found as a single group based on the majority. The validation error rate low at minimum value of K and error rate reach to peak with maximum value of K (Figs. 4 and 5).

The KNN algorithm works well for my research to identify the more accuracy on sound event detection in the forest. The output interpretation in more fast compared to the random forest algorithm and low calculation time too (Table 1).

2.5 *Deep Neural Networks (DNN)*

DNNs provided more research on sound event detection which basically presented in two methodologies. The first one Multi-Label (ML) for sound event. From this category of data, DNN extracts polyphonic material with supervised learning. Here, we need to provide the learning with different supervised leaning algorithms; simultaneously, we have to train few of elements with single-label event and acquire same polyphonic material. We join the yields of the single-mark DNNs to get a multi-label yield for each time instance. It is guaranteed that deteriorating a multi-name characterization into several binary arrangement issues will lose the connection data between various names in a solitary example. Be that as it may, the adaptability of

Fig. 3 Flowchart of KNN experimental execution on test data

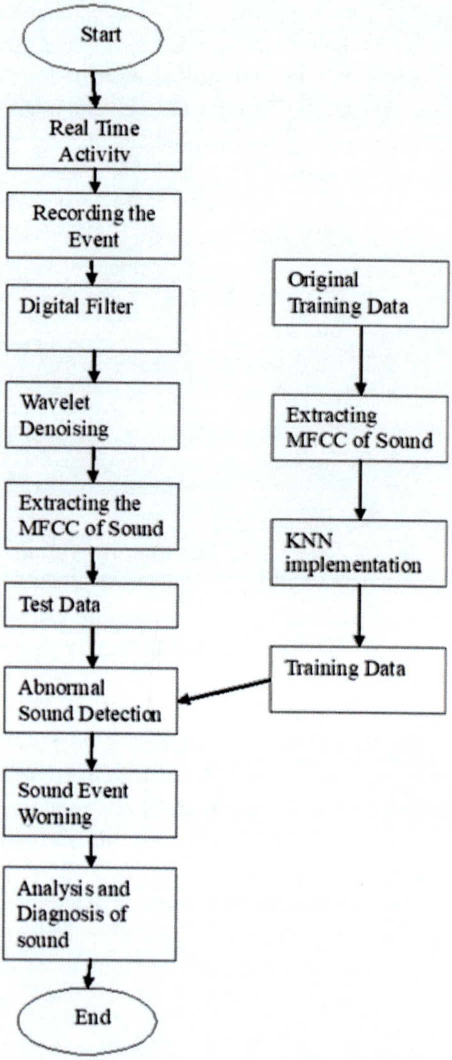

causing various arrangements of marks for various applications to can be significant and valuable to the detriment of marginally diminished precision for certain applications, particularly in SED frameworks. Second one Combined Single Label (CSL) utilizing a lot of single-label classifiers permits dynamic incorporation of new marks via preparing classifiers just for the new solid occasions rather than re-preparing the total structure. Supposedly, this is the principal work that thinks about these two profound learning approaches on polyphonic SED [7, 8]. The two techniques are investigated sensible sound material with single component.

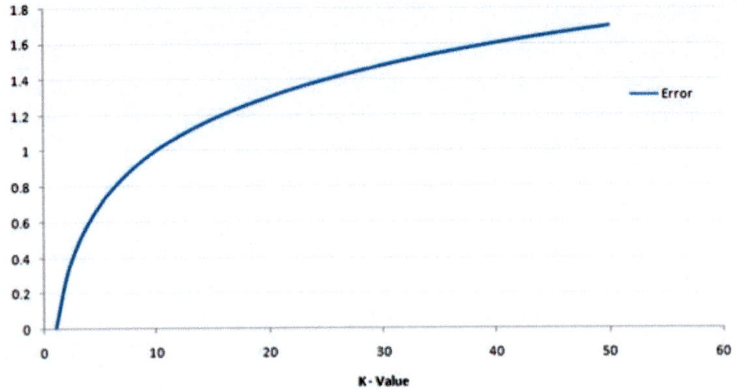

Fig. 4 Training error rate with *K*-Value

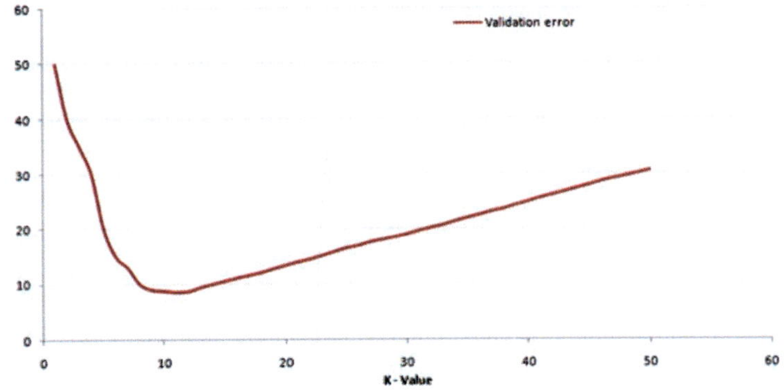

Fig. 5 Validation error rate with *K*-Value

Table 1 Accuracy rate of KNN

Name of algorithm	Ease to interpret output	Calculation time	Predictive power
Logistic regression	2	3	2
Classification and regression trees	3	2	2
Random forest	1	1	3
K-nearest neighbour	3	3	2

For each label, l of sound event DNN trains and tests irrespective of the other labels and finally provides availability from trained datasets. In the case of CSL, the input for trained set has taken from polyphonic sound signals. Here, polyphonic material only creates comparison between multi-label and combined single-label DNN and provides maximum analysis on trained data. Let consider the number of sound events are N, then we need to train the N different trained set, create the new classes based on combined groups of N different models.

In DNN, the relationship between the input, x, and the output of the first hidden layer, $h1$, is described as

$$h1 = f(W1\,x) + b1 \tag{7}$$

where $W1$ and $b1$ are the weight matrix and bias vector, respectively, and f (.) is the activation function.

Several algorithms discussed which are generally implemented in sound analysis. The sound in the real world measured by decibel (dB) in a unit level. The sound signals are waves travel in all directions from omitting point with the support of media [9]. Here, sound waves are just pressure waves in the air or any media which creates micro phonic vibrations. When the waves are travelling in the air, the sound pressure and intensity will reduce with respect to the distance. The general threshold for sound level drop is 6 dB per doubling of distance. Here, sound pressure means sound filed quality which can change their value with respect to the distance [10]. The sound intensity means sound energy quality which can change their value with respect to the distance. The sound pressure and intensity are inversely proportional to the distance.

Sound field quality or sound pressure is $p = 1/r$; sound intensity quality is $I = 1/r_2$; and the relation between pressure and intensity is $I \sim p_2$. But sound pressure and sound intensity are not equal. These values can change with respect to the distance. From the generating point, let us consider the two different distances r_1 and r_2. The pressure value will be chance when it reach from r_1 to r_2 and similarly intensity also [11]. Depends on the previous pressure value and the distance, only current pressure will be evaluate, and it is also similar to intensity.

$$p_2 = p_1 \frac{r_1}{r_2} \tag{8}$$

$$I_2 = I_1 \left(\frac{r_1}{r_2}\right)^2 \tag{9}$$

The quality of sound will r_2 reduce rapidly after some time and the waves lost their energy parallel with the distance. The some sounds are loud, and some are not. The perception of frequency is called pitch. The small wavelength of sound generates high pitch, and large wavelength of sound generates low pitch. The travelling speed of sound also one of key point in my proposal. In the forest, generally, sounds will generate simultaneously from different sources and there pitch, frequency and wavelengths. This composition of sounds will create noise for our detection for specific sounds (Table 2; Fig. 6).

The speed of the sound wave affected with temperature which may we can observe the small changes with respect to temperature change. At 0 °C, the speed of sound is 331 m/s, whereas at 20.0 °C, it is 343 m/s, less than a 4% increase. Sound waves have

Table 2 Distance law for sound field quantities

Distance ratio	Sound pressure $p \sim 1/r$
1	1/1 = 1.0000
2	1/2 = 0.5000
3	1/3 = 0.3333
4	1/4 = 0.2500
5	1/5 = 0.2000
6	1/6 = 0.1667
7	1/7 = 0.1429
8	1/8 = 0.1250
9	1/9 = 0.1111
10	1/10 = 0.1000

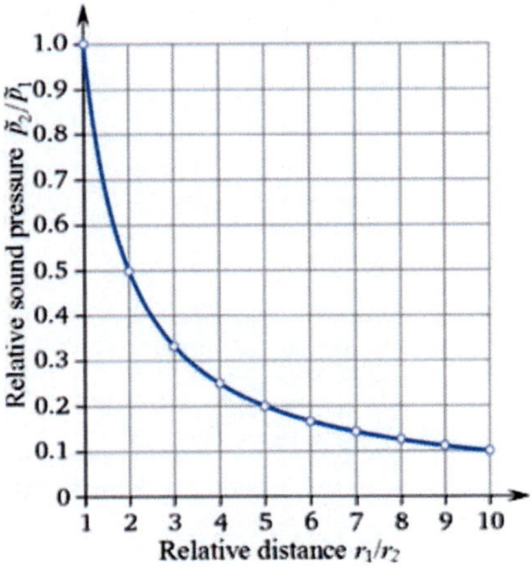

Fig. 6 Graph for relative sound pressure with distance

the behaviour of expansion and compression in the media, where they are travelling except in the vacuum space. Generally, they travel in a straight line with longitude directions. The generating of sound from the origin point with different levels called as amplitude measured with decibels. The loudness of sound increases; then, it is called expansion or rarefaction and loudness decreases; then, it is called compression [12]. The acoustic pressure is produces with compression property, louder sound produces high acoustic pressure then softer sound in the media.

3 Analysis on Sound Event in Forest Environment

In proposal, my research wants to find the different sound actions of tree cutting and vehicle transportation in area with detection constraints of road side's. The cutting of tree with axe or chainsaws generates different way of sounding in the forest. Notice rate of the sound also high with animals, birds, winds and rivers. Apart from that, we need to detect the suspected area in the forest with sound detection system. It is not a simple thing. As we discussed in the introduction, there are many barriers to identify sound in suspected area. In the existing systems to detect, the sound in general research uses MFCCs which are very efficient for identify and filter the sound [13]. Mel cepstral coefficients are a perceptual representation of the signal characterized by a non-linear scale of perceived frequency and by a number of critical frequency bands. The classification based on support vector machines (SVM) (Figs. 7 and 8) [14].

The recognition of sound identified nearly 80 dB with frequency of 9.5 kH when stand 1 m distance from cutting tree with axe. We can see the accuracy in the sound

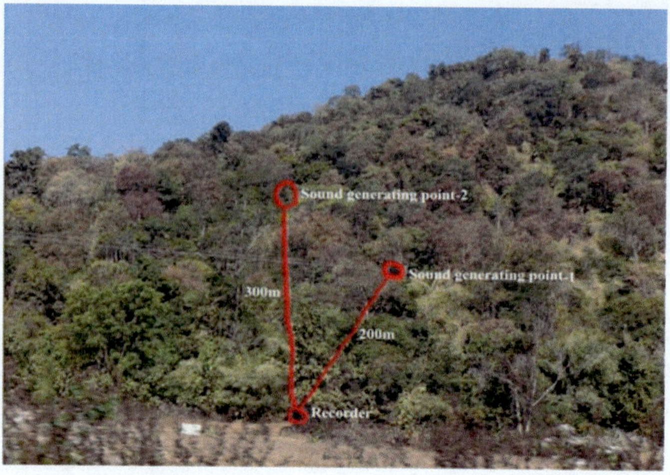

Fig. 7 A forest area of Telangana state in the India

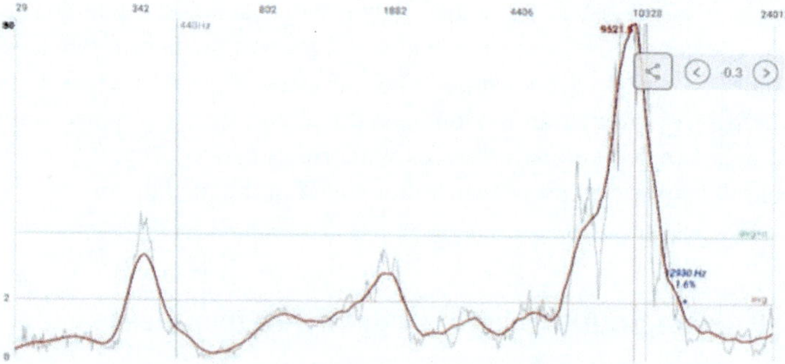

Fig. 8 Sound event detection from origin point to one metre distance

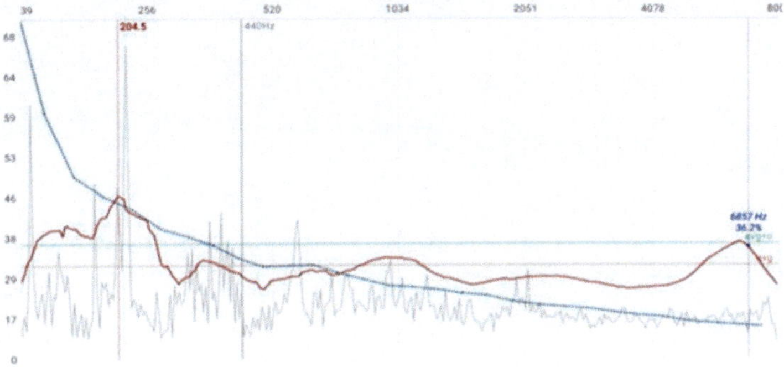

Fig. 9 Falling of accuracy when more noise created

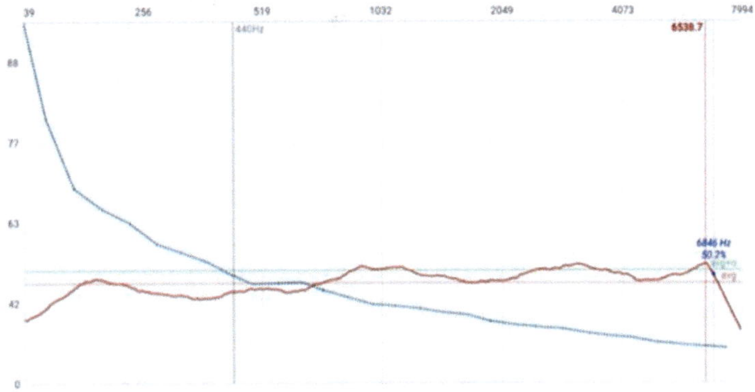

Fig. 10 Sound event detection from origin point to 200 m distance

even there is noise is in the forest when we stand very near to the act (Figs. 9 and 10).

The recognition of sound identified nearly 50 dB with frequency of 6.8 kH when stand 200 sound pressures, intensity and energy of the wave fall down to reached to 50 dB. This sound also affected by the noise. In the graph, the dotted blue line is showing the level of noise at that time of act performed which leads to reduce the accuracy. The value 50 dB is may be which helps to identify the suspected area in the forest but if there is more noise is created or composed with different sounds of same dBs, then we cannot identify the suspected area. It need efficient classification process for filter the noise and identify the sound what we need (Fig. 11).

Sometimes, on the same frequency, we identified the 25 dB of sound level when tree hits with less energy. Obviously, the frequency value it generates the less sound but the wave frequency is all most same (Fig. 12).

When a person is cutting a tree with axe, then the sound generated from the suspected area will be contiguous. But there is gap between each hit with min of two seconds. In this gaps, there are other sounds which we called as noise recorded with

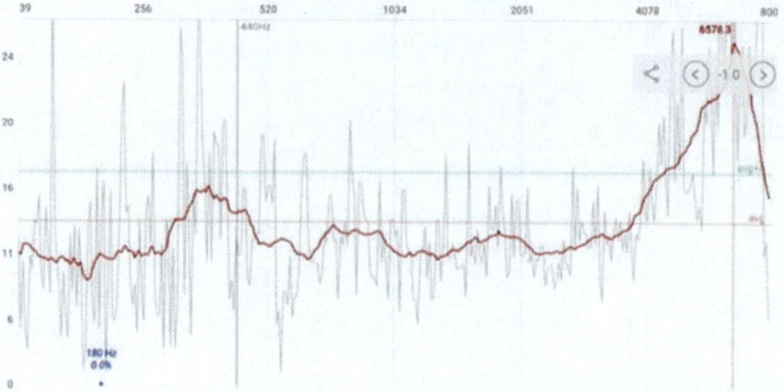

Fig. 11 Sound event from origin point to 200 m distance with less energy hit on tree

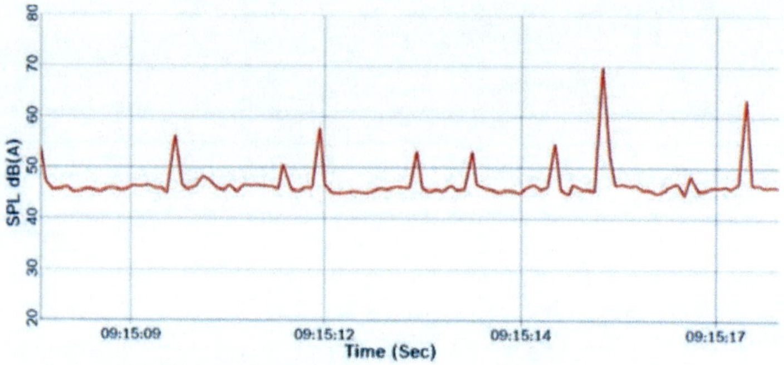

Fig. 12 General tree cutting frequency with axe by human

minimum 40 dB in the forest. In the forest, mostly noise created by wind and when I captured the sound level the wind flow is somewhat high. So we can predict that in a normal wind flow, in the forest will create 30 dB of minimum noise (Fig. 13).

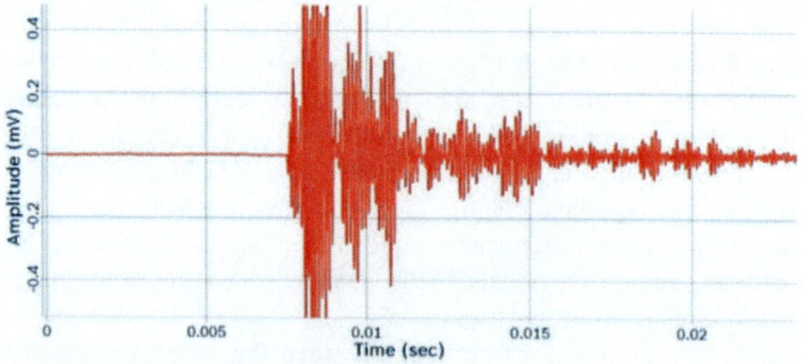

Fig. 13 This graph shows the amplitude of each hit on tree

4 Conclusion

This paper has discussed about objectives of forest protection from thieves and illegal logs to avoid the tree cutting with help of sound event detection systems. In this paper, also discussed about how far the existing algorithms helped to detect the sound event in the forest and what extends I need to research on forest protection system based on constraints and current environment of forest. Definitely, the existing algorithms need to refine or add new algorithms with respect to the forest environment to gain the accurate result. My future research will continue until find the proper solution to my objective of forest protection system.

References

1. Suman P, Karan S, Singh V, Maringanti R (2014) Algorithm for gunshot detection using mel-frequency cepstrum coefficients (MFCC). Springer Science and Business Media LLC, Berlin
2. Marcu A-E, Suciu G, Olteanu E, Miu D, Drosu A, Marcu I (2019) IoT system for forest monitoring. In: 42nd international conference on telecommunications and signal processing
3. Akcinar D, Ariturk MK, Yildirim T (2018) Speaker dependent voice controlled robotic arm. In: 2018 innovations in intelligent systems and applications (INISTA)
4. Dai Wei JL, Pham P, Das S, Qu S, Metze F (2016) Sound event detection for real life audio DCASE challenge. In: Detection and classification of acoustic scenes and events
5. Cakir E, Heittola T, Huttunen H, Virtanen T (2015) Multi-label versus combined single-label sound event detection with deep neural networks. In: 2015 23rd European signal processing conference (EUSIPCO)
6. Stowell D, Giannoulis D, Benetos E, Lagrange M, Plumbley MD (2015) Detection and classification of acoustic scenes and events. IEEE Trans Multimedia 17(10):1733–1746
7. Suciu G et al (2017) Remote sensing for forest environment preservation. In: WorldCIST, Recent advances in information systems and technologies, pp 211–220
8. Rakotomamonjy A, Gasso G (2014) Histogram of gradients of timefrequency representations for audio scene detection. Tech Rep, HAL
9. Foggia P, Petkov N, Saggese A, Strisciuglio N, Vento M (2015) Reliable detection of audio events in highly noisy environments. Pattern Recogn Lett 65:22–28
10. Battaglino D, Lepauloux L, Pilati L, Evans N (2015) Acoustic context recognition using local binary pattern codebooks. In: Worshop on applications of signal processing to audio and acoustics (WASPAA), New Paltz, NY, Oct 2015
11. Li Y, Li X, Zhang Y, Liu M, Wang W (2018) Anomalous sound detection using deep audio representation and a BLSTM network for audio surveillance of roads. IEEE Access
12. Yoo C, Yook D (2008) Automatic Sound Recognition for the Hearing Impaired. IEEE Trans Consum Electron 54(4):2029–2036
13. Zhang L, Yu S, Wang X (2014) Research on IOT RESTFUL web service asynchronous composition based on BPEL. Intelli Human-Mach Syst Cybern 1:62–65
14. Dubois D, Durrieu C, Prade H, Rico A, Ferro Y (2015) Extracting decision rules from qualitative data using Sugeno integral: a case-study. In: European conference on symbolic and quantitative approaches to reasoning and uncertainty. Springer, Berlin, pp 14–24

Comprehensive Study on Different Types of Software Agents

J. Sasi Bhanu, Choppakatla Surya Kumar, A. Prakash, and K. Venkata Raju

Abstract In recent decades, programming engineers have inferred a logically better comprehension of the qualities of unpredictability in programming. Programming structures that contain numerous powerfully collaborating segments, participating in complex problem solving, normally significant degrees more effectively and efficiently engineer than those that essentially figures an element of some contribution through a solitary string of control. Effectively and efficiently engineer programming can be achieved by using software agents. A software agent is the program which can be run in any system environment without any interface of the user or any other external software. Agent software is emerging area of research. However, the word "agent" is most frequently used knowing the fact that it is heterogeneous for research. In this paper, various software agents such as collaborative agents, interface agents, mobile agents, Internet agents, reactive agents, hybrid agents are studied.

Keywords Agent · Collaborative agents · Mobile agents · Hybrid agents · Reactive agents · And smart agents

J. Sasi Bhanu (✉) · A. Prakash
CSE Department, CMR Institute of Technology, Kondlakoya, Medchal, Hyderabad, India
e-mail: sasi.bhanu@cmritonline.ac.in

A. Prakash
e-mail: prakash15aug@gmail.com

C. Surya Kumar
Accenture P Ltd., Hyderabad, India
e-mail: suryakumar.ch@gmail.com

K. Venkata Raju
Koneru Laksmaiah Education Foundation, Veddeswaram, Guntur 522502, India
e-mail: kvraju@kluniversity.in

S. Bhattacharyya et al. (eds.), *International Conference on Intelligent and Smart Computing in Data Analytics*, Advances in Intelligent Systems and Computing 1312,
https://doi.org/10.1007/978-981-33-6176-8_28

1 Introduction

Before continuing any further, it is essential to define the meaning of agent-based system [1] and is the key point of deliberation utilized which is an operator. Specialist-based frameworks may contain an abstraction specialist, (as on account of UI operators or programming secretaries [2]); however, seemingly, the best possible lies in the utilization of agent-based system [3]. By a specialist, framework that is appreciates accompanying properties [4, pp.116–118]:

- Autonomy: The ability of the agents to interact without the help of human and other system.
- Reactivity: The ability of agents to adapt the environment and can upgrade itself at any given time.
- Pro-activeness: The ability to take the behavior changes.
- Social ability: The ability to receive and send messages among other agents (and possibly humans) via agent language.

2 Related Work and Discussion

2.1 *Collaborative Agents*

Collaborative agents are Multi-Agent Systems (MAS). MAS consolidating programming designing, propose answers for exceptionally dispersed issues in progressively changing and computational areas. It is progressively comprehended that MAS has a significant job as a product building approach, as proposed by the papers in this volume. Specialists in fields of creating operator situated systems that take into consideration operator and MAS detail and check (e.g., [5, 6]), structure, and examination (e.g., [7]), and reuse (e.g., [8]). Even though specialists are now observed as a product designing worldview [9], the value of multi-operator frameworks as a product engineering style [10] was just mostly contemplated. We inspect compositional qualities of multi-operator frameworks (and not the interior design of single specialists) through an examination between existing MAS structures. We survey shared characteristics and contrasts in structure, execution of the MAS, the subsequent qualities, shortcomings, etc. MAS-related research for the most part tends to issues, for example, the improvement of MAS, either without any preparation, utilizing specialist particular and confirmation systems, re-utilization of present MAS, for a given issue (example in [11]). MAS principally regarding their product design qualities, for example, heartiness, adaptability and flexibility, code re-convenience, and so forth. It is important to examine the connection between the design of a MAS and its usefulness to give data, whereupon one may choose both whether a MAS might be a suitable computational answer for given an issue, and assuming this is the case, on the answers of the MAS. From a Software Architecture (SA) perspective, MAS is frameworks consisting different parts, called operators. The operators are typically self-ruling.

2.2 *Interface Agents*

"Rather than client started connection through orders as well as immediate control, the client is occupied with a co-usable procedure in which human and PC operators both start correspondence, screen occasions and perform errands. The illustration utilized is that of an individual associate who is teaming up with the client in a similar workplace."

There are numerous interface operator frameworks and models, propelled by early works, arranged inside an assortment of spaces. Most of these frameworks are audited and ordered in the following area. Basic to these frameworks, not withstanding, client can operate three different types of issues: Knowing the client interacting with the client includes learning inclinations and the work propensities. If a client colleague is to help at perfect time, and correctness, at that point, then it should help us with client functioning. Anxious collaborator, continually hindering with immaterial data, would simply irritate the client and increment the general outstanding task at hand. The accompanying difficulties exist for frameworks attempting to find out about clients: Extracting the clients' objectives and expectations from perceptions and input getting adequate setting in which clients' objectives are adapted to the client's changing destinations decreasing the underlying preparing duration.

2.3 *Mobile Agent*

A program that is self-governing can travel in a heterogeneous system in its control, relocating a host and communicate with various modes of operators [12]. By choosing when to locate and where to locate. It can execute and suspend execution any time and anywhere, relocate to host and forward its execution. Portable operators have certain highlights, for example, independence, versatility, objective driven, temporarily constant, knowledge, collaboration, learning, reactivity, and so on. The highlights, they are all around adjusted to the area of portable processing [13]. For example, a portable operation will have movement from PDA to Internet to gather intrigued data for client. Since system side does not need movement on various solicitations/reactions over the low data transfer capacity association, it can get to important assets effectively. Further, abrupt association misfortunes will not influence the operator since it is not in ceaseless contact with the cell phone. A specialist can play out its assignments regardless of whether the cell phone is separated from the system. Upon the reconnection of cell phone to the system, operator will come back to it with results. On the other hand, a system application can dispatch a versatile operator onto the cell phone. The specialist following up in the interest of the application associates with the client whether cell phone is associated [13]. Mobile specialists improve the turn of events, testing, and usage of dispersed applications as a result capacity on corresponding channels cancelation and calculation rationally. They can disseminate, redistribute, and go about in customers or servers relying upon the objectives. The mobile agent systems likewise build versatility of programs that are capable to move work to a fitting area [14].

2.4 *Information/Internet Agents*

An intelligent agent (IA) is an independent, self-governing programming module that could play out specific errands for the benefit of its clients. It could likewise communicate with other canny specialists and or human in playing out its task(s). There is presently developing enthusiasm for utilizing wise programming specialist for an assortment of undertakings in differing scope of uses: individual collaborators, canny UIs, overseeing electronic mail, exploring, and recovering data from the Internet and databases, planning gatherings and assembling activities, electronic business, web-based shopping, haggling for assets, dynamic, structure, and broadcast communications. The utilizations of insightful specialists on the Internet and web and feature their possibilities [15].

Wise specialists are right now utilized for an assortment of assignments in different scope of uses: individual collaborators, clever UIs, overseeing electronic mail, exploring and recovering data from the Internet and databases, booking gatherings and assembling tasks, electronic business, web-based shopping, haggling for assets, dynamic, structure, and media communications.

2.5 *Reactive Agents*

The dominating way to deal with creating techniques for multi-operator frameworks is to adjust those produced for object-situated examination and structure: the motivation from Rumbaugh, FUSION, etc. Focal points these methodologies, the most important is the ideas, documentations, and strategies related with instance of a class-arranged examination and structure (and UML specifically) are progressively natural to a mass crowd of programming engineers. Be that as it may, there are a few impediments. To begin with, the sorts of disintegration that object-situated strategies support are at chances with the sort of deterioration that specialist arranged structure empowers. Operators are more general than specialists; they are expected to have computational assets using UNIX procedure or Java string. Specialist frameworks executed utilizing object-arranged programming dialects will ordinarily contain numerous articles (maybe millions) yet will contain far less operators. A decent specialist arranged plan procedure would urge designers to accomplish the right decay of substances into either operators or items.

2.6 *Hybrid Agents*

The single operators that interface multi-specialist framework commonly exist along continuum going from the heavyweight intellectual operators (regularly of "BDI") compare to lightweight operators with respect to restriction individual handling of the operators. Most frameworks uses specialists from a solitary situation along this range. We have effectively executed a few frameworks, where operators of altogether different degrees of inward refinement connect with each other. In view of this experience, we recognize a few distinct manners by which specialists of various types can be incorporated in a solitary framework, offer perceptions, and exercises from our encounters.

2.7 *Smart Agents*

We propose to utilize keen specialists to alleviate the issues of the absence of thinking and knowledge in things in the IoT frameworks. The thought is that everything ought to have installed thinking and insight capacities. The insight in things can be accomplished utilizing programming operators installed in things. Their capacity to reason about their surroundings can add to helpful results for people, utilizing aggregate insight strategies. Multitude insight [9] is the control that reviews marvels, whereby a framework made from numerous locally acting people shows an important worldwide conduct. Such multitude frameworks utilize self-sorting out, decentralized control components. Savvy operators can misuse these methods and their own ability to detect their environment to collaborate, learn, and adjust to arrive at a objective. This transformative point of view permits urban areas to grow new brilliant administrations misusing a keen urban framework which should be structured open, adaptable, versatile, and secure in order to execute shrewd operators that collaborate for all intents and purposes among themselves from the outside fringes up to the cloud organize. This vision is made conceivable utilizing the idea of haze figuring.

3 Implementation of Software Agent

3.1 *Overview*

As to make effective software agent for decreasing execution time, we propose an intelligent advancement strategy for programming operator called Interactive Software Agent (ISA) in light of the agent repository system for multi-agent structure which centers with respect to a basic element of repository framework plan, i.e., the reuse of existing operators put away in the repository archive.

Reuse of existing specialists: Based upon configuration measure, the operators and the repository frameworks that have just been planned and used as applications are put away and figured out how to reuse them using software agents for new operator framework. For example, the store of the archive-based operator structure clarified can be used as one of the fundamental components.

Collaboration among design and implementation of software agent: To help the age and test cycle in the bases of configuration measure, some supporting capacities are accommodated the originators. For example, an intelligent software engineering conduct over a virtual distributed environment might be valuable for the test and investigating of operators.

3.2 *Algorithm*

Step 1: Attempting to reuse the current software agent.
Step 2: Programming of operator information and capacity.
Step 3: Interactive reproduction.
Step 4: Enrollment of software agent to repository.
Step 5: Test and verification.

4 Result

See Table 1.

whereas

The quantity of reality utilized as the beginning conditions: K

The hours of inputs: X

The time required by the correction of adjustment of the I-th blunder from a participation activity start: T_{i} $(i \leq k)$

The necessary time from the activity start as far as possible on account of being errorless: $T_{\min}$

The necessary time from the activity start to the end utilizing ISA: T_a

From the above table, one can observe that there is a huge difference with ISA and without ISA. The effective and efficient result are been obtained by the ISA.

Table 1 Comparison of results with ISA and without ISA

	The number of start times of IAS	The number if inputs given to ISA	Execution time
Without ISA	$X + 1$	$(X + 1) + K$	$\Sigma T_i + T_{\min}$
With ISA	1	K	T_a $(T_{\min} < T_a < < \Sigma T_{\mathrm{i}} + T_{\min})$

5 Conclusion

This paper has given a foundation to the field of processing known as "programming operator innovation," covering an assortment of work, established in various territories. A survey of current specialist innovation prompted an assessment of utilizations to the personalization of frameworks and administrations to singular clients and procedures which offer open doors around there. The paper finished up by offering a few recommendations for future advancement of the advances referenced, specifically the requirement for expanded combination of operator innovation with existing frameworks if the best advantage is to be picked up from them.

References

1. Hyacinth S (1996) Software agents: an overview. Knowl Eng Revi **11**(3), 205–244
2. Maes P (1994) Agents that reduce work and information overload. Commun ACM 37(7):31–40
3. Bond AH, Gasser L (eds) (1988) Readings in distributed artificial intelligence. Morgan Kaufmann Publishers, San Mateo
4. Wooldridge M, Jennings NR (1995) Intelligent agents: theory and practice. Knowl Eng Revi 10(2):115–152
5. Wooldridge M (1997) Agent-based software engineering. IEEE Proc Software Eng 144(1):26–37
6. Parunak VD, Nielsen P, Brueckner S, Alonso R workshop on engineering self-organizing agents, Hakodate, Japan Integrating Swarming and BDI Agents Hybrid Multi-Agent Systems
7. Miles S, Joy M, Luck M (2000) Designing agent-oriented systems by analysing agent interactions. In: International workshop on agent-oriented. Springer, Berlin
8. Dikenelli O, Erdur RC (2000) Agent oriented software reuse. International conference on software. ebizstrategy.org
9. Jennings N (2000) On agent based software engineering. Artif Intell 117(2):277–296
10. Shaw M, Garlan D (1996) Software architecture: perspectives on an emerging discipline. Prentice Hall, New Jersey
11. Huhns M, Singh M (eds) Reading in agents. Morgan Kaufmann, San Mateo
12. Wan AI, Sorensen C-F, Indal E. A mobile agent architecture for heterogeneous devices
13. Mittal M, Bhall T. Mobile agent. researchgate.net
14. Milojicic D, Douglis F. An introduction to mobile agent programming and the ara system. In: Mobile agents and process migration—an edited collection
15. Murugesan S (1998) Intelligent agents on the internet and web. IEEE

Hybrid Acknowledgment Scheme for Early Malicious Node Detection in Wireless Sensor Networks

A. Roshini, K. V. D. Kiran, and K. V. Anudeep

Abstract Wireless sensor networks with distinct node property referred to as heterogeneous sensor node covers a large area for sensing purpose. The most appealing characteristic of sensor nodes is systematic information collection and the further transmission to a remote base station. Performance of the node is affected by the malicious nature. The sensor nodes are susceptible to errors and malicious assaults. The impacted or compromised sensor nodes can send erroneous information or inaccurate reports to the destination. Therefore, precise and timely identification of malicious and defective nodes is essential to ensure reliable network functioning. In this paper, a hybrid acknowledgment scheme (HAS) is considered for prior detection of malicious nodes in order to reduce the degree of energy consumption. The autonomous sensor node in wireless sensor network is grouped into number of clusters. The base station shares the cluster key to every sensor node within the network. The malicious nodes are then detected by receiving the acknowledgment from the destination node. The effectiveness and efficiency of the proposed system are evaluated in terms of throughput.

Keywords Hybrid acknowledgment · Heterogeneous sensor node · Malicious node · Cluster head · Data forwarding

1 Introduction

Wireless sensor networks are made up of individual autonomous systems that can record the environmental abnormalities and forward the same to the base station with the help of all intermediate sensor nodes. Responsibilities of the sensor nodes include sensing, and the abnormalities in the environments and communicating the

A. Roshini (✉) · K. V. D. Kiran (✉) · K. V. Anudeep
Department of Computer Science Engineering, Koneru Lakshmaiah Education Foundation, Vaddeswaram, Andhra Pradesh, India
e-mail: roshinicse22@kluniversity.in

K. V. D. Kiran
e-mail: kiran_cse@kluniversity.in

S. Bhattacharyya et al. (eds.), *International Conference on Intelligent and Smart Computing in Data Analytics*, Advances in Intelligent Systems and Computing 1312,
https://doi.org/10.1007/978-981-33-6176-8_29

gathered information to the destination after which the actuators take the control in taking necessary actions. Deployment of such wireless sensor networks is a great challenge which must include the various constraints and deployment rules [1].

Deployment of large number of sensor nodes faces challenges in terms of network connectivity and network coverage. Direct communication wireless sensor nodes transmit the gathered data directly to the base station without any interrogation with the intermediate nodes. Cluster-based wireless sensor networks follow CH–CH communication pattern, where data handling is done only by the sensor node and the cluster head of the respective cluster [2].

Clustering is used to stabilize the network topology and optimize the energy consumption [3]. The clustering of the sensor nodes prompts the network to go vulnerable in which the intruder imitates or compromises CHs in the network to collapse and degrade the functionality of the wireless sensor networks. These nodes are called as malicious nodes and they must be detected and eliminated earlier in order to increase the performance and behavior of the wireless sensor networks [4]. Management of wireless network to attain an attack free communication is essential.

Assume the network has individual clusters, for which cluster 1 consists of nodes N1–N7 and cluster 2 consists of N7–N12, where node N7 is a common node to both cluster 1 and 2. The node in cluster 1 sends the data to cluster head1 (CH1) which is responsible for delivering the data from nodes to sink. Similarly, nodes in cluster 2 send the data to cluster head2 (CH2) which is responsible for delivering the data to the sink.

2 Literature Survey

Mitigation of the potential damage caused by compromised nodes is done by the adaptive acknowledgment (AACK). Malicious nodes in the network are detected at the early stage. Network overhead is reduced by consistently maintaining the throughput of the network with the help of AACK. The disadvantages of using AACK method are false misbehavior report and forged acknowledgment [5].

Despite the presence of malicious node, the watchdog system increases the throughput of the network. This abnormality in the counter limit reports a note of node misbehavior by the watchdog node. In such scenario, the reliability of the link and node misbehavior are combined by the path rater of each node to detect a reliable path. Watchdog scheme fails to detect collisions, false misbehavior report, and partial dropping [1].

Malicious observer node detection system (MOD) makes use of the context-free grammar which is the primary challenge of MANETS. Malicious or normal functioning of the sensor node is detected by the CFG method [2]. Node’s passive behavior and network misuse are identified by using Fibonacci Pascal Triangle. The Fibonacci numbers are obtained by adding the elements in the increasing diagonal lines in the Pascal’s triangle. FPT is used for confidential data transmission. FPT generates dummy route to protect the data from the malicious observer [2].

An energy-efficient protocol low energy adaptive clustering hierarchy (LEACH) follows the hierarchical arrangement of sensor nodes. The protocol forwards the data from the sensor node to the cluster head (CH) and then will be transmitted to the base station or sink. Distribution of cluster head in an even manner results in increased network lifetime. LEACH experiences trouble with the geographical distribution of cluster heads that directly influences the energy consumption of the sensor node. LEACH follows asymmetric communication pattern where all the sensor nodes will be reachable to base station [4].

Intra-cluster communication is made possible only with the cluster head (CH). CH–CH communication continues till the data is given to the destination. Change in one cluster head may create an impact resulting in clustering again where after the cluster heads are reelected. MANET nodes are clustered in a hierarchical manner with multiple levels for evenly distributed energy consumption.

Hierarchical cluster formation makes along with spanning tree logic is used in cluster-based hybrid routing protocol [6]. The nodes in the clusters are organized in hierarchical fashion followed by route discovery to route the data packet from the source to destination. The advantage of following, such a routing strategy, is it makes use of link state routing to overcome scalability problem. Reducing the network view of each node, routing complexity, and routing table size could be reduced [7, 8].

Static nature of the nodes results in node stability which enables management of intra-cluster networking [7, 9, 10]. Fluctuation in the nodes membership is a result of network mobility either due to nodes or the cluster heads. Cluster head selection is also done based on a random basis and mobility. Heuristic approach is followed to determine the node's mobility on a periodic basis [7, 11].

CLAE uses public key cryptography and identity-based encryption for secure key sharing. The technique encrypts a secure key and transmits it over the insecure network [12, 13]. Key management is done by third-party central authority. Authentication and ease of access of secret keys are attained through identity-based encryption. Identities like email id, mobile number, and device number are used for key generation. CLAE shares secret keys in a decentralized manner [14].

Onion routing follows decentralized fashion that allows relay nodes to carry the packets from the source to destination rather than direct communication. IP address is hidden by bouncing the connection from the server at a random basis [15]. The drawback is that encrypted data is available at the final connection point as the last relay but it can be compensated for a non-SSL Web site [3, 16, 17].

Data forwarding is done in a greedy fashion where the network does not consider any of the traffic issues with Greedy Perimeter Stateless Routing (GPSR) in an efficient way, with the support of dynamic routing algorithms [18]. Since the node's location is shared with the neighbor nodes, the vicinity is public which remains as a drawback of GPSR [19].

Next model which includes mobility in the working where each node communicates within the group and the nodes outside the group is the reference point group mobility (RPGM). The sensor nodes in each group which are randomly distributed can be used for military applications [20]. Nodes also migrate on a random manner to new position in an arbitrary direction. After some predicted time when the groups seemed to be settled, the individual nodes of each group are allowed to move randomly in an area. RWP and RGMP are combined in such a way that the location of node in first phase becomes starting node in second phase [21, 22].

3 Proposed System

The suspicious nodes can be detected using hybrid acknowledgment scheme (HAS) as shown in Fig. 1. In this method, the nodes in the wireless sensor network are grouped into several clusters [8]. The individual cluster key is supplied to each cluster in the network by the sink. The nodes are named as N1, N2, and N3. Initially, node N1 likes to transmit a packet to node N3. It first passes the packet to the node N2 with its own cluster key. Node N2 receives this packet after checking the cluster key of the node N1. If the cluster key of the node N1 is matched with cluster key of node N2, then node N2 accepts the packets from the node N1 and sends this packet to node N3 if the destination address is not matched with its own address [12]. The node N3 follows the same packet reception procedure performed by node N2 to receive the packets from the previous node in the cluster. After receiving packet, node N3 sends the HAS signal to the node N1 via node N2 using the procedure stated above. The node N1 must receive this HAS signal with in a stipulated duration. If it do not received the HAS signal within the stipulated time, then node N1 assumes that node N2 and node N3 are suspicious or malicious nodes. Finally, node N1 immediately sends this data about malicious nodes to the sink.

The recorded working mismatch is forwarded to the sink by malicious attackers to report for innocent nodes as malicious. To overcome this, the node (N4) nearby the malicious cluster node sends the dummy packet with its own address to the node (N5) in the cluster 2 through the node in the false cluster where the node N1 delivers the malicious report to the sink [23]. If the reported node is malicious, it does not transmit this dummy packet to the source node N5, otherwise, it passes this packet to the node N5. At the same time, node N4 in nearby cluster sends the same dummy packet with

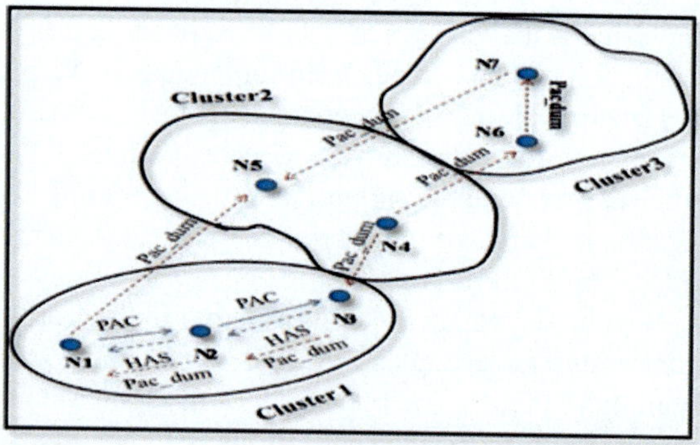

Fig. 1 Proposed HAACK system

its own address to the node N5 with an alternative routing. A false misbehavior report is generated if node N5 does not receive dummy packet from node N1.

4 Algorithm

The data should be transmitted over a specified time interval. If the total time taken for transmission is greater than the estimated time specified, then it rejects the corresponding data packet as it assumes there are malicious nodes present in the system [7]. Then, it sends malicious cluster node information to the sink. False misbehavior happens when a malicious node intentionally reports the other nodes as malicious. If false misbehavior report is false, then the nearby cluster sends dummy packet through malicious node cluster. If the dummy packet is transmitted successfully, then we can conclude that it is not a malicious node [9, 24]. If the packet is not transmitted, then malicious node is present in the system. If the false misbehavior report is trusted and accepted, then the node is allowed to further data transmission from that node.

```
Algorithm:
begin:
If(Transmission time (end-start) time interval)
 then
1. Rejects the corresponding data packet, assumes that there are
suspicious or malicious nodes
2. Sends malicious cluster node information to the sink
Else
      If(false misbehavior report = false)
              3. Nearby cluster sends pac_dum through the malicious
cluster node
If(pac_dum = transmitted) then
4. Not a malicious cluster
Else
5. Malicious cluster
      Else
    6. False misbehavior report is trusted and accepted
7. No further data transmissions through that node.
```

5 Increased Network Lifetime

The number of rounds for data gathering directly is dependent on the residual energy. Lifetime as in Fig. 1 is the key parameter which decides throughput and robustness of the network. The lifetime of the node depends on energy consumption of sensor node and remaining residual energy of the node [25]. The lifetime of M–EETRP protocol is 67.89% and other NBBTE algorithm is 35%, SNDP is 20%, and EETRP is 66%.

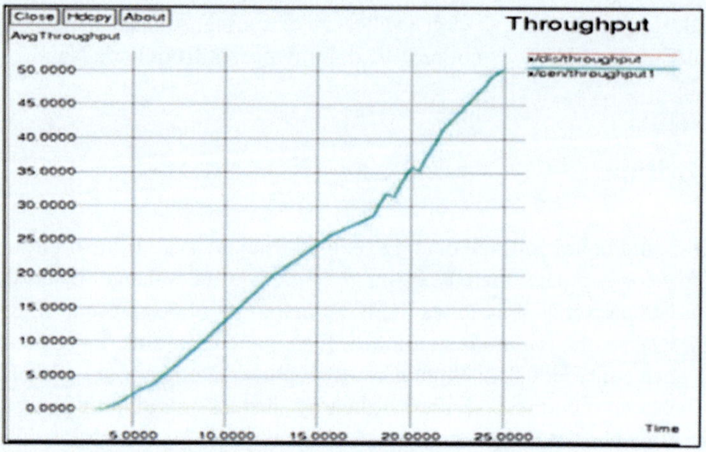

Fig. 2 Throughput graph established from hybrid acknowledgment scheme

6 Enhanced Throughput

The success rate in effective packet delivery for every 1000 packets during the transmission [13] is called throughput. It is given by:

$$\sum_{0 \text{ to } n} \text{packet received } (n) \ast \text{ packet size}/1000 \tag{1}$$

From the result, Fig. 2 AACK protocol maintains the same throughput for reducing the network overhead. We used HAS scheme to increase the throughput by reducing the network overhead by intern reducing the malicious nodes involved in a network.

7 Conclusion

The proposed solution for data loss attacks in wireless sensor networks completely isolates the malicious node in the network. This technique detects the misbehavior node in network and broadcasts the information about the misbehavior node detected to all the nodes present in the network. Mobility of the individual nodes in the network is an additional parameter. Simulation result records increased throughput in the network.

References

1. Sharma T, Tiwari M, Sharma PK, Swaroop M, Sharma P (2013) An improved watchdog intrusion detection systems in Manet. Int J Eng Res Technol (IJERT) 2(3). ISSN: 2278-0181
2. Durga Devi S, Rukmani Devi D (2019) Malicious node and malicious observer node detection system in MANETs. Wiley. https://doi.org/10.1002/cpe.5241
3. Balamuralikrishna T, Hussain MA (2019) A framework for evaluating performance of MADA-AODV protocol by considering multi-dimensional parameters on MANET. https://doi.org/10.1007/978-981-13-1921-1_16
4. Ashish Rajshekhar C, Misra S, Obaidat MS (2010) A cluster-head selection algorithm for wireless sensor networks. In: 17th IEEE international conference on electronics, circuits and systems. https://doi.org/10.1109/ICECS.2010.5724471
5. Al-Roubaiey A, Sheltami T, Mahmoud A, Shakshuki E, Mouftah H (2010) AACK: adaptive acknowledgment intrusion detection for MANET with node detection, enhancement. In: 24th IEEE international conference on advanced information networking and applications. ISSN: 2332-5658
6. Stetsko A, Folkman L, Matyas V (2010) Neighbor-based intrusion detection for wireless sensor networks. In: 2010 6th International Conference on Wireless and Mobile Communications, IEEE
7. Ahmad M, Hameed A, Ikram AA, Wahid I (2019) State-of-the-art clustering schemes in mobile ad hoc networks: objectives, challenges, and future directions, vol 7, IEEE. ISSN: 2169-3536
8. Roshini A, Varun Sai VD, Chowdary SD, Kommineni M, Anandakumar H (2020) An efficient SecureU application to detect malicious applications in social media networks. In: International conference on advanced computing and communication systems, IEEE, pp 1169–1175. ISSN: 2575-7288
9. Shaik R, Kanagala L, Sukavasi HG (2016) Sufficient authentication for energy consumption in wireless sensor networks. Int J Electr Comput Eng 6(2). https://doi.org/10.11591/ijece.v6i1.9038
10. Gali S, Nidumolu V Multi-context trust aware routing for Internet of things. Int J Intell Eng Syst 12(1):189–200
11. Anusha M, Vemuru S (2018) Cognitive radio networks: state of research domain in next-generation wireless networks—an analytical analysis. https://doi.org/10.1007/978-981-10-3932-4_30
12. Amiripalli SS, Bobba V, Potharaju SP (2019) A novel trimet graph optimization (TGO) topology for wireless networks. https://doi.org/10.1007/978-981-13-0617-4_30
13. Bhandari RR, Rajasekhar K (2016) Study on improving the network life time maximazation for wireless sensor network using cross layer approach. Int J Electr Comput Eng 6(6):3080–3086. https://doi.org/10.11591/ijece.v6i6.11208
14. Gaur SS, Mohapatra AK, Roges R An efficient certificateless authentication encryption for WSN based on clustering algorithm. Int J Appl Eng Res 12. ISSN: 0973-4562
15. Anguraj DK, Smys S (2019) Trust-based intrusion detection and clustering approach for wireless body area networks. Wireless Pers Commun 104(1). https://doi.org/10.1007/s11277-018-6005-x
16. Zhao L, Shen H (2011), ALERT: an anonymous location-based efficient routing protocol in MANETs. In: 2011 International conference on parallel processing, IEEE. ISSN: 2332-5690
17. GPSR, Karp B, Kung HT GPSR: greedy perimeter stateless routing for wireless networks
18. Guizani B, Ayeb B, Koukam A (2012) A new cluster-based link state routing for mobile ad hoc networks. In: The 2nd International conference on communications and information technology (ICCIT): communication networks and systems, IEEE, Hammamet
19. Rajakumar R, Amudhavel (2017) GWO-LPWSN: grey wolf optimization algorithm for node localization problem in wireless sensor networks. J Comput Netw Commun. https://doi.org/10.1155/2017/7348141
20. Yan Z, Mukherjee A, Yang L, Routray S, Palai G (2019) Energy-efficient node positioning in optical wireless sensor networks. Optik 178:461–466

21. Pires WR, de Paula Figueiredo TH, Wong HC, Loureiro AAF, Malicious node detection in wireless sensor networks, IEEE. https://doi.org/10.1109/IPDPS.2004.1302934
22. Kiran KVD (2018) Prevention of spoofing offensive in wireless sensor networks. Int J Eng Technol (UAE) 7:770–773. ISSN: 222752
23. Praveen Kumar D, Pardha Saradhi P, Sushanth Babu M (2018) Energy efficient transmission for multi-radio multi-hop cooperative wireless networks. J Adv Res Dynam Control Syst 10:117–122
24. Kiran KVD (2018) Performance analysis of hybrid hierarchical K-means algorithm using correspondence analysis for thyroid drug data. J Adv Res Dynam Control Syst 10(12):698–712. Special Issue, ISSN: 1943023X
25. Anusha M, Vemuru S (2016) An efficient mac protocol for reducing channel interference and access delay in cognitive radio wireless mesh networks. Int J Commun Antenna Propag 6(1):14–18. https://doi.org/10.15866/irecap.v6i1.7891

Prediction of Temperature and Humidity Using IoT and Machine Learning Algorithm

A. Vamseekrishna, R. Nishitha, T. Anil Kumar, K. Hanuman, and Ch. G. Supriya

Abstract In this paper, we analyze and predict the temperature and humidity using IoT and linear regression algorithm in machine learning. In ancient days, people use to check the climate conditions by seeing clouds or through storm warnings or by using animals they have noticed the weather conditions for many purposes like harvesting and involves many household activities. To overcome this situation, weather forecasting was found. We collect the temperature and humidity data in various places for few days using Message Queuing Telemetry Transport (MQTT) protocol. So, we initialize the collected data for 5 days in Amazon Web services (AWS) cloud. This data is stored in AWS and by using Dynamo Database (DynamoDB) the stored data is created in the form of the table and it is exported to .csv file. Hence, the data is recorded. Now by using linear regression algorithm in machine learning, we predict the temperature and humidity data. People can therefore easily monitor the weather conditions without eagerly waiting for tomorrow. This makes more easy and comfortable way to the people so that they will be able to know the climatic conditions within a short period of time.

Keywords AWS · ESP8266 · DynamoDB · Arduino IDE

A. Vamseekrishna (✉)
Department of Electronics and Computer Engineering, Koneru Lakshmaiah Education Foundation, Vaddeswaram, Andhra Pradesh 522502, India
e-mail: vamseekrishnaa3@kluniversity.in

R. Nishitha · T. A. Kumar · K. Hanuman · Ch. G. Supriya
Department of Computer Science Engineering, Koneru Lakshmaiah Education Foundation, Vaddeswaram, Andhra Pradesh 522502, India

S. Bhattacharyya et al. (eds.), *International Conference on Intelligent and Smart Computing in Data Analytics*, Advances in Intelligent Systems and Computing 1312,
https://doi.org/10.1007/978-981-33-6176-8_30

1 Introduction

Weather report is the major work done in every country and helps a lot. Weather report helped a lot in the growth of sedentary human civilization. From the past, so many years, the weather report is done only by human prediction [1]. As the present world is changing into an era of development in new technologies and implementations it is a necessary goal to trend up with weather also [2]. IoT plays a critical role in smart weather report. We are using the IoT sensors to gather the status of each and every day in the weather report. We have implemented a smart weather report using AWS which will help us to know the climatic conditions.

In the recent era, IoT is emerging rapidly throughout our life by finding its path to improve the quality of life by connecting many technologies, applications to the physical objects around us by automating the things [3]. Enormous attention has been paid toward the digitization of the physical world such as home, offices, factories, vehicles, and cities [4]. The research made by international data corporation (IDC) confirms IoT solutions in increasingly recognized as transformative to consumers, business, and governments each of them will innovate, experience, and operate in the world, where end user will fell the tangible benefits of IoT [5]. All the physical objects relate to sensing elements enabled by wireless sensor network (WSN) technologies in our daily life [6]. WSN consists of different wireless technologies such as Bluetooth (over IEEE 802.15.1), ZigBee (over IEEE 802.15.4), and Wi-Fi (over IEEE 802.11), every protocol has got it advantages and disadvantages based on speed, power, and transmission capacity [7]. The gateway can receive the data from all the sensor nodes which may use different wireless protocols and send that to cloud and it must receive the data from remote location and act according to the commands given by user which is dealing with interoperability in IoT [8]. By obtaining a common data format for the data received from the sensor nodes to transmit to cloud and converting the commands accordingly to sensor nodes which are given by the user from the remote location which solves the interoperability problems [9]. In this paper, we propose a design of bidirectional IoT gateway, with wireless protocols Wi-Fi which enables the interoperability of wireless protocols in cooperating the transformation of data [10].

The IoT-based smart weather report makes use of wireless sensor network (Wi-Fi) that gathers information from DHT11 sensor which collects the temperature and humidity data at various places, and it transfers the data through the wireless protocol [11]. We have implemented the smart weather report using the NodeMCU (ESP8266). It consists of DHT11 sensor. When IoT-based smart weather report starts, it checks the temperature and the humidity of surrounding places [12]. It will display the latest temperature and the humidity of the places on AWS. The data will automatically be updated on the AWS for every 15 min.

2 Methodology

The aim of this project is to report the weather conditions on the dashboard, in the AWS, we are going to display the last updated it means that the temperature and humidity at a place. We are deploying the NodeMCU at different places and we are going to monitor the environmental conditions from our place. The ESP8266 consists of in built Wi-Fi module which can be used to transmit sensor values to a long distance. We are going to send the data from the ESP8266 to the MQTT client, which is used for establishing the communication between the ESP8266 and the AWS. Once the data is published into the MQTT. We are going to store that data into the DynamoDB in order to use the data for the further analysis, using the timestamp. We are retrieving the data from DynamoDB and exporting the data as .csv file for prediction of the future temperature and humidity.

2.1 Open SSL

It is simple software that will be used for converting the files from one format to the other format. To establish a connection between the AWS and the NodeMCU. We are using the certificates which are of (.der) format and we are downloading the (.pem) formatted certificates from the AWS. In order to convert the certificates from (.pem) to (.der), we are using the open SSL.

2.2 MQTT

The MQTT publish and subscribe modules are used to gather and to transfer the data from the hardware communication module. By subscribing to the topic which is used in the program to get the data on to the IoT core console and publish module in the AWS is used to send the data into the required modules such as DynamoDB. We can get the message alerts in Arduino IDE monitor.

2.3 DynamoDB

It is used to store the huge amount of data which we have collected using the MQTT, DynamoDB is a NoSQL, we can store the data securely, the time to live feature is available in the DynamoDB which will be used to automatically delete the items in the DynamoDB which has been expired based on the time which has been given to it.

It is used to perform some of the actions on the data which is in the DynamoDB and to perform the back-end actions on the data. AWS is a server less computing service that executes your code in response to events and manages the underlying computation resources for you automatically. You can use AWS to expand other custom logic AWS services or build your own back-end services that run on an AWS scale, performance, and security.

2.4 API Gateway

The API Gateway is used to transfer of data from the database to the Web site. It is used to send and receive the request from the Web site. We are using the functions which are available in the API Gateway, we are linking the AWS endpoint for the processing of the requests.

2.5 Colab

Colab notebooks are used to execute code on Google's cloud servers. It helps to run large machine learning programs which uses GPUs. We used Colab to run machine learning algorithm (linear regression) to get predicted output. Firstly, in Colab, we will export the .csv file. Then, we divided the dataset into training and test datasets and use machine learning technique linear regression to predict the future temperature and humidity.

3 Flowchart

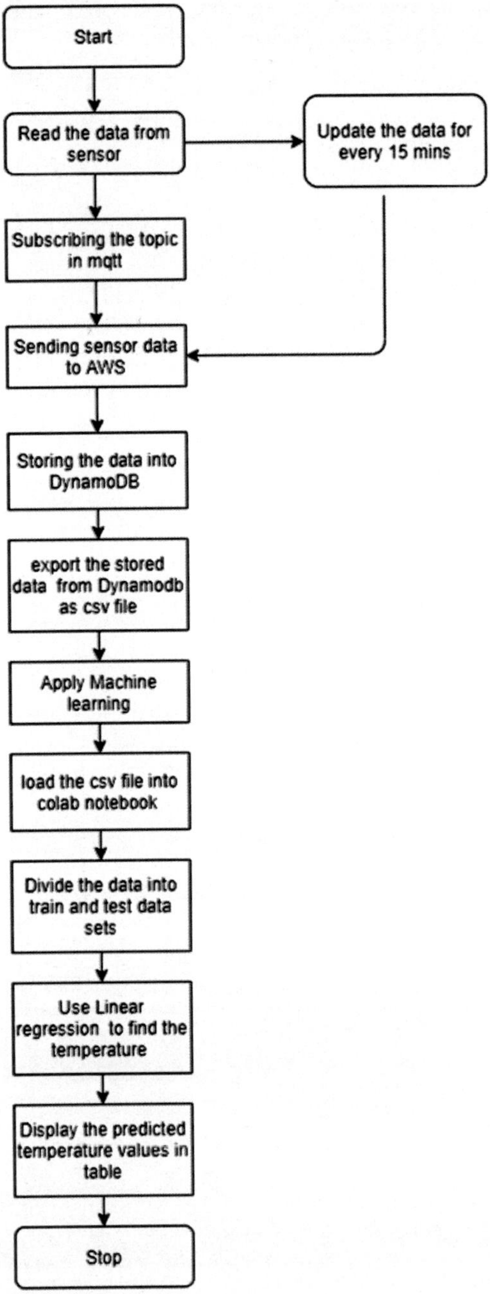
Start
Read the data from sensor
Update the data for every 15 mins
Subscribing the topic in mqtt
Sending sensor data to AWS
Storing the data into DynamoDB
export the stored data from Dynamodb as csv file
Apply Machine learning
load the csv file into colab notebook
Divide the data into train and test data sets
Use Linear regression to find the temperature
Display the predicted temperature values in table
Stop

First of all, when we subscribe the MQTT in AWS, the sensor sends the data from NodeMCU to AWS cloud. The data sent is stored in DynamoDB and it is updated for every 15 min. The stored data is exported as .csv file and loaded into Colab. We split the data into test and train datasets to perform linear regression machine learning algorithm. We display the predicated temperature in table.

4 Results

The DynamoDB we have created the fields like temperature and humidity and on another field, which is used for differentiating the places of the nodes in Fig. 1. We have stored the temperature and humidity data in the AWS cloud. The stored data is then shifted to DynamoDB which is stored in the form of tables and save the data to create table in the DynamoDB. After creation of table, go to action menu and export the data into .csv file. Then, use the .csv file in Colab to apply machine learning.

4.1 Linear Regression Model

We are using linear regression for our machine learning; we have split the dataset as train_X, train_Y, test_X, and test_Y for training and test instances in Fig. 2. We have imported the linear regression model to model and used model.fit() to fit the values into the model. We have calculated the mean value of the model. Linear regression performs a regression task. Regression models a target prediction value based on independent variables. Regression technique finds out a linear relationship between input and output, algorithm establishes the relationship between dependent

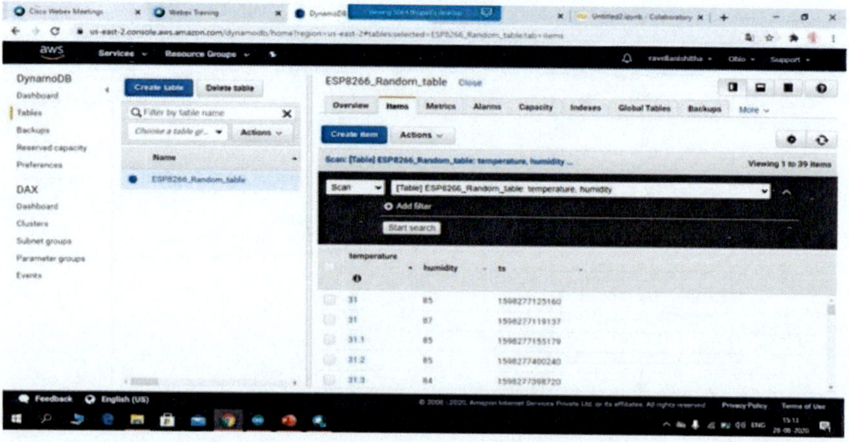

Fig. 1 Creating table in DynamoDB

Fig. 2 Applying linear regression using .csv file

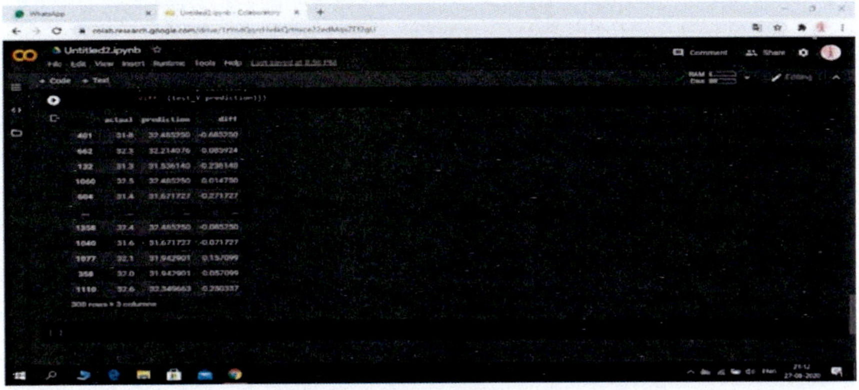

Fig. 3 Comparison between actual and predicted values

variable and independent variable, and the relationship will be linear nature. Linear regression is one of the simplest machine learning algorithms that come under supervised learning technique and is used for solving regression problems. It is used for predicting the continuous dependent variable with the help of independent variables. The goal of the linear regression is to find the best fit line that can accurately predict the output for the continuous dependent variable when compared to other machine learning algorithms.

Figure 3 shows the actual and predicted values of temperature which are printed randomly and also displayed the difference of actual and predicted values, which difference is very low, so it has high accuracy of predicted temperature values. And we printed the values of size 308 rows × 3 columns.

Figure 4 shows the code which we used, in the code, we have used aws_endpoint to make the connection with AWS cloud and also we uploaded the certificates which are downloaded from AWS cloud, then we upload the certificates to NodeMCU to make a secure connection with AWS. After uploading the code, we are connected to AWS cloud with MQTT connection.

After then, we go to AWS console, choose IoT core in search box, and click the test menu, then open and connect to MQTT gateway. We are subscribing the topic which is named as out topic and click the subscribe button in AWS cloud to get the output data of temperature and humidity from NodeMCU board as shown in Fig. 5.

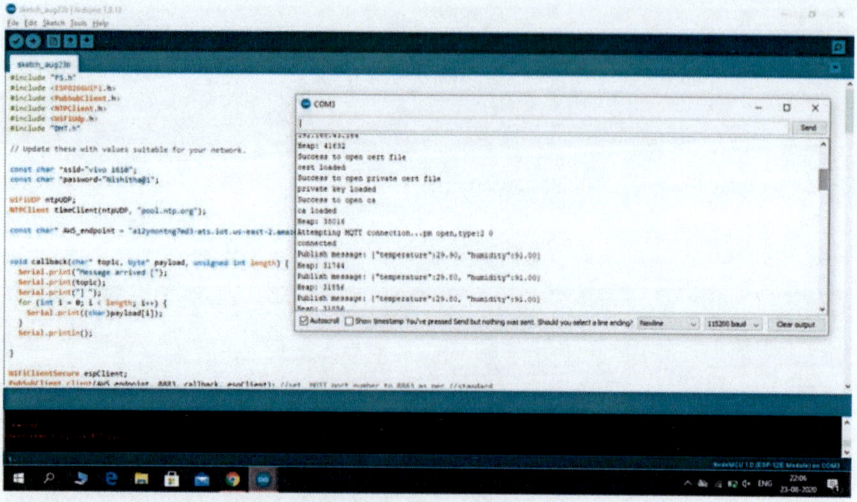

Fig. 4 Temperature and humidity output

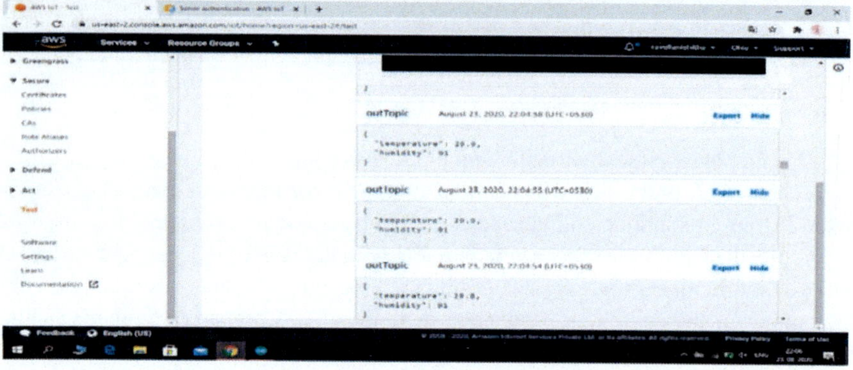

Fig. 5 Data stored in AWS cloud

5 Conclusion

We have used AWS cloud to store the data and we have used certificates to make mutual authentication with NodeMCU. The collected temperature and humidity values from NodeMCU we have stored them to DynamoDB as shown in Fig. 1. All the nodes which are placed at the different places will gather the weather conditions using the AWS and stored data will be displayed on the dashboard as shown in Fig. 5. The stored data is exported as .csv file. We use it in Colab to predict the values of temperature and humidity. We do this by splitting the data into train and test datasets. Then, we will use linear regression machine learning to train the model and to display predicted values as shown in Fig. 3.

References

1. Dabbakuti JK, Ch B (2019) Ionospheric monitoring system based on the internet of things with thing speak. Astrophys Space Sci 364(8):137
2. Krishna PG, Ravi KS, Kishore KH, KrishnaVeni K, Rao KS, Prasad RD (2018) Design and development of bi-directional IoT gateway using ZigBee and Wi-Fi technologies with MQTT protocol. Int J Eng Technol 7(2.8):125–129
3. Kommuri K, Ratnam KV, Prathyusha G, Krishna PG (2018) Development of real time environment monitoring system using with MSP430. Int J Eng Technol 7(28):72–76
4. Sastry JKR, Miriyala T (2019) Securing SAAS service under cloud computing-based multi-tenancy systems. Indonesian J Electr Eng Comput Sci 13(1):65–71
5. Dabbakuti JRKK, Jacob A, Veeravalli VR, Kallakunta RK (2019) Implementation of IoT analytics ionospheric forecasting system based on machine learning and Thing Speak. IET Radar Sonar Navig 14(2):341–347
6. Vamseekrishna A, Madhav BTP, Anilkumar T, Reddy LSS (2019) An IoT controlled octahedron frequency reconfigurable multiband antenna for microwave sensing applications. IEEE Sensors Lett 3(10):1–4
7. Allam VK, Madhav BTP, Anilkumar T, Maloji S (2019) A novel reconfigurable bandpass filtering antenna for IoT communication applications. Prog Electromagnet Res 96:13–26
8. Sucharitanjani G, Kumar PN (2019) Internet of things based smart vehicle parking access system. Int J Innov Technol Exploring Eng (IJITEE) 8(6):732–734
9. Kumari KA, Sastry JKR, Rao KR (2019) Energy efficient load balanced optimal resource allocation scheme for cloud environment. Int J Recent Technol Eng (IJRTE) 8(1S3)
10. Bhanu JS, Sastry JKR, Kumar PVS, Sai BV, Sowmya KV (2019) Enhancing performance of IoT networks through high performance computing. Int J Adv Trends Comput Sci Eng 8(3):432–442
11. Prabu AV, Sateesh Kumar G (2019) Performance analysis and lifetime estimation of wireless technologies for WSN (wireless sensor networks) /IoT (internet of things) application. J Adv Res Dynam Control Syst 11(1):250–258
12. Prabu AV, Sateesh Kumar G (2019) Hybrid MAC based adaptive preamble technique to improve the lifetime in wireless sensor networks. J Adv Res Dynam Control Syst 11(1):240–249

Forensic Investigation of Tor Bundled Browser

Srihitha Gunapriya, Valli Kumari Vatsavayi, and Kalidindi Sandeep Varma

Abstract The Tor Browser bundle is said to maintain user privacy. With many users depending on it, the research interest has grown up in investigating the Tor Browser behavior. This paper researches on the aspects of whether the user privacy is really maintained completely. The experiments conducted reveal that digital traces are left behind which can be later analyzed by the investigators. This paper presents the memory forensic experiments done and the methods used to analyze the digital artifacts left by Tor.

Keywords Private browsing · Memory forensics · Tor · Privacy · Digital artifacts

1 Introduction

Tor Bundled Browser has gained its prominence by the public and cyber criminals [1] for the anonymity feature it provides. A considerable number of privacy researchers are working on the Tor Browser to find how effective it is protecting the user's privacy. This research focuses on conducting the forensic analysis on the Tor Bundled Browser in safeguarding the privacy of the user. It also analyzes the adversaries of software and the interactions on the host operating system.

This research focuses on the Tor Bundled Browser and its activities. Static and live analyses are performed on the Tor Browser. Virtualization is used to simulate the testing environment along with predetermined browsing protocol. Both static and live analyses were performed. The artifacts of the browser like browsing information

S. Gunapriya · V. K. Vatsavayi
Department of Computer Science and Software Engineering, Andhra University, Visakhapatnam, India
e-mail: srihithagunapriya@gmail.com

V. K. Vatsavayi
e-mail: vallikumari@gmail.com

K. S. Varma (✉)
Department of Computer Science Engineering, GIT, GITAM (Deemed To Be University), Visakhapatnam, India
e-mail: skalidin@gitam.edu

S. Bhattacharyya et al. (eds.), *International Conference on Intelligent and Smart Computing in Data Analytics*, Advances in Intelligent Systems and Computing 1312,
https://doi.org/10.1007/978-981-33-6176-8_31

are retrieved and analyzed. In static analysis, the snapshots of the machines are captured and analyzed to find the leakage of the user activities such as web page titles, URL information and HTTP headers. Whereas the live analysis is done by capturing the main memory, and the artifacts are found even after removing the Tor Browser. With the live analysis, it is also observed that installation directory of the browser was captured. It also captured the device on which the browser was opened. It is observed that Tor cannot securely delete the activity within a browsing session. It is also observed that the TOR design did not consider the local attacker. This paper presents methods to collect digital artifacts and traces of evidence in the usage of Tor Browser for digital forensics.

Various sections of this paper arranged are as follows. Section 2 shows the background and related work. Section 3 explains various methods to collect digital artifacts. It also discusses the experimental setup and evidence collection process. Section 4 discusses the results. Section 5 compares the results with other existing works, and Sect. 6 concludes the paper.

2 Background and Related Work

Tor Bundled Browser was built on Mozilla Firefox. According to Sandvik [2], if any vulnerability exists in Mozilla Firefox private browsing mode, the same may exist in Tor Bundled Browser (TBB). The developer must patch those vulnerabilities. To check the anonymity of the Tor Bundled Browser, Sandvik has performed the forensic analysis with the Tor Browser on various operating systems. Even though TOR uses anti-measures, Sandvik was able to find multiple artifacts. Darcie et al. [3] performed forensic analysis of the Windows Registry and found artifacts even after the uninstallation of TOR Bundled Browser. His research proposed a methodology like the methods used by Montasari et al. [4], where the RAM dumps of the target machine are analyzed by searching and indexing the keywords to find the artifacts. Epifani et al. [5] with his work proved that a trail of evidence could be captured from the host operating system using the prefetch files. This evidence proved the importance of live forensic analysis. Dayalamurthy et al. [6] proposed that de-anonymizing the Tor users can be done using live forensic analysis on the use of Tor Bundled Browser. The research proposed a methodology to capture web graphics by using the volatility framework for memory analysis. Warren et al. [7] proposed a comprehensive methodology like the Dayalmurthy which used volatility framework for the analysis of RAM of a Windows 10, with third-party plugins installed. The artifacts like SIDs, environment variables, Tor DLLs and command line usage were captured by the methodology proposed by Warren. Tor does not write the browsing information onto the disk, and it can only be captured by the live RAM forensics. These artifacts are in the form of images and HTML files. According to Findley et al. [8], in live memory forensics of Firefox, private browsing mode captured more artifacts when the browser is open rather than when the browser is closed. Their research proved that the Firefox private browsing mode was unable to remove the artifacts after a private browser window was closed. However, they have not verified this for the Tor Bundled Browser.

Several other methods for Tor Browser analysis are proposed in [9–11].

3 Finding the Artifacts After Browsing with TOR

This section explains how the artifacts were retrieved after browsing with TOR. The paper uses the same URLs and search words to confirm the correctness of the methodology as used by existing works.

3.1 Assumptions and Pre-definitions

The forensic analysis in this paper mainly aims on finding the existence and use of the Tor Browser on the virtual machine consisting of Windows 10 operating system. This existence can be proved by capturing the artifacts from the Tor Browser on the target computer.

This paper is designed to find whether the Tor Browser is securely deleting the evidence from the RAM after the session is closed to protect its users. It is also used to detect four different moments such as

1. When the user is using the Tor Browser,
2. User has closed the Tor Browser,
3. User has removed the Tor Browser and its files,
4. User has logged out of the system.

Inspired by Montasari et al. [4], this research simulates different browsing actions performed by the user. (i.e., opening a URL, searching a text, download content, etc.)

The following operations has been performed for the experimentation.

1. The Web site www.theguardian.co.uk has been browsed in the Tor Bundled Browser.
2. Next https://support.mozilla.org has been visited in the Tor Bundled Browser, and a search operation is performed with sample text. ex:'Profile'.
3. Next "moog mother 32" keyword has been searched on Google image search in Tor Bundled Browser and downloaded the first image.
4. Next downloaded a sample image from www.duckduckgo.com in the Tor Bundled Browser.
5. Next the Tor packets have been captured while Tor Bundled Browser is open.
6. The captured Tor packets have been analyzed using network log files. This analysis helped in finding the artifacts of actions performed. ex: domain names.
7. Next, the prefetch files are opencd through command prompt to find when the Tor Bundled Browser was executed for the first time.

3.2 Experimental Setup

In this experiment, newly installed operating systems have been used on a virtual environment. VMware Workstation 15 Pro has been used to provide the virtual environment to perform the operations. Window 10 (64 bit) operating system is used in this research. Tor Bundled Browser 9.0.5 is used. Linux Reader software has been installed to read the files on the filesystem such as pagefile.sys, hex files and DAT files. The network log files also can be analyzed using Linux Reader software, which can be used to get the information of the domains visited on the Tor Bundled Browser. Network log files are also analyzed using Linux Reader software, and then we get the information of domain names of the Web sites visited.

4 Analysis of the Artifacts

The artifacts identified after the analysis of the RAM captured can be observed from the results given in this section. The artifacts can be identified from Live RAM Forensics when the Tor Bundled Browser is open and when it is closed.

Figure 1 shows the proof that user has installed the Tor Bundled Browser along with the path of installation from DAT file using Linux Reader software. It can also show some partial information of the user.

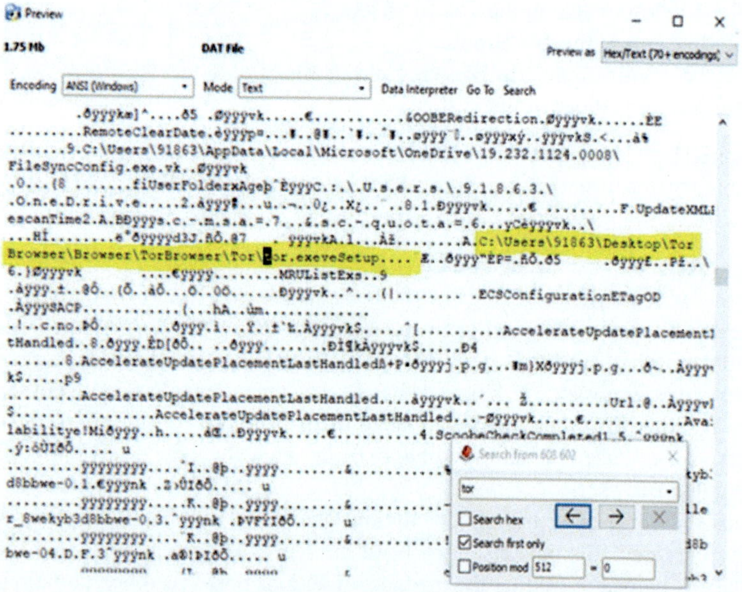

Fig. 1 Highlighted section shows the directory where Tor is installed and the user profile information

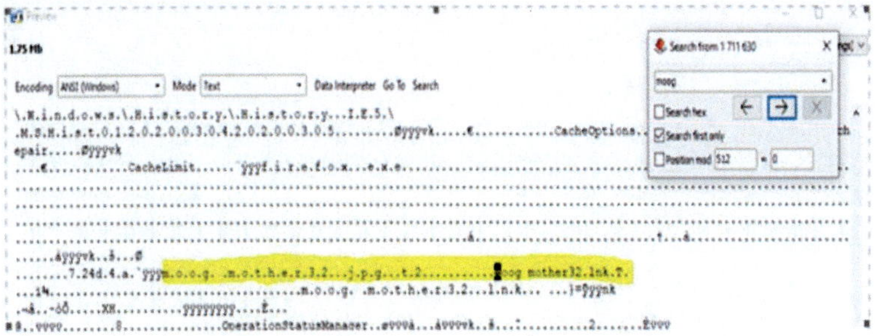

Fig. 2 Highlighted section traces of the downloaded image (moogmother32)

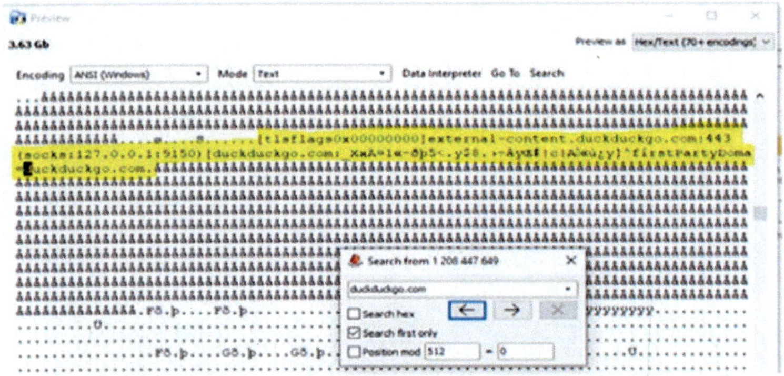

Fig. 3 Highlighted section shows traces of downloaded image (external content)

Figure 2 shows the proof of the search keyword which is used while searching the Google images. It shows that the user has searched for the keyword moogmother32.jpg.

Figure 3 shows that the user has downloaded the image from the www.duckduckgo.com. It also shows the partial traces of the downloaded image.

Figure 4 shows the public keys of the user which have been captured by the investigator which has been used by the user when using an encrypted session.

Figure 5 shows the prefetched files that have been captured during the time of execution of the Tor Bundled Browser.

Figure 6 shows the proof of the mail data of the user can be identified from the captured data. It can be observed that the data of the mail can be read in the plain text which can be used as an artifact.

For network artifacts, two scenarios are considered, and they are when the browser is opened and when it is closed. When browser is opened, smsniff tool is used to capture network packets. The network packets are combination of http packets, TCP packets, UDP packets, bridge connections and more. The http packets are collected, and the webpage visited can be created. So, the Web site visited can be easily seen. The network capture starts when the browser is opened and started any searches and

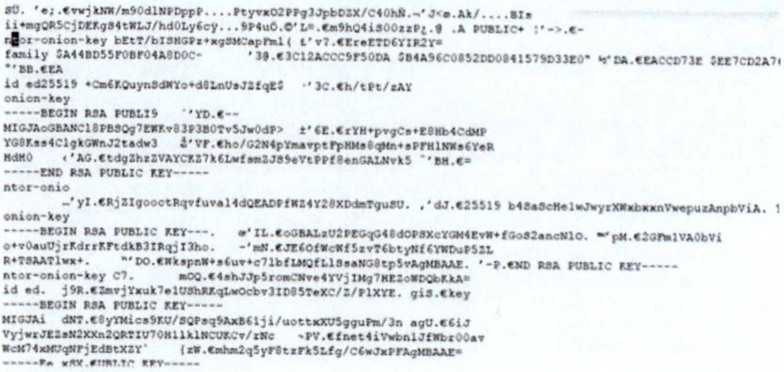

Fig. 4 Image shows the RSA public keys of the user

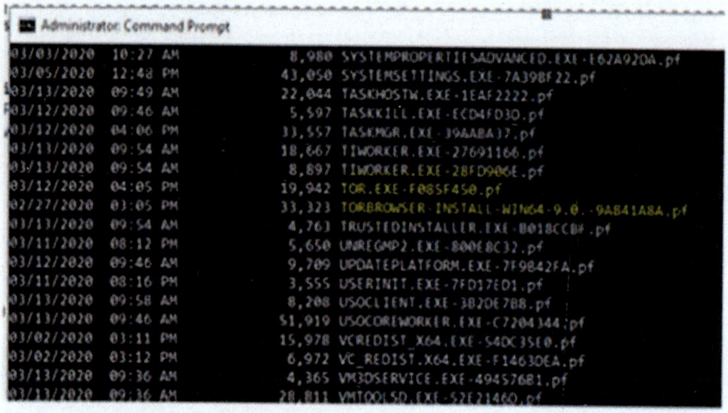

Fig. 5 Highlighted section shows prefetch file showing the time of execution of tor.exe

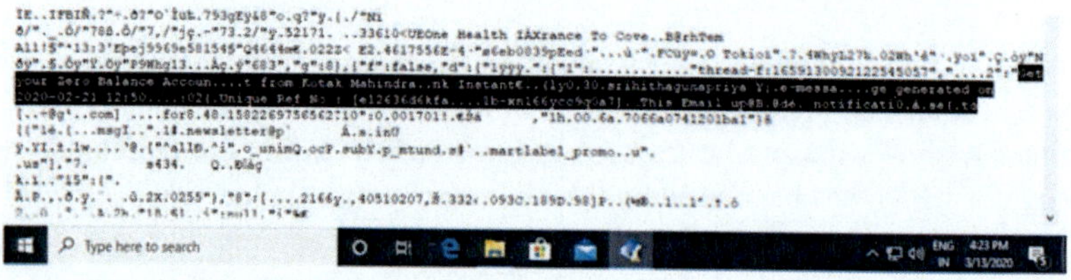

Fig. 6 Highlighted section shows the retrieved mail data

till the browser is closed or the capture is stopped. smsniff tool also gives the bridge connections as Tor network always changes its path and IP address of the system.

Second scenario considered is when browser is closed. This part of research is not addressed by any previous published works. To get the evidence when the browser is closed, we analyze the log files.

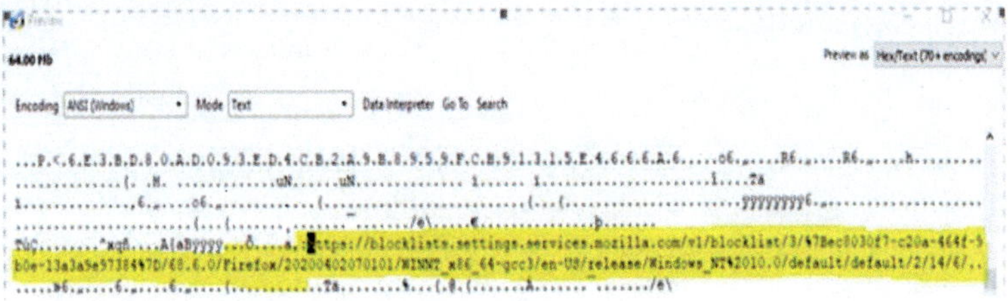

Fig. 7 Artifact showing that we visited https://support.mozilla.org

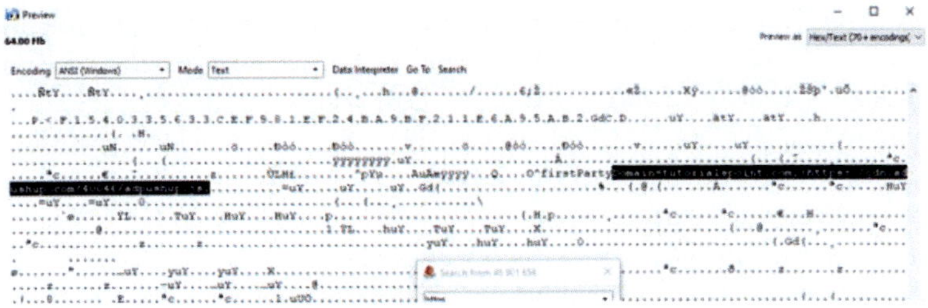

Fig. 8 Highlighted section shows artifact showing the domain name (tutorial point) visited

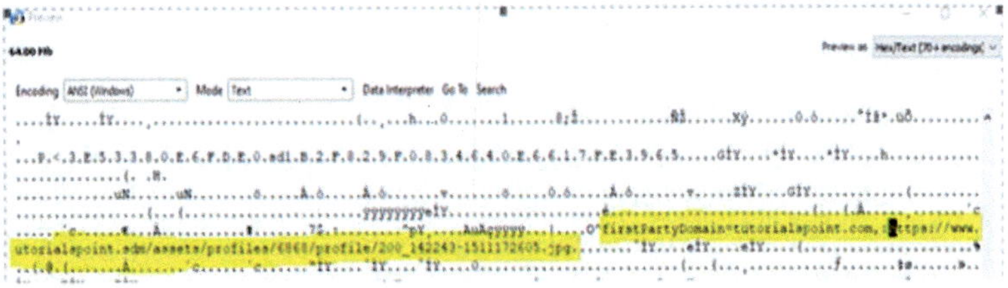

Fig. 9 URL showing the visited profile information

Network log files are analyzed to get absolute paths, URLs and domains visited by the user that are retrieved. These are the most useful artifacts that give us the recent activity of the user. Figures 7, 8 and 9 show the artifacts has been retrieved by analyzing the data that is captured after closing the Tor Bundled Browser.

5 Comparison with Other Existing Works

In this section, we compare the findings in this paper with other published works. Muir et al. [9] perform forensic analysis of TOR. They use volatility framework. This paper uses various open-source tools available. Four similar works related to our work were found. A comparative analysis was done based on memory artifacts and network artifacts found while performing forensic investigation.

Table 1 Comparison with existing works

Different works	Memory artifacts		Network artifacts
	Tor	Tor closed	
Our work	Yes	Yes	Yes
Winkler et al.	No	Yes	Yes
Atta et al.	No	No	No
Aron et al.	Yes	Yes	No
Jadoon et al.	Yes	Yes	No

Winkler et al. [6] performed memory analysis of TOR. The experiments were conducted on Windows 7. As of now, Windows 10 is the most popular and has come up with many security features. Atta et al. [10] considered general web browsing behavior. They also claim that the artifacts are removed when TOR is closed. Aron et al. [7] do not perform any artifact analysis of browsing traces in memory or hard disk. Jadoon et al. [11] perform the experimentation on Windows 8.1. They consider hard disk and memory artifacts. Our work considers memory and network artifacts. The comparison is illustrated in Table 1.

6 Conclusions and Future Work

This paper presented methods for forensics investigation of TOR Browser on Windows 10 OS. The experimentation has used open-source tools for finding the memory and network artifacts. It is found that TOR browser leaves traces in memory and network data. It is also found that the data can be linked to the user. The work is compared to four other works published in literature in the same lines. The novelty of this proposed work is that it can find the memory as well as network artifacts of TOR while it is running and even after it is closed in Windows 10.

Further, it is intended to build an intelligent system which can use the data and capture artifacts for further analysis and evidence tracking.

References

1. Dewey C (2013) Everything we know about Ross Ulbricht, the outdoorsy libertarian behind Silk Road. The Washington Post. https://www.washingtonpost.com/news/the-switch/wp/2013/10/03/everything-we-know-about-ross-ulbricht-the-outdoorsy-libertarian-behind-silk-road.
2. Sandvik RA (2013) Forensic analysis of the tor browser bundle on OSX, Linux, and Windows. Technical report. The Tor project. https://research.torproject.org/techreports/tbb-forensic-analysis-2013-06-28.pdf. The TOR Project, https://www.torproject.org/
3. Darcie W, Boggs RJ, Sammons J, Fenger T (2014). Online anonymity: forensic analysis of the tor browser bundle. Technical Report. Marshall University. https://www.marshall.edu/forensics/files/WinklerDarcie

4. Montasari R, Peltola P (2015) Computer forensic analysis of private browsing modes, in: global security, safety and sustainability: tomorrow's challenges of cyber security. In: ICGS3 2015. Communications in Computer and Information Science, vol 534. Springer, pp. 96–109. https://doi.org/10.1007/978-3-319-23276-8_9
5. Epifani M, Scarito M, Picasso F (2015) Tor forensics on windows OS. In: DFRWS EU, Dublin. https://www.dfrws.org/sites/default/files/session-files/pres-torforensicsonwindowsos.pdf
6. Dayalamurthy D (2013) Forensic memory dump analysis and recovery of the artifacts of using Tor bundle browser: the need. In: Australian digital forensics conference, pp 71–83. https://doi.org/10.4225/75/57b3c7f3fb86e
7. Warren A (2017) Tor browser artifacts in windows 10. Retrieved from SANS Institute website: https://www.sans.org/reading-room/whitepapers/forensics/tor-browser-artifacts-windows-10-37642
8. Findlay C, Leimich P (2014) An assessment of data leakage in Firefox under different conditions. In: 7th International conference on cybercrime forensics education and training (CFET 2014), Canterbury, UK. https://www.researchgate.net/publication/330925976
9. Muir M, Leimich P, Buchanan WJ A forensic analysis of TOR browser bundle. https://arxiv.org/pdf/1907.10279.pdf
10. Al-Khaleel A, Bani-Salameh D, Al-Saleh MI (2014) On the memory artifacts of the tor browser bundle. In: The international conference on computing technology and information management (ICCTIM), Society of Digital Information and Wireless Communication, p 41
11. Jadoon AK, Waseem IM, Faisal AH, Afzal Y, Abbas B Forensic analysis of tor browser: a case study for privacy and anonymity on the web

Energy and Efficient Privacy Cryptography-based Fuzzy K-Means Clustering a WSN Using Genetic Algorithm

K. Abdul Basith and T. N. Shankar

Abstract Current mechanical advancements in sensors, low-power microelectronics just as scaling down, and cordless systems administration permitted the plan and spreading of mobile ad hoc networks ready to self-governingly keeping up a watch on and furthermore controlling settings. Remote sensor networks (WSNs) can be portrayed as a self-arranged and furthermore framework parcels much less cordless systems to show physical or natural issues, total of temperature stage, sound, reverberation, pressure, and distraction. A wireless sensing unit network (WSN) incorporates an enormous amount of sensor hubs. The sensor nodes can speak among themselves the use of radio alerts. A Wi-Fi sensor node is ready with selecting up and calculating gadgets, radio transceivers, and also electricity substances. The sensing unit nodes rely upon battery power. Sensor nodes make use of more power as contrasted to a day-to-day node. Mobile Impromptu Network (MANET), it is constructed from a diffusion of self-organized and also battery-organized cell nodes, is applied notably in endless applications, collectively with navy and additionally non-public industries. Nonetheless, protection is a prime trouble in MANET directing, due to the fact the network is at risk of attacks. This paper introduces the breach detection scheme for establishing the safeguarded route in MANET. The proposed cryptography schema takes much less memory, reduces the time, gives tremendous protection, and perfectly is suitable for low stamina gadgets like cell nodes. The goal of this task is to provide safety to the Wi-Fi sensing unit place using elliptical exerciser curves cryptography on the facet of genetic set of rules.

Keywords WSN · MANET · Wireless sensor network · High efficiency · Genetic algorithm

---

K. Abdul Basith (✉) · T. N. Shankar
Department of Computer Science and Engineering, Koneru Lakshmaiah Education Foundation, Vaddeswaram, Guntur, Andhra Pradesh 522502, India
e-mail: khateebabdulbasith2020@gmail.com

T. N. Shankar
e-mail: tnshankar2004@kluniversity.in

S. Bhattacharyya et al. (eds.), *International Conference on Intelligent and Smart Computing in Data Analytics*, Advances in Intelligent Systems and Computing 1312,
https://doi.org/10.1007/978-981-33-6176-8_32

1 Introduction

Directing in MANET as a mobile self-configuring infrastructure, a bargain load much less Wi-Fi neighborhood is greater complex than one of a kind fundamental networks. A node in MANET may be both terminal node as well as router. Indeed, a node as a terminal node sends in addition to receive packets also as that node as a router will find and additionally keep a path and in addition plays programs to a vacation spot. In the opposite hand, topology on this kind of network is hollow due to nodes' wheelchair. Therefore, router-based completely transmitting systems which attempt to maintain area geography do now not paintings as it should be in MANET [1]. A WSN consists of lots of tiny and additionally occasional rate sensor nodes that are able to find bodily sensations that consist of temperature, minor, warmth and audio, in addition to remarkable deals of others. WSNs have many bundles together with militia, monitoring, residential programs, Web site vacationers manage, and so on. Because the sensor nodes can be finished in unsteady as well as inaccessible environments, converting or recharging their stamina additives is not always possible in addition to financial. Consequently, maximizing electric strength intake for lengthening the area lifestyles time is an important trouble in WSNs [2].

MANET has the dynamic geography and also the nodes gift in the community does no longer provide first-class shape to the community, and additionally finally, it may be suffering from various network moves. MANET consists of some of nodes brazenly allocated over the wireless device [3]. The info is exceeded from the supply node to the getaway node thru several collection of intermediate nodes, and also the verbal exchange numerous of the nodes can be referred as hopping. Based upon the interplay, the MANET comes beneath guidelines; they will truly be single hop network and multi-bounce community. Various directing formulas are to be had without problems on hand for establishing the directing direction among the supply in addition to the holiday spot for statistics transmission. Selecting a marked node en masse head is an entirely beautiful, however, complicated undertaking. A selection of variables can be thought about for picking the excellent hub as a bunch head. A part of these parts integrate specific of the center with noteworthy to unmistakable hubs, flexibility, power, save in musings, and also throughput of the center. In amazing determined hubs of WSN, notwithstanding MANETs have actually constricted battery and furthermore possessions [4]. Improvement of political decision will really broaden the all out handling costs of the network. So the political decision approach wants to besides hold up under as a main priority dealing with power snags of the hubs. Aim of these examinations is to discuss their particulars, decision of reclustering, and execution. In any case to the premium of records, no assessment of the CH political race flexibly accentuation to place of hub in bunch, get as certifiable with component of hubs, just as singular assortment head determination steady with political race producer has been a distant memory over to day [5]. High satisfactory of service in directing needs to make sure that selected path has a good deal and awful lot less Website online traffic, a good deal much less packet loss, best duration, as well as the maximum possible bandwidth together. Approaching to transmitting QoS is unrealistic without attention of nature in addition to dynamic geography in MANET [6]. This endeavor has attempted to apply hereditary and also blurry formulas in DSR to method to QoS in MANET directing. The preliminary part of this article will provide an explanation for the second-hand hereditary series of recommendations. Section will introduce our adjustments on DSR and additionally our method works. Section three is the thing of route updating with the supply of fuzzy. As nicely as one way or every other, we imitate our transmitting technique with the resource of NS2 as well as examine it with elegant DSR [7].

2 Related Study

Wireless sensing device networks (WSNs) are objectifying a large wide kind of sensing unit tools that may seriously talk with each extraordinary by making use of cordless networks, with constrained power together with computer of such ambience which is a tough mathematical as well as technological task [1]. These WSNs operate in that, and they will be open to aid numerous of really one-of-a-kind real all over the world plans; there could be on top of that a hard research study along with engineering trouble as a result of this truly versatility. As important, there could be no singular collection of needs that actually recognizes all WSNs, and also furthermore there may be moreover currently saying goodbye to a solitary technological selection that incorporates the entire design area. Research looks at noticing system networks ended up being prior to every little thing maintained with the supply of armed forces strategies [2]. Extremely very early research studies wind up being ended up by means of design of navy making use of noticing system networks for protection handling occasions at adjoining rates. A WSN may be commonly defined as an area of nodes that en masse gratification in as well as additionally could manage the atmospheres enabling interaction among people or PC systems as well as additionally that contains setups. Today, wireless sensing system networks are thoroughly utilized in business in addition to company areas together with, e.g., eco-friendly surveillance, environment surveillance, therapy, and method surveillance and additionally monitoring. As an instance, in an armed forces location, we have the ability to utilize Wi-Fi sensor networks to reveal activity [3]. If an event is created, the ones picking up unit nodes relish it and in addition to furthermore deliver the papers to the sink node with talking to many nodes. Utilizing WSNs developing each day and also at the same time, it comes across the migraine of power restraints with regard to controlled battery lifetime. As every node is primarily based upon electric power for its sporting activities, this has actually been included to be a vital trouble in WSNs. In nonetheless positioning, the nodes take in practically the identical amount of stamina as in energized setting, at the same time as in sleep mode; the nodes are closure to the radio to save the electric power. In order to make a totally safe and secure Wi-Fi picking up system networks, protection must be included to every node of the system [5]. The purpose is that a variable done with none defense will do not have difficulty and becomes an aspect of attack. It suggests that a safety and security and also safety need permeating using every components of format of cordless sensing unit networks. Wireless observing tool networks (WSNs) are the work to countless moves because of the likely setups, controlled alternative, in addition to open communication channel [6]. Wireless networking has actually observed a durable rate of interest, in nowadays, past due to the packages in cell in addition to distinct communications. Wireless location patterns are most likely determined right into framework Wi-Fi area designs as well as additionally ad hoc wireless community formats. Commonly, Wi-Fi networks are extended from existing confused out area. While organizing the wireless picking up gadget network, the noticing device nodes may do not have trouble released within the unreceptive atmospheres [7].

3 Proposed System

The invoked technique has been evolved to justify efficient electricity and security metrics in a mobile ad hoc network with fuzzy logic-based genetic algorithm and excessive safety problem with the elliptical curves digital signature set of rules cryptography. Our research simulation is based on NS2 tool (Network Simulator-2). It is a software program programming device to be applied to actual time networks to assess the performance of a MANET. The behavior of a MANET can be able to verify in two codes using this tool.

- Graphical representation of nodes in a MANET.
- Realizable in other suitable platforms.

This proposed work is to be applied in four steps, and the consequences have been discussed as follows.

1. Deployment of the mobile nodes: This community is proposed with 150 mobiles nodes which might be randomly generated.
2. Cluster formation: It organizes these randomly generated nodes to shape (topology). This cluster formation has been developed via fuzzy K-means algorithmic techniques.
3. Cluster head selection: By incorporating fuzzy good judgment ideology alongside genetic algorithm (GA) to pick cluster head for selected cluster. Here specially focussed to choose a greater green cluster head in MANET to degree the parameter of a MANET complements its overall performance.
4. Security and information transmission: Encrypted and decrypted for excessive and precise facts safety purpose statistics transmissions between the nodes in a given network structure. So in this work a try has been made with the aid of bringing all constraints to carry excessive safety alerts. In the information transmission procedure, the nodes live idle until an occasion takes place. On detection of the occasion, the mobile node appears within the near vicinity, understands the message, and transmits it to the CH and the usage of a multi-hop course.

This research work mainly focussed on methodologies and algorithmic approaches to improve the overall performance of a MANET in wireless communication. The work mainly concentrates on three major key factors that enhance the performance of a MANET that are to be discussed as follows:

- Performance factors of MANET network
- Overall power consumption of MANET network is to be reduced.
- By avoiding unused/unnecessary nodes to improve the network lifetime and to achieve the highest security in a network.

3.1 Energy and Efficient Cryptography-Based Fuzzy K-Means WSN Using Genetic Algorithm

The proposed scheme proposes a revolutionary routing community architecture model to gain excessive safety and carry out most energy utilization. This architecture model consists of a set number of frames of cluster with limited range of sensor nodes. This painting consists of fuzzy k approach with set of regulations for cluster formation. The major topic of these paintings is to evaluate the performance factors power intake and network lifetime in a MANET.

3.1.1 K-Means Algorithm

It is a promising and lively clustering set of guidelines. It is a classical approach for unsupervised evolutionary DM set of guidelines which resolves the clustering trouble in a smooth manner. It has famous applications in biometrics, medical imaging, and numerous new upcoming fields. It adapts the clustering strategies recognized for noticing the devices grouping. It consists of nodes regrouping inside the network to shape many clusters. The cluster formation is grounded on parameter like need cluster and the Euclidean distance for locating the nearest cluster for every node. The cluster head choice with the algorithm of OK technique is grounded on factors just like the function of cluster head to be at the cluster center on the aspect of node residual electricity.

In MANET, the clustering method using okay manner is performed on repetitive optimization of node distance to categorize. It creates a K cluster with the aid of using N nodes set.

$$Z_{\min} = \sum_{r=1}^{K} Z_r = \sum_{r=1}^{K} \left(\sum_{x_i \in n_r} d(x_i - \mathrm{ch}_r)^2 \right) \tag{1}$$

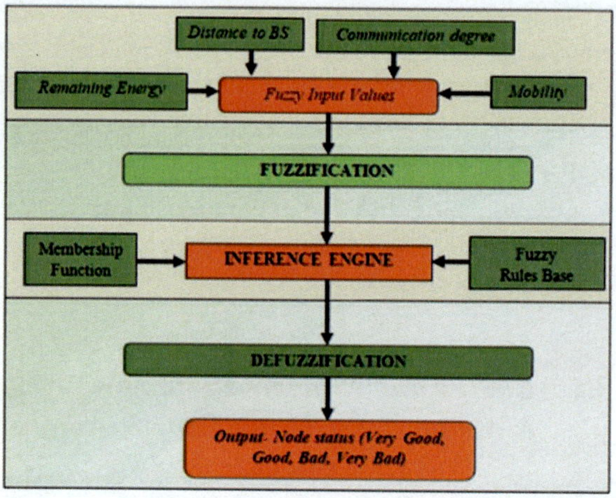

Fig. 1 Fuzzy system block

3.1.2 Fuzzy K-Means

The routing technique basically tires to optimize the ate up energy for the duration of the statistics transmission. The use of this approach with fuzzy c-manner protocol permits the node contributors linked near CH inside the network. By this technique, the strength transmitted is minimized and enhancement of the network lifetime is finished. With the attention of "*n*" nodes at a random segment generated inside a place of length M*M, the good enough manner clustering set of rules is completed for classifying the nodes to most range in MANET employer. The device of classification takes place as follows: the okay initialization, hold in thoughts OK kind of employer, and the chosen k centroids at the beginning in random locations of group fashioned it OK <*n*. In the succeeding segment, the nodes are grouped into clusters through Euclidean distance. Every node is hooked up to nearest centroid within the network. Later to calculate the centroid role in every institution, think the centroid role is various then last node in the cluster movements to their respective nearest centroid, else live same (Fig. 1).

$$Z_{\min}(K, q) = \sum_{K=1}^{K} \sum_{i=1}^{N} (\gamma_{K_i})^q d^2(x_i, C_K) \tag{2}$$

3.1.3 Genetic Algorithm (GA)

In 1975, the genetic algorithm was first proposed by Holland with the natural selection and genetic idea. It is basically a dominant search method in which the evolutionary algorithm class is applied for problem solving in various areas. Its implementation can be straight forward to give good performance to MANET's operation. The GA is primarily a straight, stochastic, and parallel method in global search as well as to provide optimized solution to the exiting problems. It can be started with randomly generated set with probable solution for an assignment known as population. Within the population, the single individual solution is called as chromosome. Each chromosome may be denoted as a string or genes array contained within solution part. It takes into consideration of fitness function for testing new structures for selecting the best population.

The graph $G = (N, A)$ specifies the underlying topology of any multi-hop network, where N is a set of nodes and A is a set of their links. Also, we can have a cost for each link (i, j) and call it as Cij. In this case, we have a source node which we named it as node "S" and a destination node with name "D". The name Iij is denoted for each link (i, j) and can be defined as follows:

$$I_{i,j} = \begin{cases} 1 & \begin{array}{l}\text{If the link from node } i \text{ to node } j\\ \text{exists in the routing path}\end{array} \\ 0 \text{ otherwise} \end{cases}$$

It is clear that diametrical elements of Iij must be "0". By using the above definition, we can formulate the SP routing solutions to syntactic optimization solution to minimize the objective function as follows:

Minimize:

$$\sum_{i=s}^{D} \sum_{\substack{j=s \\ j \neq i}}^{D} C_{ij} I_{ij}$$

Subject to:

$$\sum_{\substack{j=s \\ j \neq i}}^{D} I_{ij} - \sum_{\substack{j=s \\ j \neq i}}^{D} I_{ji} = \begin{cases} 1 & \text{if } i = S \\ -1 & \text{if } i = D \\ 0 & \text{otherwise} \end{cases}$$

And

$$\sum_{\substack{j=S \\ j \neq i}}^{D} \begin{cases} \leq 1 \text{ if } i \neq D \\ = 0 \text{ if } i = D \end{cases}$$

For each individual, the fitness value is given by the fitness function. The individual chromosome fortune depends on the fitness value. The basic differences between the GA with remaining heuristic methods are as follows.

(1) GA working rule depends on the conceivable arrangement populace while the heuristic strategies utilize one arrangement in redundancies.

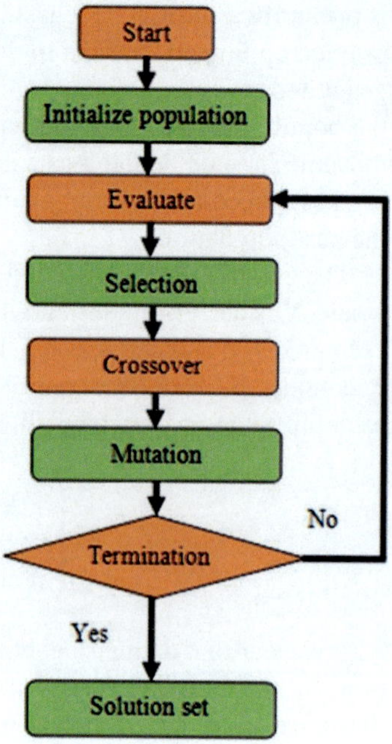

Fig. 2 Flowchart of a simple genetic algorithm

(2) GA is stochastic and not deterministic. Each and every in the GA populace gives a potential arrangement. Hardly any people's determination is done on the wellness esteem. The GA emulates the nature hereditary procedure, hybrid for trading hardly any individual hereditary information coolly for posterity (Fig. 2).

4 Results and Discussions

The broad variety of rounds contrasts from 1000 to 9000. In each round, the meaningless centers are selected for every solitary plan, and furthermore the result uncovers the decline sort of array head centers located inert in suggested strategy analyzing to various other present setups used in this activity. This is because of the determination of group head with most noteworthy lingering power with the help of intuitionist fluffy K-way-based bunching and furthermore want of best physical well-being charge basically based hubs as assortment heads in MANET.

Figure 3 represents network development with certain of time. Transmission array is specified in between the sensing unit nodes (Figs. 4 and 5). And also node 54 starts to get in touch with node 93 and also transfers the details. Figure 6 presents information communication with respective node in the network. Figure 7 discusses communication in between two nodes with equivalent time. Figure 8 describes sink

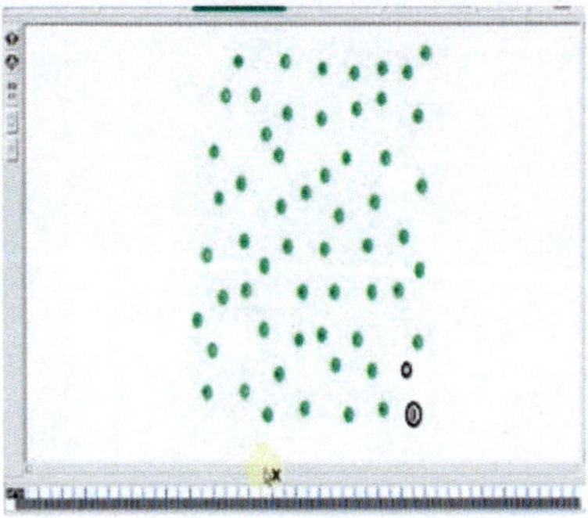

Fig. 3 Network creation

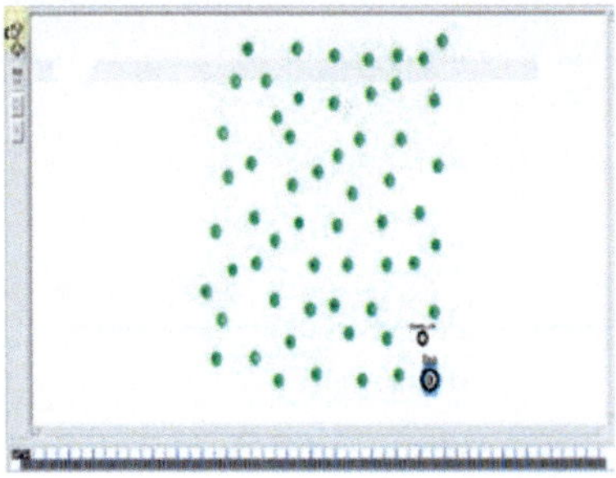

Fig. 4 Nodes representation

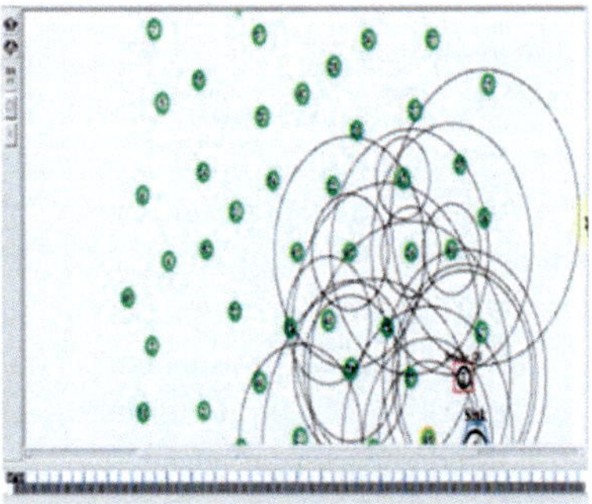

Fig. 5 Data communication

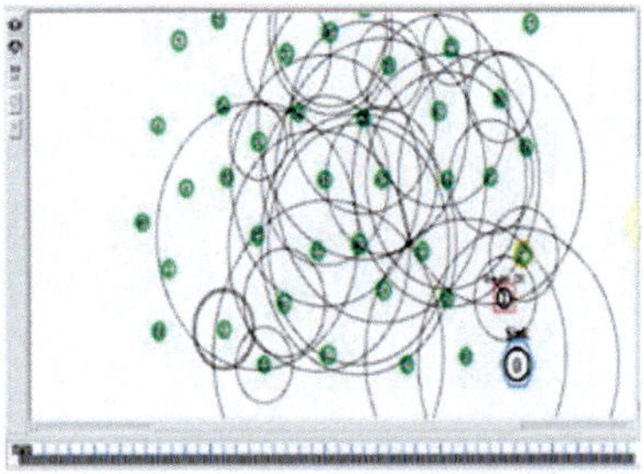

Fig. 6 Data communication with respective of node

Fig. 7 Communication between two nodes

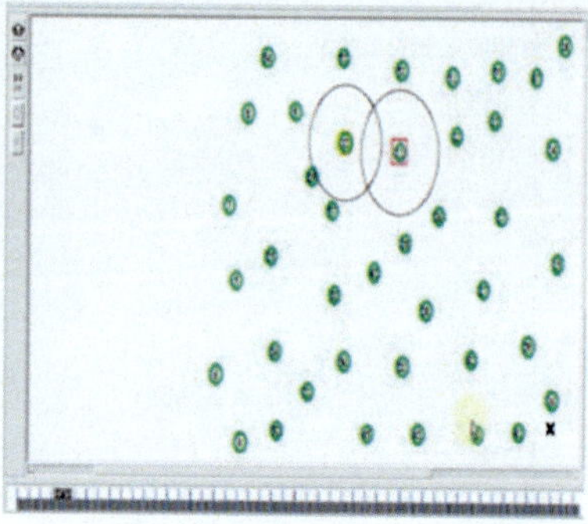

Fig. 8 Sink indication

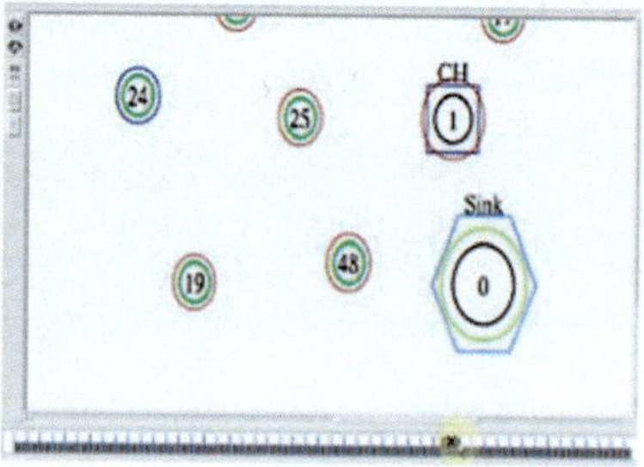

sign with matching of time sink node production. Figure 9 explains interaction in between all nodes with corresponding time. Figure 10 represents nodes indication selection signs with respective time.

The bundle dispersion convey of the each plan is discovered, and furthermore the final product notable shows that the upheld work appropriations bounty are more noteworthy kind of parcels to the based absolutely station because of the most satisfying decision of group head. This on account of the decision of team head with least steeply estimated member share extremely worth of array from the base station to number head as well as also the non-selection head density with the assistance of intuitionist muddled K-technique-based definitely bunching and also additionally

Fig. 9 Communication with all nodes

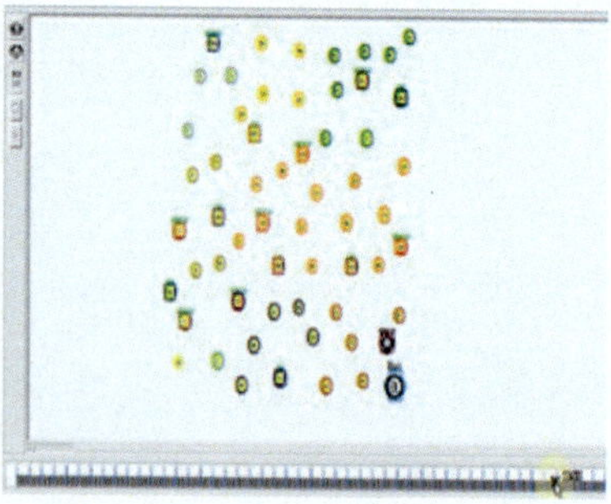

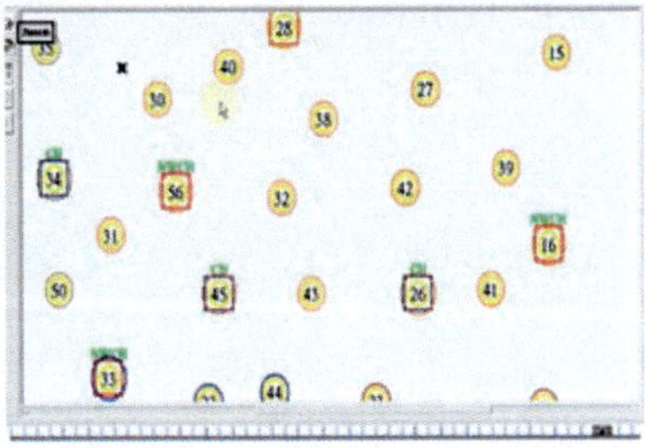

Fig. 10 Nodes indication wide range indication

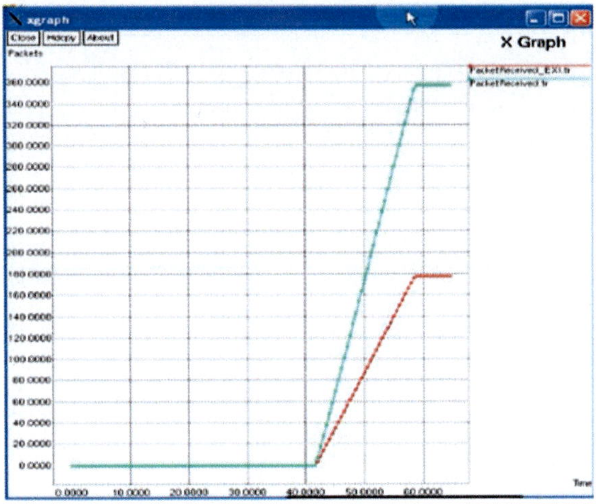

Fig. 11 Packet delivery ratio

time of appealing centers as masses in each round, political consultation of bunch head with best feasible real health expense with the array as the aspect.

Figure 11 stands for the chart detailed versus package circulation proportion versus interval considering the executed techniques. Figure 12 represents the graph plotted versus drooping proportion versus duration, Fig. 13 represents the chart plotted versus jitter versus duration, Fig. 14 represents the chart outlined versus throughput versus period, Fig. 15 means the chart outlined versus network life time versus period, and Fig. 16 represents the chart detailed versus range of nodes versus safety and security and also safety and security ratio utilizing node to node for the applied method.

5 Conclusion

In remote sensor organized, the quality limits of hubs play an essential capacity in developing such a technique for utility. The Wi-Fi sensor systems safeguard expanding and amplifying to be all around applied in loads of bundles. In this way,

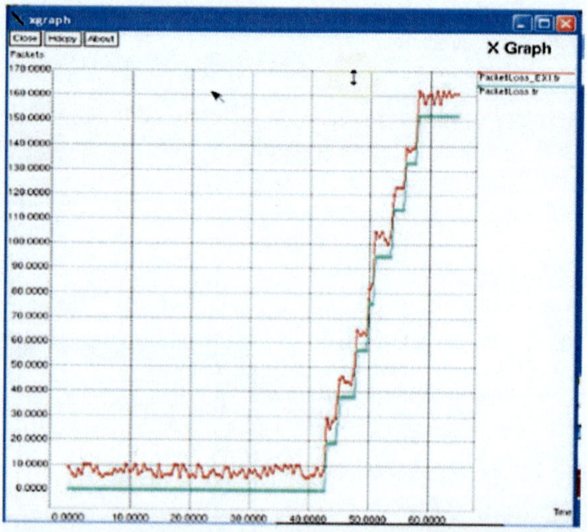

Fig. 12 Packet loss ratio

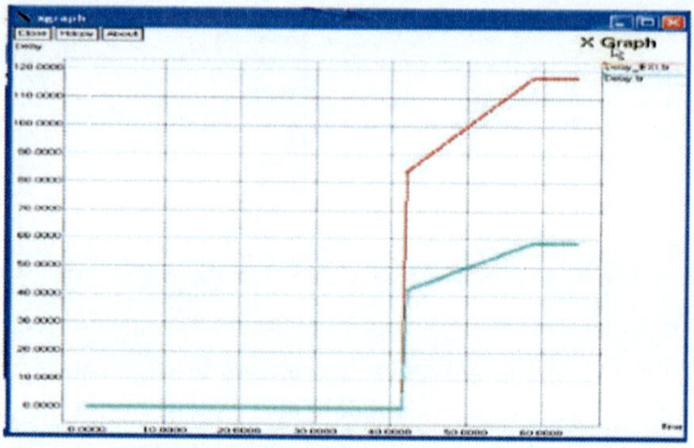

Fig. 13 End-to-end delay

the need for security will wind up pivotal. By and by, the cordless detecting unit organized experiences a lot of guidelines which comprise limited force, refining limit, and carport potential, and masses of others. There are various techniques to convey security, and one is cryptography. In the directed gadget, an intuitionist unsure alright approach based thoroughly bunching shape for sensor hubs is advanced. The political appointment of assortment head is finished with the innate arrangement of rules with the factors of routine vitality, assortment, and thickness of each hub. The hub with the overall population of things is picked typically put together absolutely and obviously with respect to the club and also non-club charge of the components. The data gave through the hubs inside the assortment does not converse with the base terminal, and they forget about it to the group head wherein the data are produced, squeezed, and furthermore long past to the base station through front or the various distinctive assortment heads. Along these lines, the proposed fine art propelled suits in word intensifying situations.

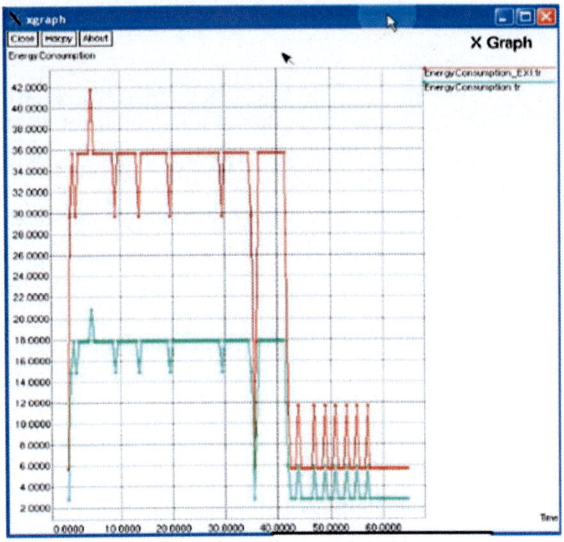

Fig. 14 Energy consumption

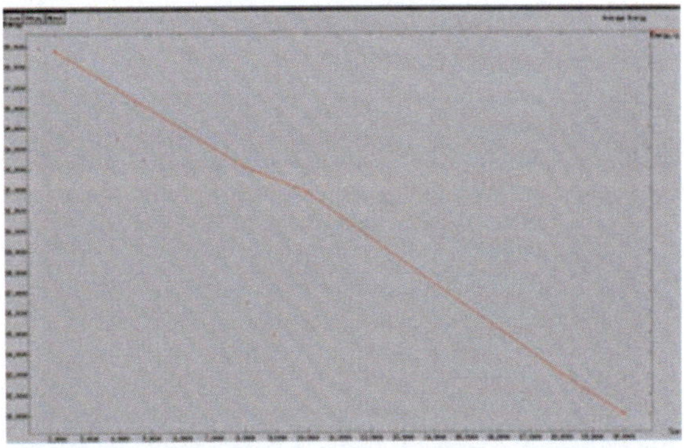

Fig. 15 Average energy

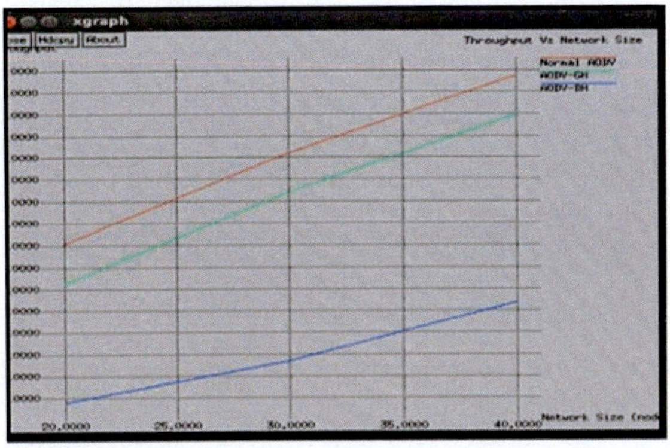

Fig. 16 Node to node power consumption

6 Future Scope

Remote sensor networks (WSNs) in which every sensor hub arbitrarily and on the other hand remains in a functioning mode or a rest mode. The dynamic mode comprises two stages, called the full-dynamic stage and the semi-dynamic stage. At the point when a referenced sensor hub is in the full-dynamic period of the dynamic mode, it might detect information bundles, transmit the detected parcels, get bundles, and hand off the got parcels. At long last, a parcel misfortune approach will be assessed.

References

1. Alakesh B, Umapathi GR (2014) A comparative study on advances in LEACH routing protocol for wireless sensor networks: a survey. Int J Adv Res Comput Commun Eng 3(2)
2. Nguyen DT et al (2012) An improved LEACH routing protocol for energy-efficiency of wireless sensor networks. Smart Comput Rev 2(5)
3. Gundalwar PR, Chavan VN (2012) A literature review on wireless sensor networks (WSNs) and its diversified applications. Int J Adv Res Comput Sci (IJARCS 2012) 3(7). ISSN: 0976-5697
4. Petre-Cosmin H et al (2010) Hierarchical routing protocol based on evolutionary algorithms for wireless sensor networks. In: 9th RoEduNet IEEE international conference
5. Heinzelman W, Chandrakasan A, Balakrishnan H (2002) An application—specific protocol architecture for wireless microsensor networks. IEEE Trans Wirel Commun 1(4):660–670
6. Heinzelman W (2000) Application—specific protocol architectures for wireless networks. Ph.D. Thesis, Massachusetts Institute of Technology
7. Smaragdakis G, Matta I, Bestavros A (2004) SEP: a stable election protocol for clustered heterogeneous wireless sensor networks. In: Second international workshop on sensor and actor network protocols and applications (SANPA)
8. Agrawal R, Motwani M (2009) Survey of clustering algorithm for mobile ad hoc network. IJCSE 1(2):98–104
9. Gerla M, Tsai JT (1995) Multicluster, mobile, multimedia radio network. Wireless network
10. Chen G, Nocetti F, Gonzalez J, Stojmenovic I (2002) Connectivity based k-hop clustering in wireless network. In: Proceeding of international conference on system science, vol 7, pp 188.3
11. Basu P, Khan N, Little TDC (2001) A mobility based metric for clustering in mobile ad hoc networks. In: Proceeding of IEEE ICDCSW, pp 413–418
12. Arima C, Hanai T, Okamoto M (2003) Gene Expression Analysis Using Fuzzy K-Means Clustering. Genome Inf 14(1):334–335

Author Index

S. Bhattacharyya et al. (eds.), *International Conference on Intelligent and Smart Computing in Data Analytics*, Advances in Intelligent Systems and Computing 1312,
https://doi.org/10.1007/978-981-33-6176-8